FUNCTIONAL
Movement
REEDUCATION

A Contemporary Model for Stroke Rehabilitation

Susan Ryerson, M.A., P.T.

Partner and Therapist, Making Progress
Washington, D.C.
Clinical Instructor and Lecturer
Neurodevelopmental Treatment Association (NDTA)
International Bobath Instructor/Tutor Association (IBITAH)

Kathryn Levit, B.S., O.T.R.

Partner and Therapist, Making Progress
Washington, D.C.
Clinical Instructor and Lecturer
Neurodevelopmental Treatment Association (NDTA)
International Bobath Instructor/Tutor Association (IBITAH)

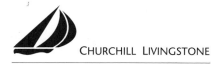
CHURCHILL LIVINGSTONE

New York, Edinburgh, London, Madrid, Melbourne, San Francisco, Tokyo

D1088756

Library of Congress Cataloging-in-Publication Data

A catalog record for this book is available from the Library of Congress

ISBN 0-443-08913-2

Distributed in the United Kingdom by Churchill Livingstone, Robert Stevenson House, 1–3 Baxter's Place, Leith Walk, Edinburgh EH1 3AF, and by associated companies, branches, and representatives throughout the world.

Medical knowledge is constantly changing. As new information becomes available, changes in treatment, procedures, equipment and the use of drugs become necessary. The editors/authors/contributors and the publishers have, as far as it is possible, taken care to ensure that the information given in this text is accurate and up to date. However, readers are strongly advised to confirm that the information, especially with regard to drug usage, complies with the latest legislation and standards of practice.

The Publishers have made every effort to trace the copyright holders for borrowed material. If they have inadvertently overlooked any, they will be pleased to make the necessary arrangements at the first opportunity.

Acquisitions Editor: *Carol Bader*
Assistant Editor: *Ann Ruzycka*
Production Editor: *Donna C. Balopole*
Production Supervisor: *Laura Mosberg Cohen*
Desktop Coordinator: *Robb Quattro*
Cover Design: *Jeannette Jacobs*

Printed in the United States of America

First published in 1997   7 6 5 4 3 2 1

Preface

Functional Movement Reeducation presents a model for neurologic treatment that developed out of clinical practice and is based on the belief that we can reeducate functional movement patterns in stroke patients. This model presents information in three areas: a system of analyzing the normal movement patterns in the trunk, arm, and leg that are important for function, a detailed description of the impairments that interfere with movement and limit function, and strategies for relating treatment techniques for the reeducation of movement and restoration of function to impairments. It is our hope that this book gives the therapy community a more comprehensive model of normal movement and movement dysfunction and allows therapists to practice with improved handling skills and greater problem solving ability.

Our therapy careers as clinicians and teachers were changed by the knowledge imparted to us by Berta Bobath in the 1970s. From her, we learned a system for treating adults with neurologic dysfunction. She taught us how to inhibit abnormal tone and to facilitate normal movement patterns. This allowed us to gain confidence that therapy could make a difference in the movement patterns of stroke patients. As years passed, we realized that changing tone did not necessarily improve the patient's ability to move or function. We realized that it was equally important to have skills to reeducate new movement patterns. We went through a phase where we challenged the idea that spasticity was a neurophysiologic phenomenon. We discovered that changes in muscle tone were not only related to "spasticity," but to changes in motor recruitment patterns and in joint alignment. This meant we had to have multiple techniques for changing tone and led to a deeper study of kinesiology and the skills and practices in orthopedic therapy. We used this knowledge to enhance our study of normal and abnormal movement and to better understand the relationship between joint alignment and biomechanics to tone and movement.

About the same time, the science of neurophysiology was growing and changing. It became clear to us that the control of movement was more complex than had been previously described and that the rationale behind the Bobath approach was out of date. Motor learning theorists were stressing the need for active participation on the part of the patient and encouraging a more task-oriented, hands-off approach to treatment. In the therapy community, there was a perceived need to reconcile the techniques of practice with the "science of the times." In this process,

Bobath and other neurophysiologic approaches were being discredited in the guise of more "scientific" treatment. Our practice and teaching led us to realize stroke patients need both hands-on therapy to reeducate muscles and, later in recovery, may benefit from task-oriented, functional practice. We recognized the need to learn from motor learning theories while retaining what was effective from older treatment models.

Throughout this period, we were running an adult neurologic therapy practice, teaching NDT continuing education courses, and lecturing on stroke rehabilitation. As our thinking evolved, we began to incorporate the results of this questioning process into our treatment and teaching. We treated our patients with much more of a reeducation focus and moved from a facilitation-inhibition model to setting and achieving functional changes. In lectures and continuing education courses, we began to use new explanations to explain Bobath treatment techniques and to provide information about alignment and biomechanics in addition to tone and abnormal movement. We became better at teaching movement analysis. We learned that teaching a manual skill is difficult but can be enhanced through increased knowledge of the patient's problems, knowledge of the process of assessment and treatment, and knowledge of the relationship between impairments and functions. In the process, we realized that our treatment and our teaching was systematic, understandable, and effective. Encouraged by mentors, peers, and students, we set out to write down what we had learned. *Functional Movement Reeducation* is the result of this professional growth.

The book project grew and grew and was infinitely harder than we expected. We have been humbled by the task. It is our intention to offer this information as a baseline—to provide a springboard for debate and research—to challenge the therapy community to either confirm or repudiate our observations about normal movement, neurologic impairments, and treatment techniques. Challenging questions have been the spark that has allowed us to grow and change throughout our careers. We hope our readers' response to this book continues to push our thinking. We reserve the right to change our minds . . . and hope for many future editions!

Susan Ryerson, P.T.
Kathryn Levit, O.T.R.

Acknowledgments

The development of the ideas and concepts in this book have been stimulated by input from many people. We would like to begin by acknowledging the contribution made by Berta Bobath to our growth as therapists and as a role model in our pursuit of excellence in our careers. While we now disagree with and have moved beyond some of the premises of her approach, we continue to use many Bobath treatment techniques in our clinical practice and in our continuing education courses. We include techniques that we learned from her in this book. We hope that she would recognize her influence in our work and approve of the direction that we have taken her theory.

We would also like to thank the following therapists who served as mentors and significant role models: Joan Mohr, who guided us into the teaching process; Lois Bly, who stimulated and encouraged "cutting edge" questioning; Janice Hulme, who pushed us to produce handouts and kept asking when the book will be published; Mary Fiorentino, who told us to trust our intuition and to get our thoughts and theories in print; Jean Hannah, who showed us how to reach beyond expectations; and Barbro Salek, who taught us to love movement.

This book would not have been possible without the insights acquired during our many years of teaching and lecturing. By instructing on the clinical level, we gained a sense for the areas in which therapists need more information, and learned how to present new information about normal movement, patient problems, and treatment techniques. The encouragement and positive feedback from the participants in these continuing education courses inspired us and provided the impetus to keep writing.

We cannot thank our patients enough for pushing us to become better therapists and for helping us develop as authors. Our years of clinical practice forced us to keep our treatment practical and focused on achievable functional goals. We also learned from our patients and their families the importance of maintaining hope and trying for movements and functions that seem out of reach. Our patients' hopes and their drive to regain function demonstrated to us how much potential for recovery exists following a stroke.

The photography in the book was produced with the assistance of Jack Hiller and Michael Soper. We are grateful for their artistic direction and their generous donations of equipment and time.

Janet Epp at Making Progress served as a valuable editor for both content and style in the preparation of this manuscript. She helped immeasurably in keeping our practice running smoothly during the many years we spent writing and photographing.

Finally, we are thankful for the on-going support of our families and friends for living with us through this project . . . and to each other . . . for our mutual respect, challenging dialogue, and friendship.

Contents

Section I. The Model for Treatment

1. Functional Movement: A Practical Model for Treatment / **1**
2. Problems Contributing to Loss of Movement and Function / **15**
3. Assessment / 55
4. Treatment Interventions to Maximize Functional Outcome / **71**

Section II. Movement Analysis

5. Trunk Movements in Sitting / **87**
6. Upper Extremity Movements / **131**
7. Upper Extremity Weight Bearing Movements / **183**
8. Lower Extremity Movements in Sitting / **227**
9. Lower Extremity Movements in Standing / **261**
10. Trunk and Extremity Movements in Supine / **317**

Section III. Functional Movement Analysis

11. Rolling / **355**
12. Sidelying to Sitting / **375**
13. Sit to Stand / **397**
14. Transfers / **415**
15. Walking / **433**

Index / **479**

1
Functional Movement: A Practical Model for Treatment

Movement is central to human life. We use movement to perform life roles, meet basic and not so basic needs, express ourselves, and enjoy ourselves. In daily life, we use many different types of movement and many different movement patterns to perform the tasks associated with self-care, homemaking, parenting, work, and leisure. Control over the basic movements necessary for function is acquired in infancy and childhood. However, we continue to develop new motor skills throughout our life span, as we add new interests and tasks to our daily routine. Our success at life roles depends at least partially on our ability to learn and to perform the movements necessary for task performance. If we can no longer perform these critical movement patterns, our performance may decline, with resulting loss of independence.

Movement is also central to the science and practice of physical and occupational therapy. The major role of these professions is to help the patient overcome disability by learning to move and function again. To be successful in this role, therapy practitioners need to understand normal and abnormal movement as it relates to functional performance. Movement science and the study of normal and abnormal movement is still being developed. Although certain areas of movement, such as gait and balance, and sports activities, such as batting and pitching, have been well studied, movement analysis of most daily activities has not yet been performed. Many therapists practicing in physical disabilities feel the need for more information about movement that relates directly to functional performance in daily living.

This book describes a model of treatment for the neurologic therapist. This system of assessment and treatment of movement problems is based on the study of normal movement and functional performance. In our treatment model, techniques of movement reeducation are used to retrain normal movement control, increase functional performance, and decrease disability in the neurologic patient. We call our treatment *functional movement reeducation* because it is directed towards the specific patterns of movement and coordination that are used in daily life for functional performance. In this book, we describe the movements of the trunk, arm, and leg that are important for functional movement, relate these movement patterns to the physical impairments and functional limitation of neurologic patients, and provide a system for treatment that increases movement and decreases disability. Our goal is to expand knowledge of normal movement and provide a new model for applying normal movement to neurologic treatment.

This chapter provides a theoretical framework for understanding how functional movements are organized and executed. It serves as an introduction to both normal functional movement and movement reeducation. In this chapter, we define functional movement and normal movement, introduce terminology related to movement that will be used throughout the book, and discuss the relationship of functional movement to movement reeducation.

FUNCTIONAL MOVEMENTS

Definitions

In this book, we are concerned with the movements used to perform daily tasks and occupations, or functional movements. The word "function" refers to a specific occupation or role. *Functional movements* are the movement patterns that are used for or adapted to a function or group of similar functions. In daily life, we use functional movements to meet basic needs, perform life tasks, and accomplish functional goals. These movements are truly "functional" when they allow us to achieve our goals and produce the desired occupational behaviors in a safe, efficient, and appropriate manner.

The movement patterns that we use to perform daily activities are relatively consistent and uniform. Most people walk, stand up, and drink from a cup using movement patterns that are similar if not identical. While movements such as rolling may vary slightly between people of different ages, body types, and fitness levels, most people accomplish these functions with one of several common variants. Since most human movement is so similar, it is possible to describe the movement patterns that are typically used to perform a task or activity. The term *normal movements* is used to identify these typical patterns of coordination. Since normal movements are the preferred patterns of coordination, they provide therapy professionals with the best model for understanding how functional movement is organized and executed. This understanding is critical for the task of movement reeducation.

Normal movements use the patterns of muscle action and joint movement that are most suited to the biomechanical and kinesiologic systems of the human body. During functional performance, normal movements use the simplest movement strategy to accomplish the task, conserving power and energy, while protecting the body from stress, injury, and loss of balance. Normal movement is possible because of the interaction between the musculoskeletal system and the central nervous system. To produce normal movement, we must be able to generate the patterns of movement in the trunk, arms and legs that are necessary for functional performance. This ability depends on biomechanical factors, such as intact alignment, and available mobility in the skeletal system, and on adequate muscle strength and control. Normal movement also depends on the ability to sequence muscle contractions and joint movements and to coordinate movements of the different body segments in the specific patterns necessary for functional movement. This ability, which we call *motor control*, is the function of the central nervous system. Problems in either biomechanical systems or in motor control can interfere with the control of normal movement and lead to deficits in selective movement and atypical patterns of coordination. In the patient with central nervous system lesions, both areas contribute to the movement and functional deficits associated with this category of pathology.

Parts of Functional Movement

Functional movement is made up of coordinated movements of trunk, arm, and leg. These movements are normal when the body has normal trunk control and normal extremity control of the arms and legs. In the section below, we discuss the contributions that the trunk and extremities make to normal functional movement and the relationship between trunk and extremity movements during functional performance.

Trunk Control

The trunk is the center of the body mass and the largest segment of the body. It plays two critical roles in functional movement. First, muscle activity in the trunk is necessary to maintain the body in a balanced and erect position against the force of gravity and to adapt to the moving extremities. This is the *postural role* of the trunk. The trunk also plays a second, *dynamic role* in daily life. The trunk functions dynamically when trunk movements are used to move the center of the body over its base or to move to a new base or posture. In this dynamic function, trunk movements contribute to or increase the functional abilities of the upper and lower extremities. *Trunk control* can be defined as the ability to perform the movement patterns necessary for functional movement and to coordinate these movements with those of the extremities. In this book, we include control of the head and neck under trunk control.

Both postural and dynamic aspects of trunk control are based on ability of the trunk to move in anterior, posterior, and lateral directions. The trunk must be able to perform these movements in patterns that require concentric muscle activity (anti-gravity control) and also in eccentric patterns in which the body moves toward the supporting surface (pro-gravity responses). These movement patterns of the trunk are critical for balance and for extremity function. When the trunk is not stable and cannot move without loss of balance, the arms and legs must be used to help stabilize the body and cannot be moved freely for function. For this reason, trunk control is an important precursor to all functional movements.

The postural role of the trunk is most significant in sitting and standing. For the body to be balanced in these positions, the trunk must be centered over the body's base of support. While little muscle activity is apparently necessary to maintain the upright posture when the body is not engaged in function, the muscles of the trunk must become more active as soon as the extremities begin to move. Movements of the extremities traction the trunk, destabilizing the balance of the body. In normal movement, changes in trunk muscle activity and small trunk movements occur automatically to anticipate and respond to these displacing forces. These muscular responses maintain the body in a stable position that is compatible with the extremity movement. For example, when we move our hands behind our body to pull off our shirt, our spine extends and our weight shifts slightly forward. Similarly, when we bring our leg up in sitting to put on a sock, we automatically shift our weight back and flex our spine to balance our trunk with the leg forward (Fig. 1-1). Changes in muscle activity in the trunk are always accompanied by compatible changes in the weight bearing extremities. This combination of trunk and lower extremity muscle activation used to maintain body stability is called a *postural response*.

FIGURE 1-1 Postural movements of the trunk automatically accompany upper extremity movements. (A) In relaxed sitting, the trunk is upright over the hips. (B) When the hands reach up and back, the spine automatically extends. (C) When the leg is lifted, weight is shifted laterally and posteriorly, resulting in trunk flexion.

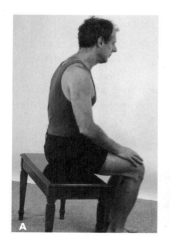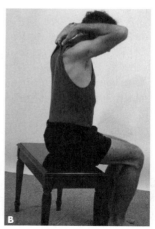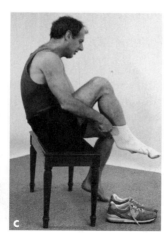

In sitting and standing, coordinated muscular changes in the trunk and lower extremities are also important components of equilibrium responses. When the body position is challenged to the extent that it is in danger of falling, muscles of the trunk contract strongly with those of the weight bearing extremities to bring the center of the body back to a stable base. In this situation, the arm muscles are often recruited as well to provide additional stability to the upper trunk. These movements of the trunk and extremities are known as *equilibrium reactions* (Fig. 1-2). Equilibrium reactions do not occur during normal functional movement. They exist as a backup system should normal postural adjustments and weight shifts fail to maintain a stable body posture during task performance, when the base of support of the body is very small, or when environmental conditions destabilize the body.

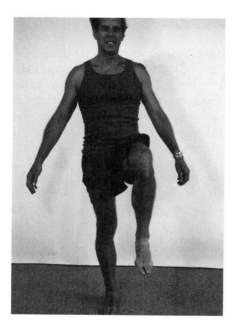

FIGURE 1-2 Equilibrium responses in the arms occur as the body's base of support becomes smaller and more unstable.

FIGURE 1-3 Dynamic movement of the trunk brings the hand closer to the shoe.

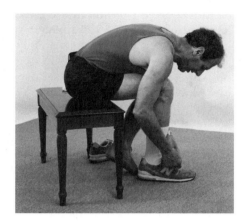

In the postural reactions described above, trunk movements occur as background movements that react to the movements of the extremities or to conditions in the environment. The trunk plays a more dynamic role when movements of the trunk are coordinated with those of the arms and/or legs in the performance of a functional movement. Trunk movements frequently combine with movements of the arm to extend the range of reach or bring the hand to a new position for function. This occurs when we move our trunk forward with spinal flexion to allow our hand to pick something off the floor (Fig. 1-3). Lateral trunk movements in sitting and standing shift weight from two legs to one, freeing the non-weight bearing leg to move. Trunk movements can also combine with those of the extremities during transitional movements, such as sit to stand and rolling. In these movements, the trunk and limbs work together to change the position of the body and move to a new base of support. The trunk movements described in all these examples result in changes of weight distribution over the base of support or changes in the base of support. We call these movements trunk-initiated *weight shifts*.

Extremity Control

Functional movements also rely on specific task-related movements of the upper and lower extremities. Both the upper and lower extremities are called upon to perform a wide variety of movements during daily life. *Skilled extremity control* refers to the ability to generate specific patterns of extremity movement required for efficient performance of a given task or type of tasks. To simplify our discussion of these movements, it is helpful to divide extremity movements into two categories: weight bearing movements and non-weight bearing movements. Both weight bearing and non-weight bearing patterns are necessary for normal movement control of the arms and legs.

Weight Bearing Movements

Weight bearing occurs when extremities are stabilized against a surface in a position where they support body weight and form part of the body's base of support. This extremity pattern is also referred to as a "closed-chain kinetic activity." During weight bearing, extremity muscles are active to maintain a stable contact with the supporting surface, to maintain good alignment of proximal over distal segments, and to lift and support the weight of the body against the force of gravity. Since the weight bearing extremities are fixed on the supporting surface, any movement of the body over its base of support results in a change in the position of the joints of the weight bearing extremity and a change in weight distribution over the portion of the weight bearing extremity in contact with the support. As body weight is shifted around the weight bearing extremities, the patterns of muscle activation in the weight bearing limb change. This allows the limb to remain stable while supporting the new distribution of weight. These changes in muscle activity represent postural adaptations in the weight bearing extremity. For example, in sitting a forward movement of the trunk to initiate standing up results in increased hip, knee, and ankle flexion in the weight bearing legs. This movement also results in a weight transfer to the feet and produces a different pattern of muscle activation in the legs as well (Fig 1-4).

The lower extremity is most commonly associated with the function of weight bearing. All of the functional movements described in this book include lower extremity weight bearing. The part of the leg that is supporting weight and the amount and type of muscle activation used during weight support will vary according to body position and functional activity. For example, in sitting the legs are weight bearing in a flexed position so that weight is taken on the thighs and feet. Since this results in a large base of support and a relatively stable body position, many functional activities in sitting do not demand a high level of activity in the weight bearing legs. In contrast, walking is an activity in which the base of support is small and constantly changing and the body is unstable. In this activity, the feet are very active as they propel the body forward, and the proximal leg muscles must be similarly active to stabilize the extended position and support the weight of the whole body. Although the legs do not work as hard to support body weight in sitting as in standing and walking, it is important to remember that leg muscles are active during trunk weight shifts in sitting, and that a loss of muscle activity in the legs will interfere with task performance in sitting.

Weight bearing is also an important component of upper extremity functional performance. In infancy, weight bearing on the arms is accomplished before lower extremity weight bearing and plays a critical role in the development of trunk control and the establishment of upright posture. While older children and

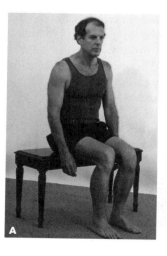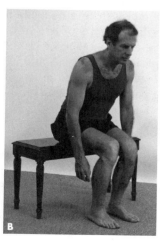

FIGURE 1-4 (*A & B*) Anterior trunk weight shift in sitting. As the trunk moves forward, weight is transferred from the hips forward toward the feet.

FIGURE 1-5 Upper extremity weight bearing on a table.

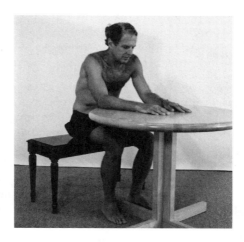

adults have little functional use for prone on elbows and quadruped positions, upper extremity weight bearing has important functional uses in sitting and standing. We use upper extremity weight bearing to support the weight of our upper bodies, to widen our base of support for additional postural stability, and to stabilize objects. These tasks are used many times during the day in self-care, homemaking, and vocational activities. As with lower extremity weight bearing, the type of activity and position of the arm will affect the amount of body weight supported on the arm and the type of muscle activity necessary to support this weight. For example, while writing at a table we often lean heavily on our non-dominant forearm. In this activity, the nondominant arm is supporting considerable upper body weight through muscle activity around the scapula and humerus (Fig. 1-5). When descending stairs, we often weight bear lightly on the railing. In this type of weight bearing, the arm is supporting little body weight but muscles at the shoulder girdle, elbow, wrist, and hand are very active to maintain the arm in a position where it can assist the trunk.

Non-Weight Bearing Movements

Non-weight bearing movements of the extremities are movements of the extremity in space. These movements are often referred to as "open-chain kinetic movements." Non-weight bearing movements are used functionally to position the extremity for task performance, to execute the movement patterns required by the task, and to return the extremity from this functional position to rest again by the body. Non-weight bearing movements are usually related directly to task performance. There is much more variability to these movements than is found in weight bearing.

Non-weight bearing movements of the arms are critical to the performance of most daily activities. During task performance, these non-weight bearing arm movements occur in sequences associated with the stages of task performance. The initial arm movements prepare for actual task performance by bringing the arms and hands into the appropriate position for the task. Subsequent arm and hand movements progress sequentially to allow completion of the task. Once the desired goal has been achieved, the arm and hand return to a position of rest by the body. Non-weight bearing movements of the leg also have important functional uses. Swing phase of gait, flexion of the leg to go up a step or put on a shoe, and crossing the leg

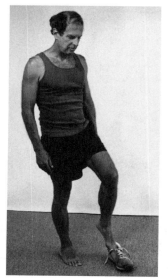

FIGURE 1-6 A non-weight bearing movement of the lower extremity in standing.

in sitting for comfort or dressing are examples of important lower extremity non-weight bearing functional movements (Fig. 1-6).

Non-weight bearing movements of the extremities can be divided into two categories: generalized movement patterns and task specific movement patterns.

Generalized Patterns of Movement These are sequences of joint movement that can be used with minor variations to perform many similar activities. These movement patterns represent the usual or typical way to move the hand or foot to a given location or place the arm and leg into a functional position. In normal movement, they involve predictable sequences of joint movement and patterns of muscle activation. An example of a generalized arm pattern is the combination of elbow flexion with shoulder flexion used for eating and drinking, brushing teeth, and shaving or applying lipstick. In the leg, unilateral stance with flexion of the opposite leg is used for similar tasks of stepping up, bringing the foot up to the hand, or moving an object out of the way. Since generalized movement patterns are not specialized, they can be easily adapted to varying tasks and situations. The acquisition of generalized movement patterns allows us to perform many similar activities easily without extensive practice or learning because the most appropriate sequence of movement can be "selected" from the generalized movement repertoire.

Task-Specific Movements These are movements of the limb that are precisely sequenced and coordinated to provide optimal performance of a given task or activity. These specialized movements are based on the generalized patterns of coordination described above but have been fine-tuned for maximal efficiency. Performance of task-specific movements is only possible when the generalized patterns of coordination from which they are derived can be executed. Since task-specific movements are highly specialized, these movement skills do not assist in the performance of other tasks or activities.

In this book, the chapters on weight bearing and non-weight bearing movements of the arm and leg focus on generalized patterns of limb movement. This was necessary to limit the number of movements to be described. But we also believe that it is possible to identify the patterns of limb movement that are most critical for functional performance and to demonstrate how a relatively small number of movement patterns in the arm and leg are used to perform many similar functions. Generalized extremity movements are the first movements of the arm and leg that are trained in movement reeducation. Once these basic movement patterns are available, reeducating specific movements is quicker and less frustrating for the patient.

Integration of Trunk and Extremity Movements

The ability to execute normal functional movements depends on coordination of trunk and extremity movements. During functional performance, our body movements combine task related movements and postural adaptations and adjustments or weight shifts. In normal movement, trunk, arm, and leg movements are well synchronized and compatible. While the upper extremities and sometimes lower extremities perform the task, postural movements of the trunk and weight bearing extremities keep the body balanced and optimally positioned by efficient task specific movements. This automatic coordination of trunk and extremity movements is only possible when trunk control and extremity control are normal. When deficits in trunk con-

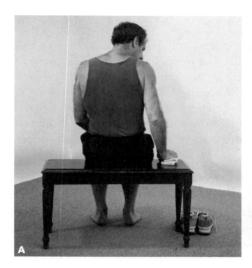 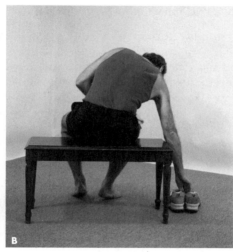

FIGURE 1-7 The demands for postural control in the trunk and legs differs according to the task. (*A*) When the arms function close to the body, small adjustments in trunk and leg position are adequate to maintain balance. (*B*) When the trunk and arm move together, the trunk and lower extremities must be more active to maintain balance.

trol or in extremity movements are present, functional movement may still be possible using movement substitutions. *Compensatory movements* are alternative movement strategies that replace normal movement patterns when problems with trunk or extremity control prevent the use of the usual pattern of coordination.

Different types of functional movements place different demands on the body for trunk and extremity control. In many functional movements, the arms execute the task while the trunk and legs remain in a stable position. When the arms are involved in task performance close to body midline, the demands for postural control in the trunk and legs are small while the need for upper extremity skill is great. In these activities, changes in spinal alignment and small weight shifts over the lower extremities are adequate to maintain a stable posture. As the arm or arms move through bigger ranges or the arms and trunk move together, the task requires greater postural control in both the trunk and weight bearing lower extremities (Fig 1-7). Task performance in standing is a still more difficult challenge to balance and requires more muscular activity in the trunk and lower extremities to maintain postural stability (Fig. 1-8).

FIGURE 1-8 Reaching in standing further increases the postural demands in the trunk and lower extremities.

Control of postural patterns and generalized extremity movements allows us to produce movement patterns that are adaptable to changes in our environments and in our bodies. Everyone has a repertoire of movement strategies that can be used to accomplish functional goals. These variations are used to modify our preferred movement patterns to meet changes in the internal and external environment. We may change the movement patterns that we use to perform a task, depending on the time of day, the place we are in, and the amount of strength or fatigue that we have in the different segments of our body. For example, most people use different patterns to stand up from a firm chair and a soft sofa. The ability to change our movement strategies allows us to respond to new situations and function in different environments. Without this ability, we can function only in a familiar, controlled environment.

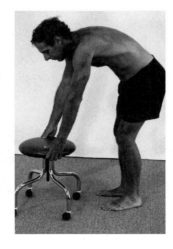

ANALYSIS OF NORMAL MOVEMENT

To simplify normal movement and make it easier to understand and apply to treatment, we have divided it into smaller segments that we call movement components and movement sequences. We use movement components to identify the normal movements in the trunk and extremities that are used during task performance. Movement sequences are used to describe the relationship between the movements of the trunk and extremities during functional movements. We also use these two categories of normal movement to assess movement problems and to plan appropriate strategies of movement reeducation.

Movement Components

The term *movement components* is used to identify basic movement patterns that are necessary for normal functional performance. In this book, we divide the body into three functional segments: the trunk, the arm, and the leg. Each of these body segments has a set of movement components that occur over and over again as we go through daily activities. Although functional movement appears extremely diverse and complex, there are probably a finite number of movement components for each body segment. These movement components represent the patterns of joint movement and muscle activation that underlie the performance of most functional activities. The movement components for each body segment differ slightly from position to position. For example, since we use our legs differently for functional activities in standing than we do in sitting and supine, we have a different set of lower extremity movement components for each of these positions. For this reason, it is necessary to describe the essential movement components for the trunk, arm, and leg in the positions of supine, sitting, and standing.

Movement Sequences

Functional movements, such, as walking or dressing, are composed of movement components of the trunk and extremities. We use the term *movement sequences* to describe specific combinations of trunk and extremity movement components that are used to perform a functional movement or complete a task. Movement sequences proceed sequentially (i.e., the movements of the different body segments occur in a specific order and with a specific temporal and spatial relationship to each other). Since there are a finite number of movement components for each body segment, the same movement components are used many times in the performance of different movement sequences. Normal variations in functional movement sequences arise when different movement components are used during the movement (e.g., the use of trunk flexion versus trunk extension to initiate the movement of sit to stand, or when the same movement components are used in a different order, such as occurs in the different patterns of rolling).

In this book, we discuss several types of movement sequences. *Transitional movement sequences*, such as sit to stand, supine to sitting, and rolling, are used to change the orientation of the body. *Mobility sequences*, such as walking or scooting, move the body in the environment. *Task-related movement sequences* are used to perform simple tasks, such as drinking from a cup or carrying a tray. More complex functions, such as eating, dressing, or cooking, can be visualized as chains of movement sequences or combinations of the three types of movement sequences. These complex functions are not discussed in this book.

Movement Analysis

In this book, we use a specific system of movement analysis to describe movement components and movement sequences. We use this system and its related terminology to both analyze normal movements and to assess our patients' efforts to move and function. To describe a movement component, our description must include the *initiation* or part of the body that starts or initiates the movement and the joint or joints that are the fulcrum of the movement, the *direction* that the body moves, and the *sequence* of joint movement that occurs. For example, to describe the movement components of extended arm forward reach, we begin by stating that the movement is initiated by the hand, the shoulder is the fulcrum of the movement, and the movement occurs in an anterior direction, and then describe the patterns of glenohumeral and scapulohumeral movement that occur as the hand moves from the side of the body to over the head.

Many movement components of the trunk and extremities result in *weight shifts* or changes of weight distribution over the body's base of support or changes in the base of support. For example, in sitting, trunk movements in an anterior direction result in weight being shifted from the ischium onto the femurs and feet. When weight shifts occur as part of a movement component, they are also included in the description. To describe movement components of a weight shift, we include the direction of the weight shift, the part of the body initiating the weight shift, and the resulting change in the position of the trunk and weight bearing extremities. Thus, in sitting, when an anterior weight shift is initiated by the lower trunk, it results in spinal extension, increased hip flexion, and a weight transfer forward toward the femurs and feet.

Movement sequences are analyzed using a similar system. Analysis of a movement sequence must include the movement components of the trunk, arm, and leg that are used to complete the function and the sequencing of those components during functional performance. Most movement sequences can be broken down into parts or stages. The movement sequences that we analyze in this book contain three phases: initiation, transition, and completion. The description of each phase must include the movement components of the trunk and extremities and the direction of the weight shifts.

The *initiation phase* is the first part of a movement sequence. A movement is initiated when the body moves to position itself for the task or changes its position relative to its base of support. Functional movements may be initiated by the trunk, the arm, or the leg depending on the goal of the activity. For example, the functional movement sequence sit to stand is initiated most frequently by a forward movement of the trunk and arms, whereas reaching for an object on the table may be initiated by the arm alone.

The second stage of movement sequence is called transition. The *transition point* is the point in the movement sequence when there is a change in the active muscle groups, the direction of the body movement, or the body's relationship to its base of support. For example, in the sequence of moving from sitting to standing, the trunk initially moves forward to shift weight from the pelvis and hips toward the feet. After the hips leave the chair, the trunk no longer moves forward but begins to move backwards to complete the movement to standing. The point in the movement sequence when the trunk has gone as far forward as it will go and is about to reverse direction is the transition point in the movement sit to stand.

The end of the movement sequence is called the *completion phase*. During completion, the body seeks to balance itself within its new base of support. For example,

Movement Components

Initiation
Direction
Sequence
Weight shift

**Movement
Sequences**

Trunk movement
components

Extremity movement
components

   Initiation

   Transition or task
    performance

   Completion

the completion phase of the movement of sitting to standing occurs when the trunk is balanced over the feet. In many functional tasks, the completion phase leads directly to a new movement sequence. For example, at the completion of sit to stand, we often start a new task or walk to a new location without a pause or rest. However, the completion of a movement sequence may signal to our body to rest or stop working, as occurs when we sit down for a rest.

In task-related movement sequences, the second or transition stage of the movement may involve one or many movements of the trunk and extremities. In a simple reaching task, the approach to the object is the initiation phase of the movement, grasp is the second or transition phase, and the return of the object to the body is the completion of the movement. However, in more complex tasks, such as drinking from a cup or brushing your hair, the second stage of the task involves bringing the object to the body and doing something with it before the task is complete. Since most functional tasks are this complex, we call the second stage of task related movements *task performance*. The description of task performance may include several distinct movement patterns.

MOVEMENT REEDUCATION

Movement reeducation is the process of teaching or training patterns of movement and functional performance that have been lost as a result of physical or other impairments. In the therapeutic literature, the term reeducation implies that the patient has the potential to acquire movement control and that the therapist can influence the patient's recovery by reteaching previously acquired movements. While these assumptions may be controversial in reference to neurologic patients, we strongly believe that both assumptions apply to neurologic rehabilitation. We call our system of treatment *functional movement reeducation* because the goal of our treatment is the restoration of those movements of the trunk, arm, and leg that are critical for functional performance. We reeducate these movement patterns to increase independence in life roles. We believe that this treatment model has the potential to both restore movement control and functional performance to patients with many different movement problems, decreasing their disability and promoting recovery from the signs and symptoms of their disease.

This book is directed toward treatment of stroke and other types of neurologic damage that result in hemiplegia, or loss of movement control on one side of the body. To reeducate functional movements for these patients we must restore movement control to the hemiplegic side and teach the two sides of the body to work together again in functional movements and actual task performance. With neurologic patients, the process of movement reeducation should begin as soon as possible, even if the patient is unable to move the hemiplegic side. In the early days of treatment the therapist used direct handling to assist the patient in the desired movements. This assisted movement allows patients to build muscle strength and control, to practice movements that they would otherwise be unable to perform, and to relearn the sequencing of normal movement. As the patient regains strength and control, the therapist withdraws her assistance until the patient is able to move independently and to use his movements functionally. In this process of movement reeducation, we are tapping into the neurologic patient's capacity for motor learning, a capacity probably based on both neurologic recovery and changes in neural organization.

FIGURE 1-9 Reeducation of a trunk movement component in sitting. This pattern of upper body-initiated lateral flexion is used to move from sitting to sidelying and to reach laterally to the floor as seen in Fig. 1-7B.

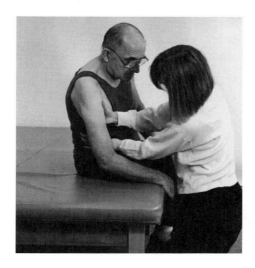

In this book, we use movement components and movement sequences to provide the model for the movement patterns to be reeducated. By training movement components, we reestablish the patterns of coordinated extremity movement in the hemiplegic arm and leg that are necessary for task completion. We also train the patterns of trunk control necessary to keep the body symmetrical, stable, and appropriately active (Fig. 1-9). The training of movement sequences and other functional patterns helps the patient learn to coordinate trunk and extremity movements and to sequence movements of multiple body segments in the correct order for functional performance. We have found that in most cases, the reeducation of movement components and movement sequences allows the patient to perform many functions and occupations, increasing functional performance and decreasing disability. This process of functional movement reeducation should be followed by task specific training and/or compensatory training to provide the patient the means to accomplish more difficult functional goals.

The distinction between functional movement and normal movement is an important one for our model of treatment. The goal of functional movement reeducation is to restore functional movements to our patients, so that they can function more independently in their life roles. Since normal movements represent the usual and preferred pattern of coordination, we believe that we should attempt to restore normal patterns of movement and functional performance. Clearly, not every patient or even most patients will recover to the extent that their movement patterns are nearly normal. However, by using normal movement as the model for movement reeducation, we ensure that each patient learns to use his available muscle strength and control to produce appropriate postural adjustments and reactions and task related extremity movements. In this way, we bring his movements as close to normal as is permitted by his pathology and help him to use these movements functionally to enhance his daily life.

2

Problems Contributing to Loss of Movement and Function

Patients with central nervous system (CNS) pathology have problems with movement that lead to functional dependence and disability. These movement problems have several typical manifestations. Neurologic patients may demonstrate a loss of movement in their involved trunk and extremities, produce atypical or abnormal patterns of movement, or develop compensatory movement strategies to replace normal movement patterns. These patients may also show changes in the quality of their volitional movement responses, affecting the speed of execution and the efficiency and appropriateness of muscle activation. These patients may also demonstrate involuntary nonpurposeful movements on their involved side during functional movements. Whenever normal movement patterns cannot be produced, the neurologic patient's system of normal functional movement is disrupted, leading to loss of independence and disability.

Although most neurologic patients have problems with movement that result in disability, they vary a great deal in the movement patterns that they generate, in the physical findings that influence their motor control, and in the level of functional independence or disability that they ultimately achieve. Thus, to assess effectively and treat these patients, physical and occupational therapists must first describe their movement problems and identify the physical impairments that contribute to these problems. In this chapter, we describe the major problems that affect neurologic patients' ability to move and function. This information is critical for assessing and treating the movement problems and for using this book. The impact that these categories have on the performance of specific movements is presented later in the book.

DEFINITIONS OF IMPAIRMENTS, MOVEMENT PROBLEMS, AND DISABILITIES

The first step in our discussion is to identify the different classifications of problems that have an impact on the neurologic patient's ability to move and function and describe the types of movement problems that relate to these problems. For this model, we will adopt the terminology proposed by the World Health Organization (WHO) for the classification of disease and disablement. *Disablement*, in this model, refers to "the spectrum of experiences associated with limitations in function."[1] Our application of this terminology to neurologic patients is similar to models proposed by Duncan,[2] Schenkman and Butler,[3,4] and Rogers and Holm.[1]

Within our model, we identify three categories of problems, representing differing levels of dysfunction related to CNS pathology, that are relevant to the therapist treating neurologic patients:

1. *Impairment*, the signs, symptoms, and physical findings that relate to the pathology. In this book, we will discuss three types of impairments: *primary impairments*, *secondary impairments*, and *composite movement impairments*. These categories of impairments are not part of the WHO model, but appear in a similar form in articles by Schenkman and Butler[3,4] and Duncan.[2]

2. *Disability*, the loss of specific functional abilities and task-related function. While disability may involve the physical, mental, emotional, and social domains,[3,4] we restrict our discussion to problems in the physical domain. These include functional limitations or loss of functional performance in gait, mobility in bed and upper extremity skills, and tasks related to activities of daily living (ADL).

3. *Handicap* is the specific social and societal consequences that disabilities and impairments have on lifestyle and occupational behavior. A handicapped person is unable to perform the majority of the essential tasks associated with a social role.[1] Examples of common handicaps that affect neurologic patients include loss of vocation, loss of community mobility, and inability to function independently at home.

The above categories represent a hierarchical ordering of the factors that influence independent function. Figure 2-1 illustrates the relationships among these levels of disablement. While the problems associated with each category become increasingly complex as we move from impairment to handicap, the model does not automatically assume that dysfunction at one level will lead to dysfunction at the next level.[1] Thus, a given group of impairments does not necessarily result in specific disabilities or handicaps, and the extent of handicap may not be proportional to the

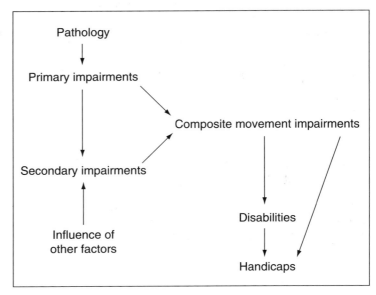

FIGURE 2-1 WHO classification of disease and disablement.

pathology and its resulting impairments. It is true, however, that patients with extensive primary impairments pose more of a treatment challenge and have a poorer prognosis for functional recovery than those patients who present with fewer initial problems.

Although disablement terminology may be unfamiliar to many therapists, we have adopted it because its use is becoming standard in academic writing, because it utilizes a common terminology that is shared with other health professions, and because it provides a systematic way of understanding the many levels of problems faced by our patients. By using this model of disease and disability, we focus our attention on both the physical findings that influence our patients' movements and the loss of function that is the end result of their CNS pathology. We believe this emphasis is an appropriate way of addressing the multiple levels at which therapy intervention occurs. The choice of this medical model also allows us to discuss treatment without reference to theoretical models of CNS organization or theories of motor learning and motor recovery.

Pathology refers to the specific type of brain damage or neurologic disease that causes the problems for which the patient requires therapy. In this book, we address the problems associated with the pathology of stroke, but our information is also applicable to other diseases or types of brain lesion, such as multiple sclerosis and head trauma. Physical and occupational therapists do not intervene at the level of pathology and, as we will see in the following chapters, brain pathology is not the only source for the problems in neurologic patients. While having a complete medical history on all patients referred to therapy is certainly preferable, it is possible for physical and occupational therapists to evaluate and treat without knowledge of the type and location of brain lesion. This is because therapy intervention is directed toward impairment and disability.

IMPAIRMENTS CONTRIBUTING TO MOVEMENT PROBLEMS

Impairments are the signs and symptoms of brain pathology. They are the cause of most of the functional limitations and movement problems that are responsible for referral to physical and occupational therapy. In this book, we discuss two categories of impairment. *Primary impairments* result directly from the brain lesion and are present immediately after brain damage. Muscle weakness is an example of a primary impairment that commonly results from brain pathology. *Secondary impairments* develop over time and in systems of the body not originally affected by the brain pathology. Their development is influenced by the direct effects of the brain lesion and by other factors, including therapy. Soft tissue contracture and changes in joint alignment are examples of secondary impairments that develop over time and influence the neurologic patient's ability to move and function.

Both primary and secondary impairments are subject to change and may continue to evolve after the initial brain damage.[1,3,4] This process of change may come about because of changes in nervous system pathology. For example, either an extension of the disease process or reduction of cerebral swelling may modify the original impairments. Changes in impairments may also arise because of complicating problems in other systems of the body, which influence the original impairments. For example, a hip fracture of the affected leg results in marked reduction in muscle strength, mobility, and independence. This change is in addition to the

Impairments
Primary
Secondary
Composite

problems of muscle weakness and hypotonia or hypertonia that result from the brain lesion. Or the original impairments themselves may improve or worsen because of the effects of learning and treatment. For this reason, the relationship between pathology and impairments does not always match, and the severity of impairments during the acute stage may not be a good predictor of the patient's status later in the rehabilitation process.

In the section below, we discuss the specific primary and secondary impairments that are most important for physical and occupational therapy. While CNS damage may result in impairments in many systems of the body, our discussion is limited to impairments that have a direct effect on the movement problems and functional limitations of the patient and are potentially responsive to intervention by physical and occupational therapists. Cognitive, emotional, and speech/language deficits may have a profound effect on the patient's function and quality of life but fall outside the scope of this book and will not be addressed.

Primary Impairments

Primary impairments are the physical findings that are associated with specific types of neurologic damage and correlate with damage to specific areas of the brain. Before sophisticated tests, such as computed tomography and magnetic resonance imaging, were widely available, primary impairments were used to diagnose neurologic damage and to localize the area of brain lesion. The primary impairments of particular relevance to the movement problems of our patients include changes in muscle strength, muscle tone, and muscle activation, and changes in sensory processing. We discuss each of these categories separately.

Changes in Muscle Strength

Changes in muscle strength represent one of the most important categories of impairments that arise from CNS lesions. CNS lesions result in impairments of muscle strength in the muscles of the affected side or in the affected body segments. The most common types of impairments in muscle strength are muscle paralysis and weakness or paresis. The patterns of weakness and paralysis observed in neurologic patients appear to correlate with specific physiologic changes in muscle fiber or in nerve conduction.[5]

Paralysis refers to the total inability of a muscle to contract for any effective use. It is the most severe type of muscular involvement that is found in the patient with brain pathology. A paralyzed muscle is unable to contract with sufficient force to produce joint movement or to provide postural stability to the body segment. When there is paralysis, the affected body segment feels floppy and heavy and the involved muscles do not resist, follow, or assist with guided movements. *Flaccidity* is the term used to describe this state of paralysis.

Paralysis may affect many muscles or be limited to selected muscles. In the acute stroke, paralysis often involves all or most of the major muscles on one side of the body, so that functional movement is absent in the involved face, trunk, arm, and leg. In less severe strokes or where motor recovery has occurred, some muscle groups on the affected side contract to produce movement while other muscles remain paralyzed and cannot be activated. When paralysis persists in even some muscles, full control of normal movement is impossible.

Primary Impairments

Changes in muscle strength

Changes in muscle/postural tone

Changes in muscle activation

Sensory changes

Muscle weakness or paresis is present when a muscle is able to contract, but the strength of contraction is inadequate to allow effective use. Weakness is characterized by either an inability to sustain contraction long enough to allow performance of a movement or tasks, or an inability to recruit sufficient force to produce the desired movement or range (Fig. 2-2). Weak muscles actively assist guided movements by the therapist and may be able to contract with sufficient strength to maintain a stable body position for a brief period. However, muscle weakness causes the body part to feel heavy because muscle strength is not adequate to fully control the weight of the body segment against gravity.

Muscle weakness may be present immediately after stroke in selected muscles of the hemiplegic side. Some stroke patients never experience full paralysis of their affected side but present immediately with muscle weakness. In degenerative diseases like multiple sclerosis, muscle weakness is often the first symptom of CNS pathology. As paralyzed muscles recover, they also pass through a stage of weakness. Weak muscles can co-exist with muscles that have regained normal strength and endurance and with muscles that remain densely paralyzed. Weakness in the muscles of the trunk also is frequently found in patients with hypertonicity in the arm or leg.

Neurologic patients may have weakness in both trunk and extremity muscles. Muscle weakness in the trunk interferes with postural control and decreases the stability of the trunk over its base of support. It also interferes with the performance of normal trunk movements necessary for functional movement sequences. This loss of trunk stability and mobility causes normal control of extremity movements and task performance to be disrupted. Muscle weakness in the arm or leg prevents use of the limb for weight bearing and functional movements in space. When these critical extremity movement components are lost, the patient's ability to function independently is often lost as well.

Muscle weakness varies depending on the starting position of the body, the length of the muscle, and the particular action the muscle is being asked to perform. In neurologic patients in particular, muscles that contract with good strength

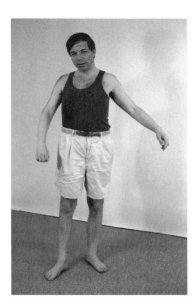

FIGURE 2-2 Muscle weakness limits functional range of motion in right hemiplegia. The patient is attempting to move both arms into horizontal abduction.

in one position or for one movement may be unable to contract if placed at a different length or asked to perform a different function. For example, the biceps muscle often contracts strongly during the movement of shoulder flexion but may contract only weakly to produce elbow flexion through partial range when the humerus is stabilized by the side of the body. Similarly, muscles that contract isotonically may be unable to work eccentrically, to be active isometrically, or to work synergistically with muscles of other body segments. For this reason, testing the strength of specific muscles using standard tests of muscle strength is usually unreliable with neurologic patients.

While loss of muscle strength is a primary impairment, it is strongly influenced by secondary changes in joint alignment and mobility, by changes in muscle and tissue length, and by problems of muscle tone and muscle activation. Muscles that are maintained in a position of constant length may have more difficulty contracting than they would in a mid-range or shortened position. The contraction of muscles is also made more difficult when soft tissue shortening or constant inappropriate muscle activity (hypertonicity) is present in the antagonist muscles. In these situations, the apparent weakness of agonist muscles may resolve when the therapist removes the mechanical restraints to muscle contraction by lengthening soft tissues or quieting muscle firing.

Impairments in muscle strength and the imbalance in strength that comes from incomplete motor return are important to physical and occupational therapists because of their effects on movement and function. Muscle weakness leads to an inability to perform movement components, movement sequences, and functional movements (movement deficits) and to the development of atypical and compensatory movement patterns. Research appears to demonstrate a relationship between muscle strength and recovery of function in selected muscle groups and functional outcome as well.[6] Several studies with stroke patients have considered muscle strength a reliable predictor of motor recovery, and other authors report increases in muscle strength coincide with improvements in performance of activities of daily living (ADL).[5]

Changes in Tone

Changes in tone are the second major type of impairment associated with neurologic lesions. These tonal changes affect both muscle tone and postural tone on the side of the body affected by the stroke or brain lesion. *Muscle tone* is defined as the amount of tension in a muscle. It is generally measured clinically by testing the amount of resistance in the muscle to passive lengthening. *Postural tone*, a special category of muscle tone, refers to the overall state of tension in the body musculature. It is used to define the body's readiness to move and its ability to resist the downward pull of gravity. Both muscle and postural tone are quantified by observation of the appearance of the muscles (i.e., their resting length and tautness), observation of body posture and limb position, and by palpation of individual muscles. Additional tests for deep tendon jerks, clonus, and clasped knife responses are also used to diagnose and quantify impairments in muscle tone. In hemiplegic patients, the tone on the affected side of the body is assessed and compared with that on the side of the body that was unaffected. Clinical measurements of tone are subjective, because no objective measurement tools are readily available to the practicing therapist.

While some neurologic patients do not show alterations in muscle tone, disorders of muscle tone are extremely common. Altered muscle tone in neurologic patients may be lower or higher than normal. The term *hypotonicity* is used to describe muscle tone that is lower than normal. Hypotonic muscles provide no resistance to passive movement and have lower than normal tension at rest and during movement. Hypotonicity is associated with muscles that are paralyzed or weak, and when hypotonia is present, it is difficult clinically to distinguish between low tone and weakness. Since tension in the affected muscle fibers is decreased, hypotonic muscles have difficulty resisting the force of gravity. This leads to the development of secondary impairments in alignment and joint stability as bones and joints are pulled out of normal alignment. Hypotonicity occurs most commonly in the acute stage but may persist throughout recovery in some of the muscles of the involved side (Fig. 2-3).

Hypertonicity is the term used to describe muscles that have greater than normal muscle tension and increased resistance to passive lengthening. In hemiplegia, hypertonicity is associated with the flexor muscles of the upper extremity and the extensor muscles of the lower extremity (Fig. 2-4). Hypertonicity may be located in muscles that the patient can actively contract. When this increased muscle stiffness is used by the patient to accomplish a function, hypertonicity can be described as increased "active stiffness" in the affected muscle groups. This type of hypertonicity commonly occurs in patients in whom incomplete motor recovery leads to atypical patterns of muscle activation. Hypertonicity may also develop in muscles that are weak or paralyzed but have been maintained in a constant position of shortness because of changes in biomechanical alignment. In this case, the positional shortening results in a "passive stiffness" of the muscle. When active or passive stiffness persists for long periods, muscle shortening or contracture of muscle will develop.

Spasticity is a special type of hypertonicity. The spastic muscle has an abnormal increase in velocity-dependent resistance to stretch and hyperactive tendon jerks. It may also demonstrate a mild to moderate increase in length-dependent stiffness and the clasp-knife phenomenon. While the scientific literature distinguishes between spasticity and hypertonicity, clinically these terms are used

FIGURE 2-3 Right hemiplegia with hypotonia.

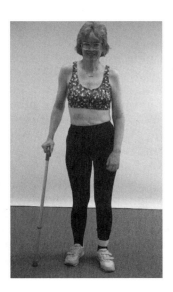

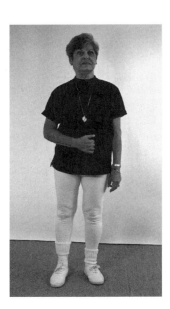

FIGURE 2-4 Right hemiplegia with hypertonia.

almost interchangeably. In this book, we will use the term hypertonicity to describe the increased muscle tension that is associated with unnatural body postures and limb positions, changes in the quality of volitional movements, and the development of atypical patterns of coordination. We prefer to use this term, because many hypertonic muscles may not truly fit the scientific definition for spasticity. True spasticity, such as occurs with massive brain damage, is probably not responsive to therapy, but hypotonicity and hypertonicity do respond to specific handling techniques and may be altered within a treatment session and on a long-term basis.

Neurologic patients show variations in how muscle tone is distributed on the affected side. Brain injury is associated with immediate or rapid onset of hypertonicity. Most stroke patients initially show hypotonic muscle and postural tone in their affected trunk and limbs. As time after the stroke increases, these stroke patients often begin to exhibit gradual tonal fluctuations and increasing hypertonicity in some of the muscles on the affected side. During the process of recovery, many variations in muscle tone develop. In some patients, muscle tone is consistent in the involved trunk, arm, and leg. These patients may have hypotonic muscle tone throughout the involved side, or hypertonicity throughout the side. Other patients have variations in the tone on the involved side. They may have hypertonic extremities with hypotonic trunk muscles, hypertonicity in the arm and lower tone in the trunk and leg, or a hypotonic upper extremity and hypertonic lower extremity. Tonal properties may also vary from muscle to muscle in an extremity. Either increased muscle tone in the proximal muscles of the extremity with decreased tone in the lower arm or leg or the reverse of this distribution are common in hemiplegia.

Variations in muscle tone may be partially explained by the type of brain lesion. For example, parietal lobe lesions are associated with hypotonia and decerebrate rigidity is found in massive closed head injury. But in many patients, muscle tone changes or evolves from its original state as the patient begins to move and develop compensations for changes in muscle strength, control, and body alignment on one side of the body. Fluctuations in muscle tone in individual patients can be observed with changes in body position, during the performance of certain movement patterns or activities, and during stressful or emotional situations. Over time, these tonal fluctuations occur less frequently and muscle tension becomes permanently increased on the hemiplegic side. The fact that increases in muscle tone develop over time and are associated with selected activities suggests that muscle tone is influenced by factors besides the original brain lesion.

From our clinical practice, we have identified three different mechanisms that contribute to the development of hypertonicity:

1. Changes in length-tension relationship: Muscle tension is increased in certain two-joint muscles when changes in orthopedic alignment result in changes in the length-tension relationship of the muscle. A common example of this occurs in the biceps brachii muscle. Increased tone in the biceps muscle develops mechanically when an anterior subluxation of the humeral head places tension on the long head of the biceps. The anterior displacement of the humeral head in the glenoid fossa increases mechanical tension at the proximal end of the biceps muscle, causing elbow flexion and often forearm supination. When the humeral head is repositioned posteriorly in the glenoid fossa, the tension on the hypertonic biceps muscle is relieved and the elbow may be passively extended (Fig. 2-5).

2. Postural Instability: Muscle tension increases when poor trunk and extremity control make the body unstable or insecure. Increased hypertonicity in the arm is often associated with postural insecurity and can be seen as an atypical balance strategy (Fig. 2-6). Similarly, hypertonicity in the leg may occur as a type of balance response when the upper body is unstable (Fig. 2-7). Handling techniques by the therapist that provide normal postural alignment and stability to the trunk and involved leg quickly remove the patient's need to recruit muscle activity in the hemiplegic side for balance. As the body becomes more stable, hypertonicity in the hemiplegic arm or leg decreases, so the the extremity returns to a normal resting position.

3. Active Recruitment: Muscle tension increases during volitional movement when the pattern of muscle activation is inappropriate. In this type of hypertonicity, the increase in muscle tension occurs when the patient activates the wrong

FIGURE 2-5 Anterior subluxation of the glenohumeral joint results in hypertonicity in the biceps muscle. (A) The resting position of the arm. (B) The therapist repositions the shoulder joint. (C) Mechanical tension in the biceps muscle is reduced so that the elbow may be passively extended and the forearm pronated. (D) The resting position of the arm after treatment.

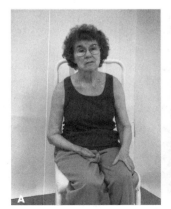
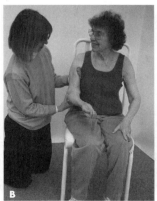
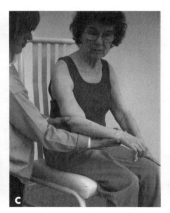
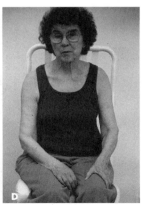

FIGURE 2-6 Flexor hypertonicity of the hemiplegic arm increases during sit to stand. *(A)* As the patient prepares to stand, the hemiplegic left arm is extended and relaxed. *(B)* Flexor tone increases in the arm as the patient pushes with his uninvolved arm. *(C)* Flexion of the hemiplegic arm increases as the body approaches the upright position. *(D)* While standing independently with the quad cane, the arm remains flexed. Body position is asymmetrical and precarious, with minimal weight, on the hemiplegic leg. *(E)* After treatment, body position is more symmetric, the hemiplegic leg supports increased weight, and flexor hypertonicity in the hemiplegic arm is noticeably decreased.

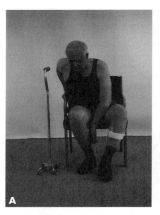
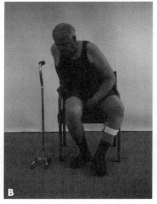
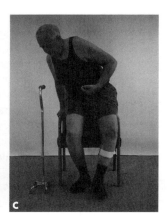
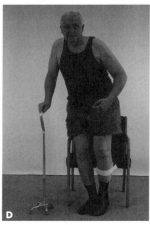
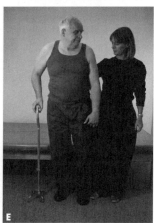

muscles for the task being performed or activates these muscles with inappropriate force (Fig. 2-8). This pattern of hypertonicity is often trained in treatment. For example, the patient with muscle weakness in the hemiplegic leg learns to lock the knee during stance by firing the quadriceps muscle and later is unable to stop the muscle from firing. Or it may be acquired because incomplete motor return and sensory changes affect the patient's ability to use the appropriate muscle groups. In either case, muscles that are activated inappropriately often cannot be quieted, creating unwanted and persistent muscle firing.

Any of the types of hypertonicity described above will eventually become part of the patient's learned movement repertoire. When muscles are constantly maintained in a state of inappropriate tension, changes in tissue length and mobility develop as secondary complications. It is difficult to distinguish between hypertonicity and soft tissue shortening or contracture without the clinical skill necessary to inhibit hypertonicity. To assess the extent to which abnormal limb position is due to hypertonicity, the therapist must decrease or "normalize" the tension in the hypertonic muscles. Once muscle tone has been decreased, soft tissue length and joint mobility can be assessed (Fig. 2-9). Techniques for reducing tension in hypertonic muscles are described later in the book.

Although the relationship between abnormal muscle tone and loss of movement control is controversial,[7] we believe that both hypotonicity and hypertonicity have a significant effect on the neurologic patient's movement patterns. Hypertonus is associated with stiff limbs and inappropriate muscle firing. These problems interfere with the production of normal movement and result in atypical movements and functional limitations. Reducing tension in the hypertonic muscle allows reeducation of normal patterns of muscle activation and functional movement without the mechanical restraints that hypertonicity place on joint alignment and muscle extensibility. Similarly, excessively low tone interferes with readiness for movement and the ability to generate sufficient force to overcome the influence of gravity and produce movement. Low-tone patients cannot move their involved trunk and limbs in normal patterns without treatment to increase postural tone in the trunk and stimulate weak extremity muscles to contract. Thus, when the presence of abnormal muscle tone interferes with the production of normal movement patterns, the therapist must combine techniques to change muscle tone with techniques of movement reeducation.

For tonal changes to last, treatment must address the underlying cause of increased tension. When flexor posturing of the arm is a result of poor trunk and lower extremity control, lasting changes in arm position and muscle tension can not be achieved until the trunk is more stable and symmetrical and the lower extremity gains control of movement and stability in weight bearing. On the other hand, if upper extremity changes in muscle tension are caused by poor alignment of the scapula and shoulder joint, treatment of the shoulder to restore resting alignment and normal mechanics during movement will achieve relatively quick changes in arm position. These changes are long lasting when balanced muscle activity in the trunk, scapula, and glenohumeral joint maintains the shoulder joint in normal alignment. If hypertonicity in the limbs is caused by excessive muscle activation or inappropriate coactivation of muscle during active movement, treatment must stress quieting unwanted muscle activity and reeducation

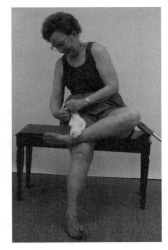

FIGURE 2-7 Hypertonicity in the hemiplegic leg occurs as a balance reaction.

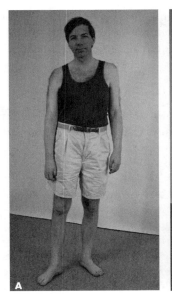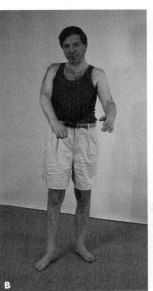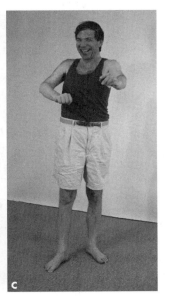

FIGURE 2-8 Increased muscle tone during active movements of the hemiplegic arm. (A) Before movement, the hemiplegic right arm is extended by the side of the body. (B) The patient initiates the movement of shoulder flexion. (C) As he attempts to raise his arm higher, more muscles are actively recruited and muscle tone increases excessively.

FIGURE 2-9 Hypertonic flexor muscles of the hemiplegic right arm before and after treatment. (A) The flexed adducted position of the arm before treatment. (B) After treatment, there is a definite change in the amount of elbow flexion and adduction, but the arm still lacks full elbow extension. The atypical resting position of the arm is caused by soft tissue contracture.

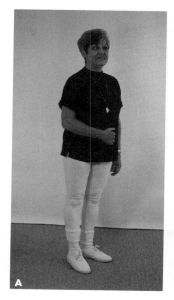 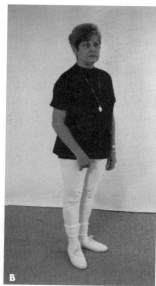

of muscle firing in correct sequences and with appropriate strength of contraction. The process of changing tone in the treatment setting prepares the patient to participate actively in treatment. It also helps the patient learn to modulate muscle tone to prepare for movement and to maintain appropriate muscle tone during movement.

In our experience, permanent changes in muscle tone are possible. Both hypotonic and hypertonic hemiplegic patients can achieve more appropriate muscle and postural tone through treatment by physical/occupational therapists. These changes in tone occur when the appropriate causes for increased tone are addressed in treatment and when the patient acquires new patterns of movement and coordination to replace atypical movements. Normalizing muscle tone rarely results in more normal movement patterns without being followed by movement reeducation. For this reason, changing abnormal muscle tone should be seen as a necessary preparation for movement reeducation, not the primary goal of treatment.

Changes in Muscle Activation

The third type of primary impairment that affects control of movement is called *change in patterns of muscle activation*. Changes in muscle activation are present during movement when the neurologic patient activates the wrong muscles for the task being performed, changes the sequence of muscle activation, or activates too many muscles with inappropriate force. These changes affect the coordination of muscle synergies and interfere with the performance of functional movements. They can be considered to be changes in *motor control*, or the ways that the brain directs the organization and sequencing of movement. Disturbances in muscle activation arise primarily from the brain lesion[3,4] but may also be strongly influenced by sensory impairments, by secondary problems, such as changes in alignment, and by treatment. Since these patterns develop as the patient attempts active movements, we believe that this category of impairments may be based as much on learning, practice, and therapy as it is a direct result of the lesion and motor recovery.

Several types of movement problems relate to changes in muscle activation. *Inappropriate patterns of muscle activation* occur when the patient activates the wrong muscles for the task being performed, or when muscles are activated in the wrong sequence for the desired movement. These inappropriate patterns of muscle activation represent a deviation from established muscle synergies and normal patterns of coordination. Inappropriate patterns of muscle activation changes most commonly substitute strong muscle groups for muscles that are weak or paralyzed. Often stronger proximal muscles are substituted for weak distal muscles, with the result that movement patterns are initiated from the wrong part of the body. For example, when elbow and wrist extensors are weak, the patient may substitute shoulder elevation and humeral abduction with flexion of the elbow and wrist to lift the hand. We call this change in movement sequence *an inappropriate pattern of initiation* (Fig. 2-10). In other cases, the patient may substitute a strong muscle group for a paralyzed muscle, even when the action of this muscle is inappropriate to the intended function. For example, when toe extensors and ankle dorsiflexors are weak, the patient may use toe flexors for a balance response in standing. We call this an *inappropriate muscle substitution* (Fig. 2-11).

Excessive cocontraction occurs when the patient activates too many muscles during movement performance, so that both the correct muscles and additional inappropriate muscles are simultaneously contracting. This overactivity usually occurs in the extremities, where it leads to cocontraction of muscles on both sides of the joint (Fig. 2-12). Inappropriate coactivation of agonist/antagonist muscle groups has "been demonstrated in gait, dynamic movements, and under static conditions."[5] Once the muscles have been activated, the patient may be unable to stop the muscle firing and return the body part to a position of rest. Cocontraction of muscles on the involved side leads to hypertonicity, muscle shortening, and to permanent changes in the resting posture of the trunk and extremities.

Excessive force production during movement is present when the patient activates muscles groups too forcefully or with inappropriate effort for the desired movement. This pattern of muscle activation, often incorrectly labeled spasticity, is instead an

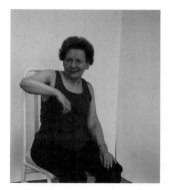

FIGURE 2-10 Inappropriate initiation of arm movement component. The patient is activating shoulder elevators and abductors to reach the arm forward, instead of initiating the movement from the hand and wrist.

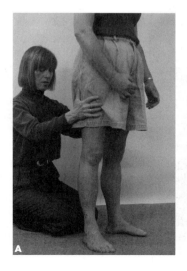 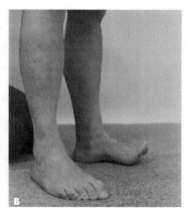

FIGURE 2-11 Inappropriate muscle activation in the hemiplegic right leg. *(A)* The therapist shifts the patient's weight backwards to activate a balance reaction in the muscles of the feet and ankles. *(B)* The toe muscles in the left foot contract appropriately to lift the front of the foot. In the hemiplegic foot, the toes flex and claw into the floor.

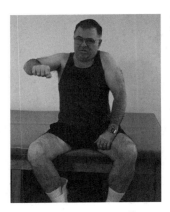

FIGURE 2-12 Excessive effort and muscle cocontraction are used to lift up the hemiplegic arm.

inappropriate change in force production during voluntary muscle contraction. When force or effort is excessive, the movement pattern is slow and the moving segment is stiff. Frequently, this pattern of excessive effort cannot be sustained long enough to complete the movement through the full range. As the muscles fatigue, they suddenly cannot sustain their high level of contraction and the moving body segment falls back to its starting position. Excessive force production often coexists with weakness and low tone and with the problems of cocontraction discussed above. When the pattern of excessive force production is reinforced, it leads to sustained inappropriate muscle activity and stiff extremities.

Changes in patterns of muscle activation always result in atypical and/or inefficient patterns of movement and coordination. As atypical patterns of muscle activation develop, they become part of the patient's movement repertoire. The patient uses these abnormal patterns of muscle activation to stabilize body position, move trunk and limbs, and attempt functional movements. They are often associated with hypertonicity, with loss of muscle length, and with changes in posture and alignment, all of which interfere with normal patterns of muscle sequencing and firing. Specific movement problems that are associated with changes in muscle activation are discussed further in this chapter, in the section on Atypical Movements.

Movement reeducation may have a powerful effect on problems with muscle activation. The process of movement reeducation described in this book emphasizes normal patterns of muscle activation, normal sequencing of movement patterns, and appropriate force production during muscle activation. When this is done from the early days of rehabilitation, treatment will establish both the sensory and motor basis for normal movement and prevent atypical patterns of muscle firing from being learned. When this type of assistance is not part of early treatment, the motivated patient may acquire and practice these atypical firing patterns. Once the neurologic patient has acquired atypical patterns of muscle activation, the process of movement reeducation must involve both the quieting of inappropriate muscle activity and the training of normal sequences and intensities of muscle activation and normal patterns of coordination. The process of unlearning undesirable movement patterns is often frustrating to the patient but can be ultimately successful.

Sensory Changes

Sensory impairments and difficulties with processing sensory information accompany the impairments of muscle strength and tone described above. Sensory impairments are important to the therapist because of the important role sensation plays in body image and body awareness, movement planning, and motor learning. Diminished sensation affects the patient's ability to feel and correctly interpret information from his involved side, his ability to learn movement patterns on his affected side, and his ability to plan and execute movements automatically. Sensory deficits also play an important role in the development of pain. Impairments of the sensory system that are common after neurologic damage include deficits in sensory awareness, deficits in sensory processing and interpretation, and deficits in sensation affecting the planning and execution of movement.

Deficits in Sensory Awareness

Deficits in sensory awareness occur when information from the sensory receptors of the involved side cannot be perceived or identified by the patient. This problem usually affects the tactile, proprioceptive, and kinesthetic systems. It influences the patient's ability to "feel" his involved side and respond to sensory information from that side. Sensory deficits may also involve the visual system, when visual field cuts remove the involved side of the body from visual regard, and the vestibular system, when abnormal head and neck posture interfere with normal labyrinthine responses. Patients with severe sensory deficits ignore or "neglect" their involved extremities or even deny that they are part of their body. Less severe deficits are more common and are associated with complaints that the involved side feels "numb" or "asleep."

Sensory deficits are most severe in patients with dense flaccid paralysis and hypotonia. They have their greatest effect on movement and function in the early days after stroke. In the acute phase, afferent sensory information from muscle, joint, and tactile receptors on the involved side is limited, since the patient is unable to move his limbs actively or change his body position. As the patient begins to participate in treatment and regain active motor control, the experience of moving and being moved increases sensory input from the involved side. Some sensory impairments may resolve or diminish at this time. For this reason, poor sensation in the acute flaccid patient should not automatically be considered a bad prognostic sign.[8] However, in many patients, sensation continues to be decreased or sensory return stops before it reaches the distal portions of the extremities. In these patients, residual sensory loss continues to influence posture and movement of the hemiplegic side and the response to treatment.

Sensory deficits influence control of movement and treatment in several ways. Patients with poor sensation are less aware of asymmetries in their body posture and make fewer attempts to spontaneously move or use their involved extremities for function or weight support. In treatment, they often have difficulty understanding the movements that the therapist is trying to teach them, and may be unable to independently reproduce movement sequences when the therapist's handling is removed. Patients with good motor recovery and persistent sensory deficits appear to forget about using their involved arm or leg for function when not in therapy, and may use compensations to avoid use of the involved side. Fine motor coordination of the hand is also affected by decreased sensitivity and patients are forced to rely on vision to compensate for tactile deficits.

Deficits in Sensory Interpretation

Deficits in sensory interpretation affect the patient's ability to correctly perceive, interpret, and respond to sensory input from the involved side. Deficits in sensory interpretation make the patient unsure about what is happening in his body. When sensory interpretation is affected, the patient is overly sensitive to sensory input from therapy, so that the therapist's touch or assistance is confusing to his body. He may misinterpret sensory information as painful if the therapist's handling provides too much sensory input or stimulates too many sensory systems simultaneously. Patients with problems in sensory interpretation are often fearful of therapy and movement, because they place demands on the patients processing abilities that exceed their capacity.

Deficits in sensory interpretation are most apparent in the acute patient, in whom they contribute to the state of general confusion and disorganization that is common in these early days.[8] These deficits often resolve when therapy helps the patient relearn to organize sensory information. The therapist does this by keeping sensory input consistent, limiting the number of sensory systems that are stimulated, and using verbal explanations to help the patient understand what he is feeling. Patients who do not regain the ability to correctly process sensory input avoid movement, protect their involved side from handling by the therapist, and often progress to chronic pain.

Deficits in Kinesthetic Memory

A third kind of sensory deficit relates directly to the kinesthetic system. Deficits in kinesthetic memory affect the neurologic patient's ability to plan and execute normal movements. *Kinesthetic memory* refers to the body's sensory knowledge of normal movement: what it should feel like and how it is correctly executed. It includes information about the sequencing of joint movements, about timing and speed, and about the amount of muscle strength necessary to achieve the desired result. Sports psychologists hypothesize that sensory feelings or kinesthetic memories for normal movement are stored in the brain. These kinesthetic memories allow us to replay movements in our imagination and recognize them when we feel them again.[9] This information is available as part of the motor programs that generate most everyday functional movements and specialized motor skills.

When neurologic patients have deficits in kinesthetic memory, they lose two important parts of kinesthetic awareness: the knowledge of what normal movement should feel like and the "muscle memory" for the patterns of muscle activity used in the movements of daily life. These losses contribute to both the abnormal quality of their movements and the atypical movements that they develop. Deficits in kinesthetic memory probably explain why some patients with good motor recovery and muscle strength in their involved side do not spontaneously regain normal patterns of movement. In treatment, active-assistive movements play an important role in reestablishing the sensation of normal movement and kinesthetic information about how normal movements are executed. These kinesthetic memories can then be used by the patient to mentally plan and rehearse normal movement patterns of his involved side and to mentally compare his independent performance of movements with the normal model provided by the therapist.

Secondary Impairments

Secondary impairments are not directly caused by the nervous system lesion but occur as a consequence of the primary impairments and other environmental influences. They may involve systems of the body that were not originally affected by the lesion, or present additional complications in the systems that were originally affected. As they develop, secondary impairments influence each other and the primary impairments as well, so that they may modify the initial level of impairment. Secondary impairments have an impact on the patient's level of disability by contributing additional physical problems that affect his ability to generate normal movements.

Physical and occupational therapists treat two categories of secondary impairments. The first type of problems develop because of factors that are outside of the therapist's control. For example, the patient may fall and fracture his hip or develop phlebitis in his leg or pneumonia. These problems complicate the patient's clinical picture and must be addressed in treatment but are not a direct consequence of his rehabilitation program. These secondary impairments are not discussed in this book.

Secondary Impairments

Orthopedic changes

Changes in muscle and soft tissue length

Pain

Edema

The second type of secondary impairment does develop as a direct consequence of the patient's primary impairments and the type and goals of the therapy that he receives. These predictable problems are often preventable by prompt therapeutic intervention. Included in this category of secondary impairments are changes in orthopedic alignment and mobility, changes in muscle and tissue length, edema, and pain. These problems are discussed individually below. Since these impairments further complicate the patient's problems, they will have to be addressed in treatment whenever their effects interfere with treatment goals. For this reason, prevention of secondary impairments is an important goal of all stages of rehabilitation.

Orthopedic Changes in Alignment and Mobility

Primary impairments in muscle strength, muscle tone, and muscle activation often lead to *secondary orthopedic changes*. These orthopedic changes include changes in alignment and changes in joint mobility. Since normal movement patterns require normal posture, normal joint mechanics, and normal joint mobility, these orthopedic changes exert a strong influence on the patterns of movement that can be produced. Secondary orthopedic changes also change the normal resting length and position of muscles, influencing muscle strength and muscle tone. If joint alignment is severely changed or joint mobility compromised, normal movement patterns cannot be produced. These undesirable orthopedic changes lead directly to atypical and/or compensatory movements and loss of functional performance.

Changes in Alignment

In the neurologic patient, changes in alignment are the first type of problem that develops in the orthopedic system of the body. Included in the category are both alterations in the normal resting postures of bones (e.g., changes in the spinal curves) and changes in the normal mechanical relationships in joints (e.g., change in glenohumeral joint alignment caused by movement of the scapula into a resting position of downward rotation). Alignment changes may develop relatively quickly, as in shoulder subluxation, or slowly and progressively, as in midfoot pronation that develops with increasing ambulation. Changes in resting alignment or posture occur in the low-tone acute patient, when the pull of gravity and the weight of the paretic limbs exert traction on the spine and ribcage and on the scapula/glenohumeral joint and pelvis. They also develop in patients with incomplete motor recovery. In these patients, use of available muscles is not balanced by contraction in the paralytic antagonist muscles. This atypical pattern of muscle use will exert destabilizing pulls on the trunk and limbs and alter the relationship between body segments.

Changes in posture and alignment are found in the trunk and extremities. In the trunk, exaggerations of the spinal curves, excessive spinal flexion or extension, and asymmetries between the two sides of the body leading to C-curve and S-curve scoliosis patterns are all common postural deviations. These abnormal trunk positions interfere with the production of normal weight shifts and postural responses and influence movement patterns in the arms and legs.

In the arm and leg, changes in alignment develop in proximal areas connecting the limbs to the trunk and in the distal segments. Alterations in extremity alignment lead to unnatural limb positions with incompatible relationships between proximal and distal limb segments (Fig. 2-13). For example, a typical flexed posture of the arm may combine shoulder internal rotation with elbow flexion, forearm supination and wrist flexion with radial deviation, a pattern that does not occur in

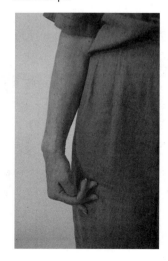

FIGURE 2-13 Abnormal resting alignment in the hemiplegic forearm, wrist, and hand, with incompatible proximal/distal relationships.

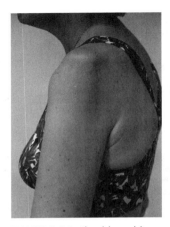

FIGURE 2-14 Shoulder subluxation.

normal movement. Unnatural limb positions change the starting position for movement. They quickly lead to problems of muscle shortening and contracture that will block passive correction of alignment without additional therapeutic input to lengthen the shortened tissues.

Changes in resting posture also place the articular surfaces of joints in unnatural positions and change the mechanics of joint movement. Shoulder subluxation, or partial separation of the humerus from the acromium fossa, is one of the first changes in alignment to develop after stroke. It develops when the weight of the hypotonic arm pulls the scapula out of alignment on the ribcage, unlocking the humerus from the glenoid (Fig. 2-14). When the shoulder joint is subluxed, passive movements of the humerus will not be accompanied by appropriate scapular rotation. Normal shoulder rhythm will not be possible until the scapula is repositioned on the ribcage and the humerus is reseated in the fossa. Similar problems of joint malpositioning may lead to the creation of a new axis of movement during weight bearing. In the foot, shortening of the achilles tendon leads to a superior glide of the calcaneus. When this foot is placed in weight bearing, the heel is not in contact with the floor and body weight is shifted forward to the midfoot. Poor alignment during weight bearing places inappropriate stress on joint capsules and muscle tendons, leading to changes in joint mobility and to pain in these joints and capsules.

Change in Joint Mobility

Change in joint mobility is a second type of orthopedic impairment that develops in neurologic patients. This category includes both joint hypermobility and hypomobility. *Hypermobility* is used to describe joints that have excessive play or laxity and greater than normal range of motion. In neurologic patients, hypermobility is found in joints that sublux because of hypotonia and muscle weakness (e.g., the shoulder). It is also quite common in the joints of the lower extremity, including the hip, knee, and midfoot, because of the stretching that is placed on the joint capsules by weight bearing on the leg with poor alignment (Fig. 2-15). Hypermobility in the wrist and hand may also be created by poor alignment during weight bearing and by aggressive passive range of motion. Hypermobile joints present a handling problem in treatment, because the joint must be realigned and stabilized during reeducation of movement. The therapist must take particular care to provide joint stability during weight bearing so that body weight does not place additional stress on lax joints and capsules.

Hypomobility is present in joints that are excessively stiff and have less than normal joint mobility available for active and passive motion. Hypomobility generally develops in joints that are maintained in a set position or that move infrequently and through small arcs of movement. It is most common in patients with severe muscle weakness resulting in poor balance and limited ability to move their involved trunk, arm, or leg. These patients spend most of their days sitting in a chair. They develop hypomobility in segments of the spine and ribcage and in the joints of the pelvis and hips. (Fig. 2-16). Hypomobility is also a common problem affecting the scapulothoracic joint of the arm in patients with many different types of muscle tone and motor control, as most range of motion exercises move the shoulder joint but neglect the scapula. Other common reasons for hypomobility include pain and mechanical blockages to full joint movement that are created by changes in joint position.

Hypomobility is always accompanied by soft tissue tightness. These restrictions develop simultaneously and should be considered as two parts of the same prob-

FIGURE 2-15 Hypermobility in the midfoot is associated with severe pronation of the hemiplegic foot during weight bearing.

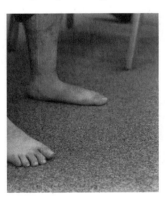

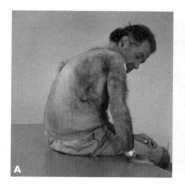 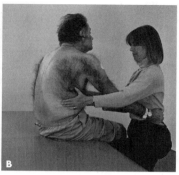

FIGURE 2-16 Loss of normal trunk alignment. *(A)* Excessive trunk flexion in sitting. *(B)* The therapist tries to increase extension in the spine. Joint hypomobility prevents her handling from producing a change in spinal position.

lem: restricted range of motion. In treatment, range of motion restrictions respond best to active and active-assisted movements that are localized to the areas of decreased mobility. The therapist should select movements of the trunk and extremities that encourage movement in the stiff joints and ask shortened soft tissues to lengthen. For example, to increase mobility in the thoracic spine in a patient with an exaggerated kyphosis, the therapist may use upper and lower trunk-initiated anterior and posterior weight shifts. While restoring mobility to stiff joints must be part of any treatment program designed to retrain normal movement, the process of movement reeducation will achieve both tissue lengthening and joint stretch while increasing movement control. Specific joint mobilization is almost never necessary in neurologic patients and may actually be harmful if increased joint mobility is achieved without teaching the patient how to move and control his increased joint flexibility.

Secondary changes in orthopedic alignment and mobility can be prevented or minimized by careful treatment. In patients with severe low tone and weakness, the therapist can minimize shoulder subluxation and collapse of the hemiplegic hand or foot during weight bearing by manually supporting the joints at risk or by the use of slings, splints, braces, and other positioning techniques to preserve good mechanical relationships. At the same time, the process of movement reeducation will help strengthen weak muscles, balance patterns of muscle activation and maintain muscle length and joint mobility. If these techniques are used from the early days of treatment, many patients will not develop shoulder subluxation or other alignment changes. When significant alignment problems are already present, the therapist must try to restore normal alignment before attempting to reeducate movement, and to maintain this alignment during movement reeducation.

Changes in Muscle and Soft Tissue Length

In neurologic patients, muscles and soft tissues on the involved side lose length and flexibility as a secondary complication of changes in muscle tone and muscle strength. These changes in length affect muscle and tendon, skin, fascia, and connective tissue. Muscles that have lost length and flexibility feel stiff or hard and may have palpable knots or lumps within the muscle belly. The tendons on these shortened muscles are prominent and feel taut and wiry to palpation. Very tight tendons often "bow string" or bulge away from the underlying bone (Fig. 2-17). Shortening in muscles and tendons is accompanied by similar changes in the surrounding skin and fascia, which become tight and adhere to the muscles, tendons, and bones

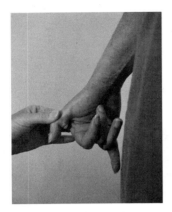

FIGURE 2-17 Shortened tendons across the wrist are prominent and pulled away from the underlying bone.

below. Mobility of the skin is lost in some or all directions, and the ability of individual muscles to be rolled away from adjacent muscle groups is similarly affected.

Several stages of length restrictions can be differentiated. *Contracture,* the most severe restriction in length, describes muscle and soft tissue that has lost passive extensibility so that the full excursion of muscle length is no longer available. Before full contracture, less severe patterns of tightness are found in which the muscles and tissues provide initial resistance to passive lengthening but respond to treatment to allow normal muscle length and tissue mobility. The term *muscle or soft tissue restriction* is used to describe this situation. Loss of muscle and tissue length develops progressively with time, and muscles and tissues that are not systematically lengthened in treatment or through active movement will gradually shorten and develop contractures. Extremity muscles that cross two joints (e.g., wrist and finger flexors) are the most common muscle groups to develop significant restrictions.

Problems with muscle and soft tissue shortening develop in patients with different patterns of impairment. Patients with low tone and severe weakness develop restrictions in trunk and extremity muscles from lack of active movement on their involved side. Splints and braces are often used to preserve good alignment in these patients. However, if the splints are not removed and tissues moved, muscles will shorten with associated joint stiffness in splinted position. Shortening and contracture also frequently develop in muscles that are hypertonic or that are inappropriately active. Sustained tension and inappropriate muscle contraction in these muscles leads fairly rapidly to shortening and ultimately to contracture. Muscles that are maintained in a shortened position by changes in joint alignment also quickly lose length and flexibility. While the shortened muscles have the most obvious changes in tissue elasticity, it is important to remember that the muscles on the opposite side of the joint are also maintained in a static position and will resist length changes as well.

Besides the problems of muscle and tissue shortening, changes in joint alignment and resting posture also cause muscle bellies to shift to new resting positions. When bones move to a new resting position, they take the origins or insertions of muscles with them, resulting in changes in the resting position of the muscle. We will use the term *muscle shifting* to describe the displacement of muscle bellies that accompanies changes in alignment. For example, in the hemiplegic arm, an abnormally flexed resting position with elbow flexion, pronation, and wrist flexion causes the flexor muscles of the forearm to roll medially. Similarly, poor joint positioning can cause tendons to slip over bone and acquire new angles of pull. For example, prolonged wrist flexion often causes the ulnar wrist extensor tendon to slip to the flexor surface, where it reinforces the pattern of wrist flexion. The shifting of muscle bellies causes unfamiliar hollow areas over bones that give the appearance of muscle atrophy. However, when boney alignment is restored and the muscle belly rolled back to its initial position, these hollow areas disappear.

Changes in muscle and tissue length and muscle shifting pose significant treatment problems because they interfere with movement reeducation. Loss of length forms a mechanical block to joint movement, to re-establishing normal alignment, and to increasing muscle strength in opposing muscle groups. Muscle and tendon shifting holds the bones in abnormal alignment, and because of altered line of muscle action interferes with normal movement. This category of secondary problems is preventable with treatment designed to maintain tissue elasticity and resting alignment of bones and joints. Problems develop rapidly if this is not incorporated into treatment or the patient's home program. When soft tissue restrictions develop, they respond best to soft tissue/myofascial techniques combined with a stretching program that uses movement to restore length. Sustained stretch through use of casting rarely produces lasting changes in tissue length and often contributes to the development of pain, skin breakdown, tendon tears, and joint hypermobility if tight tissues are held in their end range.

Other Significant Secondary Impairments

Pain

Pain is a common problem that has a great influence on the neurologic patient's patterns of movement and participation in therapy. Pain is significant because it induces protective responses that alter the posture of the body and lead to disuse of the painful extremity and avoidance of movement. When pain occurs during treatment, it creates distrust of the therapist and resistance to or noncompliance with the treatment program. Pain during or after therapy is never necessary or desirable, and the avoidance/elimination of pain is one of the most important goals of responsible treatment.

In neurologic patients, pain develops from different causes and in different locations. Pain may result from primary and secondary impairments and from external factors, such as a fall resulting in trauma to the body. Pain may be localized to specific joints, muscles, and tendons or diffusely distributed over an extremity. Each case must be individually evaluated to determine the factors contributing to pain, its type and location, and the relationship between pain and movement. The types of pain that most commonly affect movement are described below.

Joint Pain Joint pain is pain that is localized to a joint. It occurs during movements in which normal joint mechanics are disrupted. Both active and passive movements, weight bearing movements, and movements in space may be painful. In neurologic patients, joint pain is most common in the shoulder joint but may also occur in the wrist and hand, and in the hip, knee, or foot. Movement causes pain in these joints when the articular surfaces of the joint are not correctly aligned before the movement begins. Thus, shoulder subluxation is associated with joint pain during passive motion when the humerus is not lifted back into the glenoid fossa before the arm is moved.

Joint pain also is triggered when normal joint mechanics do not take place during the movement. This condition may exist when full joint motion is blocked by tight muscles or when atypical movement patterns are used to substitute for loss of muscle strength. For example, tight muscles between the scapula and rib cage frequently block upward rotation of the scapula, resulting in shoulder pain at 90 degrees of flexion from loss of scapulohumeral rhythm. Knee pain may occur in the hemiplegic leg, when loss of hip abductor stability and ankle dorsiflexion range result in strong recurvatum during stance. Joint pain should initially resolve immediately when normal alignment and joint mechanics are restored. If the painful motion is repeated without corrections in mechanics, the joint will become chronically painful. In a situation of chronic pain, the affected joint may be painful in all positions and to touch.

Muscle Pain Muscle pain results when a muscle or group of muscles is lengthened past its comfortable length. It may develop in weak or flaccid muscles, in muscles that are hypertonic, or in muscles that are shortened or contracted. It is particularly common in two-joint muscles, where a change in joint alignment in treatment may result in the muscle's being lengthened at both ends. Muscle pain may extend down the length of the limb if several muscles are simultaneously lengthened. For example, pain in the pectorals, biceps, and extrinsic flexors of the forearm is common when a tightly flexed and internally rotated arm is moved into a position of shoulder abduction/external rotation, elbow extension with supination, and wrist extension. A similar pull down the back of the leg and ankle may occur when tight hamstrings and gastrocnemius muscles are simultaneously stretched. Muscle pain is also associated with the prolonged passive muscle stretching that occurs in flaccid limbs. For example, pain in the deltoid muscle may develop in a flaccid arm from the pulling that the weight of the arm exerts on the muscles that run over the shoulder. Muscle pain is described as an uncomfortable feeling of "pulling" or "stretching" along the length of the muscle or muscles being lengthened. It is relieved when the amount of muscle length is decreased or the tractioning weight of the body segment is removed. Since lengthening tight muscles is a common treatment goal, muscle pain is most often provoked by aggressive or prolonged stretching during treatment. It is also associated with prolonged stretching in a splint or cast.

Pain from Altered Sensitivity Pain from altered sensitivity occurs in patients with impairments in sensory interpretation. This pain is triggered when the CNS misinterprets sensory information as painful. It is most common in acute patients and in patients with poor sensation and severe weakness in their involved side. Pain from altered sensitivity usually occurs first during a treatment session that has bombarded the nervous system with input from tactile, proprioceptive, and kinesthetic receptors. This dramatic increase in sensory information from the hemiplegic side may exceed the capacity of the brain to correctly interpret these sensory messages. When the processing capacity of the brain is reached, further sensory input is perceived as painful.

The therapist may diagnose hypersensitivity pain by ruling out joint or muscle pain. She should check to see that her handling is not causing joint pain from poor alignment or muscle pain from excessive stretch before suspecting a hypersensitive response. The patient's description of the pain provides another clue. Patients usually are vague in describing this type of pain or its location. Descriptions such as "it just doesn't feel right" or "I want you to stop now" are typical in this situation. When pain from hypersensitivity is suspected, the therapist must carefully limit the sensory input from her handling. At the same time, she should increase verbal descriptions of the sensory aspects of her treatment, so that the patient can learn to monitor and interpret sensation from the involved side. If this care is not taken, sensory confusion will persist, and the patient will often progress to associate all touch and movement with pain.

Shoulder-Hand Syndrome Shoulder-hand syndrome and related chronic pain syndromes in other body parts can develop out of any of the types of pain described above. While shoulder-hand syndrome is associated with specific risk factors, in our experience the initial problems usually can be traced back to instances of severe pain in therapy. Chronic pain situations develop when treatment continues to include movements and activities that are painful to the patient. The saying "no pain, no gain" is an example of a treatment philosophy that leads to unnecessary suffering during treatment and to pain that lasts outside of treatment and interferes with life tasks and sleep. Extreme pain may also arise from situations such as falls that occur outside of therapy. This pain may become chronic when treatment exacerbates the pain from the injury or does not attempt to manage and remove this pain.

Since pain from any source will interfere with active therapy, it is important that therapists attain sufficient knowledge and manual skill to be able to move patients without causing pain. To avoid causing pain, the therapist needs to understand normal movement and normal joint mechanics and to acquire treatment techniques to provide normal alignment and normal mechanics during passive and active assistive movement. A skilled therapist also develops manual sensitivity for joint and tissue mobility. This enables her to recognize the "end feel" of joint and soft tissue restrictions to motion and to stop before she exceeds available range and length.

When pain is already present, treatment must be directed toward removing the pain. This process begins with a careful assessment of the type of pain and its causes and the range of movement that is painfree. From this assessment, the therapist selects treatment techniques that eliminate the causes of pain, restore normal alignment and mobility to the affected body segment, and prepare for painfree reeducation of functional movements. When the therapist uses this system, most types of pain associated with primary and secondary impairments should gradually resolve. If the therapist lacks the skills to implement this treatment, she should refer the patient to another therapist rather than continuing or exacerbating the painful condition and causing the patient unnecessary suffering.

Edema

Edema in the hemiplegic arm and leg is a common problem in neurologic patients. It develops as a consequence of the primary loss of movement and muscle tone and from other factors relating to illness and hospitalization. Edema most commonly develops in the hand and/or foot during acute hospitalization. The initial development appears to be related to dependent positioning of the distal limb and to the disruption of muscular contributions to venous return caused by paralysis and decreased muscle tension. Edema also frequently develops around intravenous sites, where the intravenous fluid infiltrates the adjacent tissues. Although it is most common in the acute stage, edema may develop at any time. It often persists for long periods, spreads from the hand and foot to involve more proximal segments of the arm and leg, and responds poorly to treatment (Fig. 2-18).

Edema is a significant problem because of its effect on range of motion and joint and tissue mobility and because of its association with pain. Edema places the skin and connective tissues on prolonged stretch and, by filling the spaces around the joints, blocks joint movement. When edema persists for prolonged periods, it acts as a kind of glue, bonding skin to tendon, fascia, and bone. As tissues lose mobility and joint movement is restricted, the patient develops joint and tissue stiffness and loss of range of motion. Statistically, the presence of hand edema is associated with the development of shoulder pain and shoulder-hand syndrome. Similar relationships have been observed clinically in the foot and leg. Pain may initially develop in the edematous limb from the pressure that swelling places on the tissues and blood vessels or from trauma to the tissues caused by forced passive motion exercises.

Edema, with or without associated pain, will interfere with movement and the retraining of functional movement patterns. For this reason, it must be eliminated as part of treating the affected body segment. When edema is soft and pitting to the touch, deep pressure and manual pumping can express the fluid proximally, where it can disperse and be picked up by venous and lymphatic drainage systems. Edema

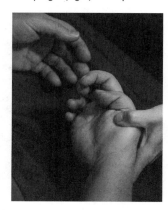

FIGURE 2-18 Edema in the hemiplegic (right) hand palm.

Composite Impairments

Movement deficits
Atypical movements
Compensations

that is firm and resistant to palpation cannot be manually expressed so easily, because the fluid is more consolidated and adhesions have developed between skin and underlying tissues. This edema must be softened and subcutaneous adhesions loosened before it can be expressed from the affected areas. In our experience, manual treatment is the only effective way to eliminate edema. Elevating pillows and compressive gloves are of little benefit at any stage of treatment, and the difficulties of putting an elastic glove on a swollen flaccid hand far exceed any benefits. Since the treatment of edema is time consuming, it is most efficient to treat it aggressively when it first appears and is still soft and pitting. An edema management program that involves the patient and/or family member as well as therapist will eliminate the problem most quickly.

Composite Movement Impairments

The impairments discussed in the previous section are significant to therapists because they influence the movement responses and level of functional independence of the patient. In this section, we will examine the specific movement problems that result from the interaction of primary and secondary impairments. Composite movement problems fall into the category that Sahrman has called *movement dysfunction*, or "imbalance or insufficient movement of body segments, limbs or the whole body." We have called this category *composite movement impairments* because we believe that the typical movement problems and functional limitations that we see in our patients result from multiple factors. These factors include the combined effects of primary and secondary impairments, motor recovery, and treatment. For physical and occupational therapists to have the greatest influence on their patient's ability to move and function, this is an important area for treatment.

Three categories of composite movement impairments affect neurologic patients: movement deficits, atypical movements, and compensatory movements. *Movement deficits* are the specific types of normal movement that cannot be performed. *Atypical movements* are abnormal or aberrant movement patterns that develop because of the impairments and motor deficits. These are movement patterns that deviate from the normal patterns of coordination. *Compensations* are alternative movement strategies that substitute for normal movement patterns in the performance of a function. These movements are necessary because of the effects of the primary and secondary impairments and the movement deficits that result from them. Figure 2-19 illustrates these three categories of movement impairments. Before we look at these categories, we will review the process of motor recovery and its influence on movement.

FIGURE 2-19 Categories of impairments.

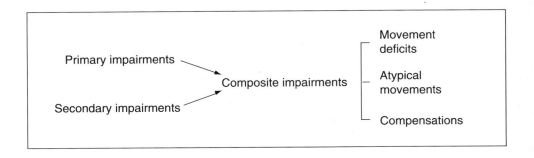

Motor Recovery

Motor recovery is the term used to describe the reemergence of muscle strength and movement control in previously paralyzed or severely weakened muscles. Motor recovery probably occurs primarily from changes in brain pathology. In the early days after stroke, reduction of cerebral edema may result in rapid improvement in motor function; later improvements may be related to neuronal reorganization that allows use of redundant pathways or establishes new neural pathways. Motor recovery is a significant predictor of functional outcome, because when muscular control returns, the patient has the potential for full functional recovery as well. Although motor recovery is most often accompanied by similar improvements in other primary impairments, the status of secondary impairments may not be altered by improved motor status. Thus, secondary impairments often interfere with full use of available movement patterns.

Complete motor recovery occurs when motor return progresses sequentially to all affected muscle groups, so that the patient regains strength and motor control in all muscles. This small group of patients has no residual problems with muscle strength, although recovery may take weeks or months. Most patients with complete motor recovery learn to activate their muscles in normal patterns of coordination and regain full functional use of their involved trunk and extremities. However, a few patients with full recovery of muscle strength continues to use atypical or compensatory movements. This occurs when primary and secondary impairments block normal use of available muscle strength.

While most neurologic patients experience partial recovery of motor control, most do not fully regain control of posture and movement on their involved side. *Incomplete motor recovery* exists when recovery stops before strength and control in all affected muscle groups have been regained. When motor recovery is incomplete, a condition of muscle imbalance exists between muscle groups that are active and capable of normal movement and those muscle groups that remain paralyzed or are too weak to contribute to movement. Patients with incomplete motor recovery can perform some movement patterns normally, either because they rely on muscles that were unaffected by the lesion or because of motor recovery; other movements cannot be performed or are performed with atypical coordination because of the partial loss of muscle control.

There are three kinds of incomplete motor recovery. Each is associated with predictable patterns of atypical movement and compensation. These patterns of incomplete recovery are also associated with secondary impairments. The pattern and extent of motor return directly affect the patient's movement deficits and play a significant role in the types of movement deviations and functional limitations that develop.

Incomplete distal recovery is found when motor return progresses from proximal to distal but stops before full strength and control of the distal muscles of the arm and leg have been achieved. This pattern of recovery is generally balanced between agonist and antagonist muscles, so that patients with this recovery pattern can control both flexors and extensors in the trunk and proximal limb segments. Recovery stops before muscle strength in the lower arm and/or leg has been completely regained, leaving residual weakness or paralysis in distal muscle groups, such as ankle and toes or wrist and finger muscles. Many times, recovery patterns in the hemiplegic arm and leg are similar, but some patients have full recovery in one extremity and residual distal paralysis in the other.

Motor deficits in the distal muscles of the extremities result in atypical movements and loss of hand function in the involved arm and atypical movements and problems with gait and balance in the leg. Patients with this pattern of recovery must rely on compensatory movements and adaptive equipment to replace distal muscle control during function. Splints or braces may be necessary to prevent the development of alignment problems and tissue tightness in the hand or foot.

A similar pattern is seen in a much smaller group of neurologic patients whose motor recovery begins distally and proceeds proximally. This pattern of recovery is called *incomplete proximal recovery*. In this group of patients, motor recovery begins in the distal muscles of the arm and leg and stops before control of proximal extremity muscle groups is complete. For example, patients with this recovery pattern are able to use the hand functionally for grasp and manipulation but lack the movement control at the shoulder and elbow necessary to reach or position the hand in space for functional use. This inability to move at the shoulder and elbow limits the functional use of the hand to positions close to the body. A similar pattern of proximal weakness with distal control is also found in the leg.

Unbalanced motor return occurs when motor recovery progresses in an uneven pattern across the affected side. These patients do not regain symmetric control of both agonist and antagonist muscles of the trunk, arm, or leg, although they recover strength in some trunk muscles and strength in some proximal and distal muscles of the limbs. Typically, this pattern of return shows preference for the flexor muscles of the arm and extensor muscles of the trunk and leg, while the antagonist muscle groups remain weak or paralyzed. Patients with unbalanced motor return must use their available muscles for postural stability and movement, even when this results in muscle firing that is very different from normal patterns of muscle activity. This use of available muscles results in atypical movements in the involved trunk, arm, and leg. As the patient continues to use these atypical movements in daily life, he inevitably develops asymmetric trunk and limb postures and secondary problems with alignment and muscle length.

When motor recovery is extensive, the patient's capacity for normal movement is vastly enlarged. However, good motor recovery does not always result in normal movements. Significant movement problems can persist in patients with good motor recovery when secondary impairments in the musculoskeletal system interfere with normal biomechanics, when sensory deficits in kinesthetic memory have left the patient without a perceptual sense of how to move, or when atypical and compensatory movements are so strongly ingrained into the patient's movement repertoire that he is unable to use more efficient patterns. In these cases, the patient may recover normal movement if treatment is able both to eliminate the causes for his persistent movement problems and to retrain more normal patterns of coordination.

Movement Deficits

Movement deficits are the specific muscle actions, movement components, and movement sequences that the neurologic patient is unable to perform because of the effects of primary and secondary impairments. They are the "missing pieces" of movement control that the patient needs to regain to be able to move normally. Movement deficits are present whenever recovery from impairments is incomplete.

They are also present when the severity of primary and secondary impairments make it impossible for the patient to use his existing muscle control to produce the movements necessary for function. Movement deficits lead directly to functional limitations and disability unless the patient can learn to compensate for his deficits and impairments when performing life tasks.

Movement deficits are a direct result of loss of muscular strength and control on the hemiplegic side. Loss of muscle control exists in the muscle groups that the patient cannot activate with sufficient strength or control to produce functional movements. We call the affected muscles *muscle deficits*. Most often, deficits are found in muscles that do not recover from their initial level of impairment and remain paralyzed. They may also be muscles whose action is blocked by secondary impairments. For example, deficits in the anterior tibialis muscle exist when the muscle does not contract to produce ankle joint dorsiflexion. This loss of muscle control may be present because the anterior tibialis muscle is weak (primary impairment) or because contracture in the gastrocnemius muscle limits available range of motion in ankle dorsiflexion (secondary impairment) (Fig. 2-20). When muscle deficits are present, the patient is unable to produce the specific actions or joint movements that these muscle groups perform as prime movers or to use these muscles synergistically in functional movements.

Muscle deficits lead directly to *deficits in movement components in the trunk and/or extremities.* When some muscles cannot contract on the hemiplegic side, the patient is unable to perform the movement components that require the action of these muscles. *Loss of trunk control* is present when critical trunk movement components cannot be performed because of loss of muscle control. Loss of trunk control affects both the postural and dynamic roles of the trunk. Loss of postural control in the trunk is present when the trunk muscles are not appropriately active to maintain trunk alignment and background postural adaptations during movements of the extremities. Loss of control of trunk movements exists when the patient is unable to move the trunk in the patterns necessary for function. For example, control of trunk extension is necessary for functional move-

FIGURE 2-20 Muscle deficit in the anterior tibialis muscle, resulting in loss of ankle joint dorsiflexion during swing. The ankle and toe muscles are not contracting as the patient initiates a step with the hemiplegic right foot.

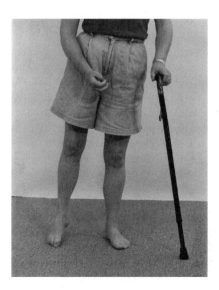

ments such as sit to stand, walking, and reaching. When control of trunk extension is lost on the hemiplegic side, the trunk assumes an asymmetric position that interferes with normal performance of these function (Fig. 2-21).

Loss of extremity control exists when the movement components necessary to position the arm or leg correctly for a function cannot be performed. Deficits in extremity movements involve both weight bearing movements and movements in space. For example, loss of muscle control at the hip and knee interferes with weight bearing in the hemiplegic leg and has a devastating effect on function and movement in sitting, standing, and walking. In the arm, movement deficits limit the ability of the arm to move in space and interfere with bilateral and unilateral coordination patterns. Because of the complexity of fine motor patterns in the hand, even loss of movement that is restricted to muscles of the thumb and fingers can have a devastating effect on functional use (Fig. 2-22).

Most neurologic patients have movement deficits that result in loss of movement control in the hemiplegic trunk, arm, and leg. Since functional movements are made up of movement components of the trunk and extremities, deficits in movement control in any of these areas result in an inability to perform functional movements and movement sequences with normal patterns of coordination. *Deficits in coordinated movement* are present when the patient is unable to perform the functional movements or movement sequences because of loss of trunk or extremity movement. For example, loss of ability to roll from supine to the uninvolved side may be present when the patient is unable to produce the appropriate movement components in the trunk, arm, or leg.

Movement deficits lead directly to compensation and functional limitation. When the motor patterns are missing, the functions that rely on those patterns of movement cannot be performed normally. Motivated patients may learn to accomplish some movements and function with atypical movements or compensatory patterns. But no satisfactory movement substitution may be available for complex patterns of coordination in the arm or leg, with the result that these movements cannot be performed any more. When the patient is unable to perform a necessary

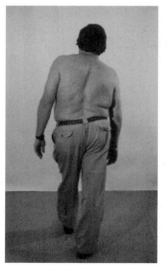

FIGURE 2-21 Loss of upper trunk alignment and stability during walking. The trunk laterally flexes with the concavity on the hemiplegic side as the patient steps with the left foot.

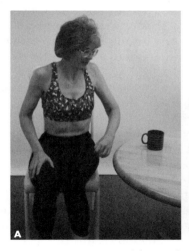 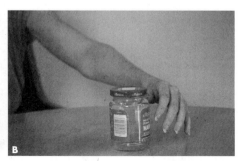

FIGURE 2-22 Movement deficits in the hemiplegic arm and hand. *(A)* Arm: the patient lacks control in elbow extension and forearm supination necessary to bring the hand to the cup. *(B)* Hand: muscle deficits in the thumb and fingers prevent the hand from being opened for grasp.

functional movement with a normal, atypical, or compensatory strategy, he is forced to rely on the assistance of others or to give up this function or role.

The presence of movement deficits is evident from observation of the neurologic patient's patterns of posture and movement. The precise distribution of muscle deficits is identified by careful assessment of movement control on the hemiplegic side. Once the assessment has identified the movement patterns that the patient is unable to perform, movement reeducation is directed toward movement deficits. This process of assessment and treatment is described in detail in Chapter 3 and 4.

Atypical Movements

The presence of atypical movements is the second major type of composite movement impairment found in neurologic patients. Atypical movements are movements that deviate from normal preferred patterns of coordination. These movements are atypical because they use patterns of muscle activation and sequences of joint movement that do not follow normal muscle synergies or biomechanical rules. In this book, we use the term to describe patterns of movement and coordination in the hemiplegic trunk, arm, or leg that are commonly used by neurologic patient but do not occur in normal functional movement. Atypical movements of the involved side are produced as the neurologic patients attempts to perform movement components, movement sequences, and functional movements. They are present whenever motor recovery is sufficient to allow some movement to take place, but primary and secondary impairments prevent the normal pattern from being executed.

Several types of atypical movement are characteristic of neurologic pathology. *Atypical trunk/extremity* movements occur when the patient volitionally activates muscles to move trunk, hemiplegic arm, or hemiplegic leg. This type of atypical movement is most obvious when the patient attempts to perform a specific movement component, so that his movements can be clearly compared with the expected nor-

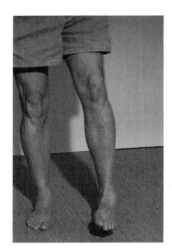

FIGURE 2-23 Atypical movement of the hemiplegic leg. The unbalanced activity of the anterior tibialis results in strong supination of the foot during swing.

mal pattern. For example, in normal stepping, ankle dorsiflexors and toe extensors are active synergistically to keep the foot in a neutral position while the foot moves forward. An atypical stepping pattern results when the anterior tibialis muscle is activated without the synergistic activity of the toe extensors and peroneals (Fig. 2-23). Similarly, atypical movements are present in the arm during movement and during more complex patterns of coordination requiring hand function (Fig. 2-24).

Atypical movements of the involved arm or leg may also occur as unwanted accessory movements during functional movements. In this case, the atypical movement of the extremity is an involuntary movement, such as the posturing of the hemiplegic arm during walking that is outside the volitional control of the patient (Fig. 2-25). Since these involuntary movements occur most frequently when balance is challenged, they can be thought of as abnormal balance reactions. We refer to this type of involuntary atypical movements as *atypical extremity posturing*. Atypical extremity posturing is troublesome to neurologic patients because it contributes to the abnormal appearance of the body and interferes with functional activities, like donning an overcoat. For this reason, elimination of this problem is frequently listed by patients as a goal of treatment.

A more complex type of atypical movement occurs when the patient is unable to normally coordinate and sequence trunk and limb movements. We call this category *atypical patterns of coordinated movement*. Atypical patterns of coordinated movement are used to execute movement sequences and functional movements. Neurologic patients frequently have problems sequencing movements of the trunk with those of the extremities. This creates difficulty in movements like sit to stand, in which movements of the trunk and legs have to be correctly sequenced. In normal sit to stand, extension of the leg occurs after the trunk has moved forward and the hips have lifted off the chair. If the legs extend too early in the movement sequence, the body is unable to achieve a full stand (Fig. 2-26).

Another common problem during movement sequences and functional movements is related to the need for trunk and extremity patterns to be compatible. Neurologic patients often are unable to activate the correct trunk and limb movements during a functional movement. For example, to initiate rolling from the upper body, the normal pattern combines flexion of the trunk with a forward flexion movement of the upper extremity. If the arm does not come forward as the trunk initiates rolling, the resulting movement pattern is abnormal because the trunk/extremity patterns are incompatible (Fig. 2-27).

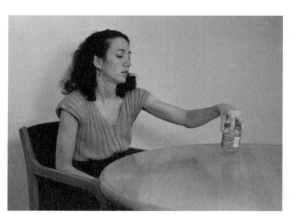

FIGURE 2-24 Atypical pattern of hand function in the hemiplegic arm.

FIGURE 2-25 Involuntary posturing of the hemiplegic arm and atypical weight bearing pattern in the hemiplegic leg during walking. The therapist has her hands on the patient to assist in balance but is not attempting to change the patient's gait pattern. The severe hyperextension in the knee, flexion of the trunk, and the amount of weight placed on the cane all suggest that balance is precarious, contributing to the flexed posture of the arm.

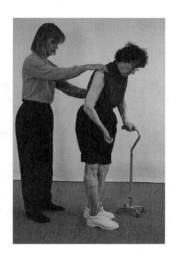

Atypical movement patterns develop as a consequence of primary and secondary impairments. Most atypical movements are probably related to the patterns of motor recovery that lead to uneven strength between agonist and antagonist muscles or between proximal and distal muscle groups. When motor recovery is incomplete, the patient uses the muscles that are available to him to produce movement on his involved side. These movements reflect the distribution of muscle strength on the involved side and the muscle deficits that prevent him from using a more normal pattern. Atypical movements may also be related to other primary impairments. Deficits in kinesthetic memory often leave the patient unsure about how normal movement is sequenced. Patients with these sensory impairments often initiate movements incorrectly and have difficulty coordinating movements of the trunk and extremities. Atypical movements that are characterized by excessive effort and cocontraction seem to be related to primary deficits in muscle tone and muscle activation. Problems in these areas may cause the patient to produce atypical movement patterns, even when motor recovery is extensive and he has the possibility of a more normal movement.

FIGURE 2-26 Atypical sequencing of trunk and leg movements during sit to stand. The patient has extended her hemiplegic leg too early in the movement sequence, with the result that the pelvis cannot come forward to complete the stand.

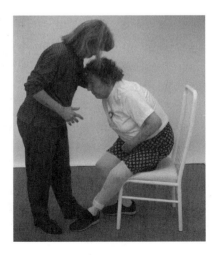

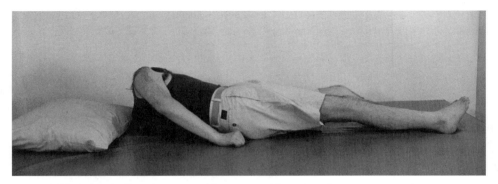

FIGURE 2-27 Atypical rolling characterized by incompatible trunk and arm movements. As the patient initiates rolling toward the uninvolved side with his upper trunk, the hemiplegic arm remains behind the body instead of moving forward as the trunk flexes and rotates.

Secondary impairments, such as changes in alignment and muscle length, also lead to atypical movement patterns. When body posture or joint position deviates from normal alignment, muscle length and mechanical advantage are disrupted, and even contractions by the correct muscles may result in abnormal movement. Atypical movements that result from secondary impairments are the easiest to remove. Once treatment has restored normal alignment and mobility to the body segment, the patient is able to use his existing movement control to produce normal movements with minimal retraining. Often these secondary impairments coexist with severe primary impairments so that removing secondary blocks to normal movement is only one aspect of the treatment process.

Atypical movement patterns are undesirable because they replace normal patterns of movement and coordination. Once they are part of the patient's movement repertoire they are extremely difficult to remove and may prevent the acquisition of more appropriate movements. Use of abnormal movement patterns is also undesirable because of the stress these movements place on joints and soft tissues. Atypical movements, such as knee recurvatum, may allow the patient to support weight on his hemiplegic leg and to walk, increasing his independence. However, over time, this pattern destroys the ligaments of the knee, leading to the development of permanent undesirable secondary impairments. Unfortunately, the use of atypical movements is often trained in therapy as a way of increasing function, without regard for the long-term consequences of this act. In our opinion, training the patient to use atypical movements is wrong and should not be practiced by responsible therapists.

Since the use of atypical movements interferes with normal movement, removal of these movement patterns from the patient's repertoire is an important goal of movement reeducation. Although both patient and therapist want to eliminate these movements, they cannot be eliminated by telling the patient not to move until he can do so properly, because they are strongly related to his need to move and function. In our experience, atypical movements only begin to disappear when the patient is able independently to use more normal patterns of movement and when the mechanical blocks to movement no longer interfere with normal muscle activation. Until those conditions have been met, the motivated patient will use atypical movements to meet functional objectives. Thus, while eliminating atypical movements is a valid therapy outcome, it is accomplished through meeting goals that establish normal patterns of movement and should never become the primary goal of treatment.

Compensations

Compensations are movement substitutions that replace normal movements to accomplish a functional goal or task. They are acquired when the normal movements cannot be produced because of existing impairments. Compensations are new sequences of movement that are adopted to reduce disability. Sometimes these patterns are clearly one-sided movements that do not involve use of the hemiplegic side. An example of this type of movement occurs when the patient sits up by pulling on the side of the bed leaving his hemiplegic side behind (Fig. 2-28). At other times, the movements are simply inefficient versions of the normal pattern (e.g., when the hemiplegic patient pivots almost a full circle rather than sit down toward the involved side). Patients may use compensatory strategies even when they possess sufficient motor control to perform the movements in a normal pattern. For this reason, compensations are not reliable indicators of the patient's motor control.

Compensatory strategies develop because of movement deficits that prevent the use of the normal movement pattern. Deficits in trunk and postural control lead to instability during the movement and to problems with the coordination of trunk and limb movements. When postural problems are present, the patient learns to compensate by holding himself stable with his uninvolved side and using adaptive equipment, such as quad canes and reachers, to avoid moving the trunk over the involved side or shifting weight to the hemiplegic leg (Fig. 2-29). Similar compensations develop when the necessary motor patterns are not available in the extremities to allow the normal pattern to be executed. For example, the patient who can not accept weight on his hemiplegic leg learns to move from sit to stand with all his weight on his uninvolved leg. Compensatory movement strategies develop quickly to substitute for movement deficits in the leg, because the patient is motivated to

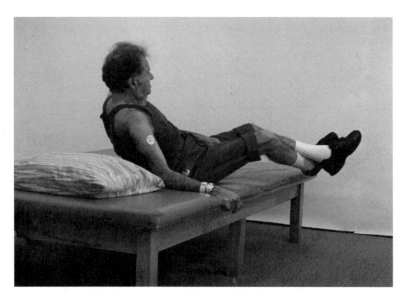

FIGURE 2-28 Sitting up from sidelying without use of the hemiplegic side.

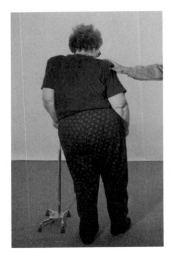

FIGURE 2-29 Use of the quad cane during ambulation contributes to asymmetry in the trunk and poor weight shift to the hemiplegic side. The therapist's hand is for guarding only.

stand and walk. When severe movement deficits are present in the arm, the patient is often unable to produce movements that assist function. For this reason, most upper extremity compensations involve one-handed adaptations. Compensatory strategies are also necessary when secondary impairments block normal patterns of coordination. For example, changes in alignment and restrictions in joint and soft tissue mobility interfere with normal mechanics, forcing movement substitutions.

Therapists use compensatory training to increase functional performance when the patient is unable to perform a critical functional movement in the normal way. Compensatory training enables the patient to learn a new way to accomplish a functional goal, reducing functional limitations and disability without a corresponding change in impairment. However, compensatory strategies are not all equally adaptive or desirable, and some compensations may actually contribute to the development of secondary impairments and atypical movements. To distinguish between desirable and undesirable compensations and to present the model for compensatory training that will be used in the rest of the book, we divide compensations into two categories: bilateral compensations and undesirable compensations.

Bilateral Compensation

When compensatory training is necessary, we believe it should use movement patterns that adapt the normal movement pattern and use both sides of the body in the movement to the full extent possible. We call this type of compensatory strategy a bilateral compensation.

Bilateral compensations closely approximate the normal pattern of movement and incorporate the involved trunk, arm, and leg into movement sequences and tasks. They use the patient's existing motor patterns to the full extent possible and leave open the possibility of further use of the involved trunk and limbs should motor return continue. The use of the involved side in even limited ways during functional performance helps the patient psychologically to believe he is getting better and perceptually to integrate this side into his body scheme.

Undesirable Compensation

We call compensations that do not resemble efficient normal movement patterns or do not use bilateral movement responses *undesirable compensations.* Typically, undesirable compensations use movement strategies that are very different from normal movements. They most frequently rely on movements of the uninvolved side and on atypical movement responses in the involved trunk, arm, or leg. Since these movements are not based on normal coordinated sequences that efficiently position the body over its base of support, balance is often a problem, and they require more steps and greater energy expenditure to perform. The use of undesirable compensations leads to "neglect" of the involved side, asymmetric patterns of posture and movement, and spasticity in the trunk and extremities. Once established in the patient's motor repertoire, they are extremely difficult to unlearn. One-sided compensatory strategies that are acquired early in rehabilitation often persist, even when there has been recovery of muscle function that could allow a more normal and efficient pattern to be used.

Undesirable compensations are often trained in therapy when the therapist wants to meet a functional goal without reestablishing the normal movement components necessary for task performance. They may also be acquired by the highly motivated patient through independent experimentation. In some cases, these typical compensations are easier for the patient to learn than the bilateral type, which requires use of the involved side, and they do allow independent movement and function. However, in the long run, use of these patterns often increases the severity of impairments and may significantly limit functional use of the involved trunk and limbs. In our opinion, this type of compensation should not be trained by therapists except as a last resort.

We believe that bilateral compensatory training is an important part of treatment that should be integrated into the process of retraining normal movement. Bilateral compensations are the most efficient way to retrain movement because they use patterns that are familiar to the patient through past performance. They develop strength in weak muscle groups through controlled use of both sides of the body. They also improve balance and postural control by training normal combinations of trunk movements and extremity movements. When acute patients are trained to use bilateral compensations from the earliest days of rehabilitation, the development of atypical patterns of coordination and of postural asymmetries is greatly reduced. By teaching bilateral compensations appropriate compensations from the early days of treatment, the patient learns simultaneously to compensate for his impairments, to use the available movements of his involved side to contribute to function, and to overcome his disabilities. In the treatment portions of the chapters in Section II, we provide specific examples of bilateral compensations to demonstrate how compensatory training is combined with other treatment goals and activities.

DISABILITIES AND HANDICAPS

The impairments and movement problems discussed in the previous sections are important because they result in diminished functional performance and dependence in important life roles as well as loss of control of movement. Disabilities and handicaps are terms that describe effects that pathology, impairments, and movement problems have on functional independence and lifestyle. Disabilities and handicaps define problems in performance; they are used to identify how well the patient is able to perform in his various life roles. We have added the category of functional behaviors to identify areas in which functional performance has not been affected by the brain pathology. The box below illustrates the relationships between these categories.

Disabilities

Disability is the term used to represent functional limitations that relate to restrictions in movement and task performance. Disabilities occur as a consequence of primary and secondary impairments and movement dysfunction. When loss of movement control occurs in any part of the body, the functions that require those movements cannot be performed normally. Some movement patterns can be relearned using a different movement strategy or compensation, but others cannot, leading to loss of functional performance. When the patient cannot perform a large number of tasks necessary for independent functioning, disability results. Common areas of disability in neurologic patients include locomotor tasks (walking, stairclimbing), mobility tasks (rolling, sit to stand), and upper extremity tasks (dressing, grooming). These areas are often placed into broad categories, such as activities of daily living, homemaking, social roles, occupational behavior, and leisure activities.

Functional Limitations

Disabilities
Handicaps

Functional Abilities

Intact abilities
Compensations

In neurologic patients, disabilities are balanced by the presence of *functional behaviors*. These are the movements and functions that the patient can still perform. Intact functional behaviors are based on the available normal movement patterns that were unaffected by the lesion and impairments. They are enhanced when normal movement patterns are reestablished through motor recovery and treatment and when the patient acquires compensatory movement strategies that increase his level of function. When functional behaviors increase, disability decreases. Therefore, treatment will have its greatest influence on disability when it provides improved movement patterns that allow the patient to accomplish specific functional goals and tasks.

Handicaps

Handicaps are the last and broadest category of the disablement hierarchy. Handicap is the cumulative effect of impairments and disability on the lifestyle and occupational behaviors of the patient. They reflect the extent to which impairments and disabilities interfere with life roles. Handicaps depend not only on the patient's specific problems and disabilities but also on environmental constraints that may be outside the control of the patient but have a considerable influence on his ability to assume his former life roles. Thus, they reflect both problems intrinsic to the patient (i.e., what he is unable to do) and extrinsic to the patient (i.e., problems in the social and physical environment that limit his access to life roles).[10] Environmental barriers in the home, workplace, or community and factors such as social isolation and economic dependency often play as significant a role in limiting final outcome as physical limitations and disabilities. While physical and occupational therapists have important roles to play as patient advocates in confronting extrinsic barriers that create handicaps and in providing specific training for overcoming specific movement deficits related to occupational and social behaviors, these roles are outside the realm of this book and will not be discussed. The information in this book is targeted to the impairment and disability level of disablement.

Patients with similar types of impairments may suffer different degrees of disability and handicap. It is important to remember that there is not always a cause and effect relationship between impairment and disability, or between disability and handicap. Differences in disability between patients with similar impairments probably relate to how well the patient uses his available movement control and to the effectiveness of the compensatory patterns that he develops to overcome his movement deficits. Differences in handicap between similar patients are probably related to differences in the demands of daily life and occupation. Older retired adults may have less handicap associated with their impairments than a younger employed individual who need specific motor behaviors and mobility skills for job performance.[2] Both disability and handicap are also highly influenced by motivation, personality, and premorbid level of function. Motivated and intelligent patients may achieve significantly higher levels of independence than patients with similar levels of impairment but less drive.

THE ROLE OF THERAPY IN TREATMENT OF DISABLEMENT

Our purpose in this chapter is twofold: (1) to identify the problems of the neurologic patient that are responsible for loss of functional performance and movement dysfunction and (2) to categorize this information in a manner that clarifies the interrelationships between the problems and leads to a systematic approach to assessment and treatment. The length and complexity of the information in the chapter demonstrates the enormous number of factors that must be considered in treating neurologic patients. It explains why there is controversy in neurologic rehabilitation about which problems are most relevant to treat and whether treatment should address the impairments or disabilities. This chapter is our attempt to answer these questions. We have included information on the problems that we consider most relevant to address in treatment. To restore functional movement patterns to neurologic patients, we believe that treatment must operate on the impairment and disability levels.

We believe that treatment of primary and secondary impairments is important. Treatment of impairments may be directed toward changing or eliminating the impairment directly or toward minimizing its effect on function. Therapy can influence impairments in three ways:

1. Therapy can prevent or minimize the influence of secondary impairments through attention to the physical condition of the musculoskeletal system. This is accomplished by treatment that addresses alignment, muscle and tissue length, and biomechanical principles to prevent the development of mechanical blocks to movement, such as joint malalignment and soft tissue contracture. When these problems are already present, they may be decreased or eliminated through appropriate treatment strategies.

2. Therapy can influence the status of primary impairments through direct interventions, such as strengthening weak muscles, reducing hypertonicity, and retraining abnormal patterns of muscle activation. The purpose of this type of intervention is to increase muscular control in the involved side and prevent or minimize the development of atypical movement patterns and spasticity. When spasticity and atypical movement patterns are present, intervention at this level is designed to restore a state of muscle tension that will allow normal movement and the reeducation of more normal patterns of movement and function.

3. Therapy can guide and organize the recovery of motor control through the teaching of normal movement patterns. This type of treatment is targeted at movement deficits by retraining the movements of daily life. Treatment of movement deficits ensures that available movement components are used in patterns of activation and coordination that are as close to normal as possible. By focusing on those muscles and muscle synergies that are most important for function, it may encourage the reestablishment of neural pathways that control these patterns of coordination and prevent the development of atypical movements. While it may be controversial to state that therapy can affect motor recovery, we believe that treatment that focuses on normal movement allows the patient to make the most of whatever movement control he regains, seems to stop the development of very abnormal movement patterns, and encourages progressive proximal to distal recovery.

Because treatment of impairments may not result in improved function and decreased disability, we believe that a second level of treatment intervention must be targeted at the disability level. Treatment at this level is designed to help the patient regain both functional performance in life tasks and control of generalized patterns of movement that promote safety, energy efficiency, and a feeling of self-efficacy. Treatment at the disability level includes three intervention strategies:

1. Therapy should help the patient devise compensatory movement strategies that allow functional movement and task performance. These compensations should include bilateral movements and closely approximate the normal patterns whenever possible. Compensations must be trained from the earliest days of rehabilitation to give the patient the opportunity for independence in basic ADL and mobility tasks. As motor performance increases, these initial patterns should be modified with further training that includes more active use of the involved side. At later stages of rehabilitation, compensatory training involves solving problems of environmental accessibility and specific homemaking or occupational tasks.

2. Therapy can increase task performance and decrease disability through intervention at the level of movement deficits, training functional movement sequences in the trunk and extremities that are important for many tasks. Movement reeducation that focuses on postural adjustments and trunk movements in sitting and standing will have a generalized effect on balance that will result in safe function in these positions. Similarly, retraining of weight bearing and movement patterns of the extremities allows the extremities to participate more in all movements and functions. Treatment that improves generalized movement control gives the patient movements that he can apply to specific tasks and daily needs. When movement succeeds at this level, the patient will report to the therapist on movements or tasks that he has been able to accomplish on his own for the first time.

3. Therapy can retrain normal performance of specific tasks and movements. Because neurologic patients have often lost the kinesthetic memory for normal movements in basic tasks, they may not use their available motor control for task performance unless these movements are introduced and practiced in therapy. Practice of functional tasks and movements ensures that the patient integrates new patterns of movement into daily life.

The ultimate goal of physical and occupational therapy is increased functional performance and decreased disability. The interrelationships between impairments, movement problems, and disabilities are extremely complicated, and the contributions that each makes to the patient's functional limitations are difficult to isolate. The extent to which therapists succeed in increasing function and decreasing disability depends both on their understanding of how the patient's impairments are limiting his functional performance and their success at minimizing the physical contributions to disability and increasing the availability of appropriate movement patterns and compensations. For treatment to succeed in producing a genuine change in function, it must address those impairments, movement problems, and functional limitations that all contribute to the patient's disability. The process of assessment and treatment of these three levels will be discussed in the next two chapters.

REFERENCES

1. Rogers J, Holm M: Accepting the challenge of outcome research: examining the effectiveness of occupational therapy practice. Am J Occup Ther 48 (10):871–876, 1994

2. Duncan P: Stroke rehabilitation. Phys Ther 74 (5):399–406, 1994

3. Schenkman M, Butler R: A model for multisystem evaluation, interpretation, and treatment of individuals with neurologic dysfunction. Phys Ther 69 (7):538–553, 1988

4. Schenkman M, Butler R: A model for multisystem evaluation treatment of individuals with Parkinson's disease. Phys Ther 69 (11):923–943, 1988

5. Bourbonnais D, Vanden Noven S: Weakness in patients with hemiparesis. Am J Occup Ther 43 (5):313–319, 1989

6. Bohannon R: Is the measurement of muscle strength appropriate in patients with brain lesions? Phys Ther 69 (3):225–228, 1989

7. Sahrman SA, Norton B J: The relationship of voluntary movement to spasticity in the upper motor neuron syndrome. Ann Neurol 2:460–465, 1977

8. Carr J, Shepherd R: A Motor Relearning Programme for Stroke, 2nd Ed. Aspen Systems Corp, Rockville, MD, 1987

9. Wanless M: The Natural Rider: A Right-Brain Approach to Riding. Simon & Schuster, New York, 1987

10. Jette AM: Physical disablement concepts for physical therapy research and practice. Phys Ther 74 (5):379–386, 1994

SUGGESTED READINGS

Horak F: Assumptions underlying motor control for neurologic rehabilitation. p. 11–27. In Lister M(ed): Contemporary Management of Motor Problems. Proceedings of II Step Conference. Bookcrafters, Fredericksburg, VA, 1991

Sahrman SA: Diagnosis by the physical therapist. Phys Ther 69:969, 1988

3
Assessment

Assessment is the process of collecting information about impairments, functional limitations, and disability for the purpose of treatment planning. This chapter describes a process for assessing movement problems and relevant impairments in neurologic patients. Our assessment is directed toward the problems and impairments discussed in the previous chapter. However, the process of movement analysis, problem solving, and goal setting that we outline could also be used to assess movement dysfunction from other types of pathology.

THE PURPOSE OF ASSESSMENT

A good assessment is critical to the planning and implementation of effective treatment and to providing the documentation of progress necessary for treatment to continue. Three reasons for performing a full assessment are to establish baselines, to understand trunk and extremity relationships, and to document therapy efficacy.

Establishing Baselines

Assessment establishes a baseline level of functional limitations, movement problems, and impairments. By identifying the movement deficits and relevant impairments, the therapist is able to structure therapy toward those areas that will have the biggest impact on improving function and safety.

Understanding Trunk-Extremity Relationships

Assessment enables the therapist to understand the relationships among the problems of the trunk, arm, and leg. In central nervous system (CNS) damage, there are strong connections between the problems of the different parts of the body. The therapist must completely assess the trunk and extremities to fully understand how the problems are interrelated and to use that understanding to plan effective treatment.

Documenting Efficacy of Therapy

Assessment allows documentation of the efficacy of therapy. By writing notes that indicate the initial problems, the treatment directed to improving those areas, and the ensuing improvements in movement and function, the therapist is able demonstrate the impact of treatment on impairment and disability. Documentation of this type is critical to ongoing insurance reimbursement for therapy, for publishing research case studies, and for the professional growth of the individual therapist. It also helps the patient, his family, the physician, and other health professionals understand the process of therapy, by demonstrating the relationships between problems, therapeutic exercises and activities, and improvements.

THE PROCESS OF ASSESSMENT

Assessment Information

The goal of assessment is to gather information on the patient's ability to move and function. To gain a complete picture of the problems contributing to disability, five major areas must be assessed. These areas are discussed separately below.

Functional Level

Assessment of functional level identifies the patient's functional abilities and functional limitations. Functional abilities are areas where the patient is able to function independently. These areas do not need to be addressed in the initial stage of treatment, although they may be approached later in rehabilitation when learned compensations are no longer necessary. Initial treatment will be directed toward eliminating some or all of the functional limitations.

Intact Motor Abilities

Assessment of intact motor abilities identifies the movement patterns that are performed normally. These movement patterns are available to the patient to use for function and will not require treatment. Movement patterns are normal when the alignment and mechanics of body segments are appropriate, muscle strength is adequate to move the body against gravity, and the patterns of muscle activation are sequenced appropriately for the task. Therefore, the presence of normal movement gives the therapist critical information about joint alignment and mobility, muscle strength, and coordination.

Movement Deficits and Compensatory Patterns

Assessment of movement deficits and atypical or compensatory patterns identifies the movements that cannot be performed (i.e., the movement deficits) and the movements that can only be performed with atypical or compensatory patterns. Movement deficits need to be reeducated to increase movement control and functional performance. Undesirable compensatory movements interfere with normal movement and must be replaced with either normal movements or more appropriate compensations.

Relevant Impairments

Neurologic patients have many impairments, only some of which directly contribute to functional limitation and disability. *Relevant* primary and secondary impairments are those that are responsible for the individual patient's movement deficits and compensations. The effects of these relevant impairments will have to be minimized or eliminated as part of treatment to improve motor performance.

Response to Manual Therapy

During the assessment, the therapist will manually touch and move the patient's trunk and limbs. This manual portion of the assessment is used to form a subjective estimate of potential for improvement that is based on the patient's response to the therapist's touch and handling. Subjective estimates of potential are used to establish realistic goals for treatment and to determine the handling techniques that will be most useful in treatment.

Data Gathering

To gain a complete picture of the patient's movement repertoire and relevant impairments, these five areas must be assessed for the trunk, arm, and leg. A full assessment includes assessing movement problems in the positions of supine, sitting, and standing, during important functional movement sequences such as rolling, supine to sit, and sit to stand, and in ambulation, and specific upper extremity tasks. Because of the amount of time necessary for conducting a complete assessment, it is rarely possible to assess all of these components during the initial session with the patient. In the first visit, the therapist must quickly identify the functional limitations that are most restrictive to the patient's life and assess the movement problems and impairments that relate to these functional needs. In each subsequent treatment session, the therapist will add additional pieces of information to that collected in the initial evaluation.

It is also important to recognize that not all assessments will be conducted in the same way. The scope of an assessment will vary greatly according to the level of independence of the patient, the setting in which assessment and treatment are to be delivered, and the purpose of the assessment. An acute stroke will require a different assessment than the higher functioning patient who wants to walk without a cane, or the patient with a painful shoulder who is hoping to be free of pain. Similarly, physical and occupational therapists may begin their assessment of the same patient in very different positions or focus on different movements and body parts because of different functional goals and professional concerns. Thus, while all assessments require that problems of the trunk, arm, and leg be evaluated, the amount of attention devoted to each area will vary according to the anticipated focus of treatment.

The Stages of Assessment

The assessment process can be divided into five stages. Although the amount of time spent in each area may vary, all are important parts of the collection of data. The five parts are each performed on the trunk, arm, and leg, and in the body positions most relevant to function. In some cases this information can be collected quickly. When the patient's problems are more complex, several sessions with the patient may be necessary before a complete clinical picture has been obtained.

The Parts of Assessment

   I. Initial impressions and establishing rapport
  II. Observation of movement
 III. Hands-on assessment of movement problems
  IV. Assessment of relevant impairments
   V. Problem solving and goal setting

Part I: Initial Impressions and Establishing Rapport

In the initial part of the assessment, the therapist gathers general information about the patient's level of functioning and the areas of functional limitation to be addressed in treatment. Much of this information is available through the patient's chart and conversations with nurses, other health professionals, and family members, but it is important to elicit similar information from the patient. The therapist also shares with the patient her assessment goals and a description of the process for the rest of the assessment.

Because therapy is an interpersonal art as well as a science, the skill of the therapist at least partially depends on the relationship she establishes with her patients. Many patients are fearful or anxious during their initial contact with a new therapist. The early minutes of the assessment provide an opportunity for the therapist and patient to get to know each other and to discuss the purpose of the assessment. During this time, the therapist may learn a great deal about the patient's problems from his perspective and gain insight into what will motivate him to participate in therapy. In all settings, the therapist should take this time to establish rapport and trust with the patient and to identify the patient's goals and concerns (Fig. 3-1).

The first minutes of the assessment are also time to observe the patient without his being asked to perform. Initial impressions of the patient's posture, movements, balance, judgment, and level of independence help the therapist identify areas of apparent difficulty to assess later. The more skillful a therapist becomes in observation, the more quickly she will be able to focus the rest of her evaluation on significant problems and plan appropriate treatment.

Part II: Observation of Posture and Movement Control

During the second part of the assessment, the therapist uses observation to analyze and identify the patient's available patterns of posture and movement. Her goal is to identify postural deviations and problems, such as atypical movements, movement deficits, and compensations, that affect movement performance and

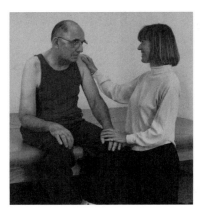

FIGURE 3-1 Establishing rapport. The first minutes of assessment are spent getting acquainted and discussing the purpose of the assessment. Many patients are fearful or apprehensive when meeting a new therapist.

to identify areas where motor performance is functional. To gain a picture of how the patient moves, the therapist asks the patient to perform specific movements of his trunk and limbs in a position such as sitting or standing or to combine trunk and limb movements in a functional movement pattern, like sit to stand or rolling. The patient may also be asked to perform a specific functional task (e.g., putting on a shirt or climbing stairs) so that the therapist can observe specific task performance. The therapist selects the movement patterns to be assessed on the basis of the patient's level of functional independence and the goals of therapy. It will probably be necessary to assess both movement patterns, such as trunk movements in sitting, and task performance (putting on a shirt) to get a complete understanding of the patient's control of movement.

As the patient attempts to move in the desired patterns, the therapist analyzes the resulting pattern in terms of the initiation of the movement, the direction and magnitude of the weight shift, the posture and tone of the trunk and extremities, and speed, coordination, and balance during movement. Movement analysis is based on careful observation of the body as it is moving and a description of what is observed. The patient's posture, movement patterns, and quality of movement are compared with the ideal efficient or normal patterns of movement, and deviations are identified. A complete description of a movement should include observations of the following:

1. The starting position of the body and the base of support. Asymmetries in weight distribution, postural deviations, and obvious differences between the two sides of the body should be noted.

2. The initiation phase of the movement, including the body part that moves first, the direction of the movement or weight shift, and changes in the base of support.

3. The transition point of the movement, if appropriate for the movement sequence, including the position of the body, the base of support, and the new direction of movement.

4. The completion of the movement, describing the position of the body and limbs and the base of support.

5. The range of movement control.

6. The qualities of the movement pattern, such as the speed, smoothness, and ease of moving.

This part of the assessment shows the therapist how the patient moves independently. The therapist should refrain from physically assisting the patient during this phase of the evaluation. The therapist uses verbal directions and demonstration to convey to the patient the specific patterns desired (Fig. 3-2). When difficulty with a certain movement pattern is identified, the therapist should give additional information to the patient to see whether he can improve his performance. Sometimes providing more specific demonstration or verbal cues will help the patient produce the desired movement, indicating that the potential for more normal movement patterns is present. When loss of muscular control or orthopedic limitations block the desired movement, the additional descriptive information will not improve performance.

While the patient is moving independently, the therapist must be close enough to the patient to assist him should loss of balance occur. The acute patient will often lose his balance during the performance of trunk weight shifts and transitional movements. Impulsive patients and those with poor insight may attempt move-

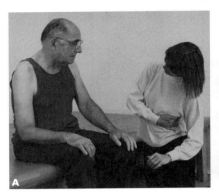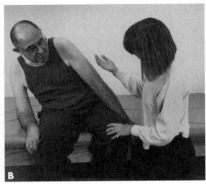

FIGURE 3-2 Observation of movement. (A) The therapist demonstrates the desired movement pattern. In this case the patient is being asked to perform a lateral trunk weight shift initiated from the upper body. (B) The patient attempts to perform the movement. His trunk does not show the desired pattern of lateral flexion, and his upper trunk rotates backward as he moves laterally.

ments that are too difficult or that can not be performed safely without assistance. In other instances, a patient will decline to perform movements that are frightening or cause pain. When either the patient or the therapist has a concern about safety, the therapist should not insist on repeating the movement until she is ready to assist the patient manually during the next part of the assessment.

Part III: Hands-On Assistance

During this part of the assessment, the therapist uses her manual skills to attempt to correct problems in alignment, modify atypical and compensatory movement patterns, and provide assistance to movement patterns that could not be performed independently. The goal of this section of the assessment is to determine the cause/causes for the movement problems identified previously and to use the patient's response to handling to obtain further information about his problems and potential for improvement. Since the handling techniques used for this phase of the assessment are similar to or the same as those used during actual treatment, this portion of the assessment is often confused with treatment. However, in an assessment, the duration of the handling is briefer than in a treatment session, and the handling is used to acquire information rather than produce functional changes.

The therapist uses manual handling several ways to assess problems of movement. These methods are described individually in the section below. In each case, the therapist uses her hands to change some aspect of the patient's posture or movement with the goal of observing whether this change helps the patient move more normally. By gathering information in this way, the therapist will discover which corrections are most effective in changing the patient's atypical movement patterns. She will also gain information about the types of impairments that are blocking normal movement. This information will be used to ensure that treatment is directed at the major causes for the patient's movement abnormalities.

Correcting Alignment

The therapist may use her hands to correct abnormal alignment. When changes in alignment affect the starting position for movement, the therapist should attempt to realign the body parts and restore normal posture and biomechanical relationships. For example, she may select hand placements that allow her to reestablish symmetry in the patient's spine and rib cage, restore equal weight distribution to the lower extremities, or realign the upper extremity on the trunk, depending on the area being assessed. In the process of discovering the corrections necessary to reestablish normal alignment, the therapist also gathers information about the causes for the atypical positions of the trunk and limbs. Shortened muscles and soft tissues and joint stiffness stop the structures from being moved fully in the desired direction. When the therapist attempts to correct alignment in this situation, full correction is impossible. Changes in muscle tone and muscle activation may also interfere with the therapist's attempts to reestablish normal alignment. When spasticity or active muscle contraction are used to maintain the body in an asymmetric posture, the therapist feels resistance to her attempts to correct postural asymmetry. Low tone in the limb girdles and trunk creates asymmetric postures that do not resist realignment. The therapist feels the weight of the flaccid limbs in her hands.

The therapist should maintain the corrected alignment while the patient attempts to move. Often the abnormal starting position of the body makes the execution of certain movement patterns difficult or impossible. When underlying motor control is present, realigning the body will make it possible for the patient to produce the movements that were blocked by the asymmetry in body alignment. For example, the weight of the flaccid arm may cause flexion in the upper trunk, affecting performance of trunk movements in sitting. When the therapist supports the heavy arm, the patient may be able to sit in a more appropriate position and actively control his trunk during sitting weight shifts (Fig 3-3).

Assisted Movement

In this manual technique, the therapist assists the desired movement. The therapist assists the movement patterns that the patient was unable to perform independently. This may be done by helping the correct part of the body to initiate the movement or by moving the body segment through the desired arc of movement. The therapist places her hands on the patient's body in selected spots that provide mechanical leverage to the desired movement.

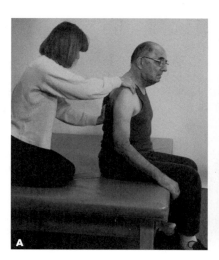 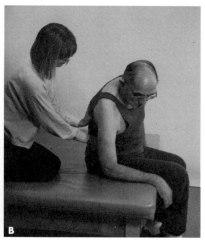

FIGURE 3-3 Correcting alignment and repeating the movement. (A) The therapist uses her hands to increase extension in the upper trunk and make the two sides of the upper trunk more symmetric. (B) Her hand near the patient's spine stops the backward rotation of the upper trunk.

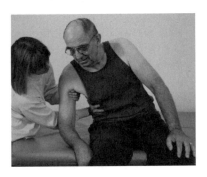

FIGURE 3-4 Assisting the desired movement. The therapist's hands assist the patient to tuck his rib cage and move his shoulder girdle laterally and down. This hand placement produces the desired trunk pattern.

Manual assistance may serve several functions. First, it provides sensory information about the desired movement pattern, giving the patient a model to reproduce. Second, the therapist is performing part of the task, allowing weak muscles to fire during the movement without having to move as much body weight. The therapist repeats the movement several times, asking the patient to "help me move" after the second repetition. If the therapist feels the patient assist the movement in the desired fashion, she should identify this for the patient and encourage him to repeat it. After several repetitions of the assisted movement, the therapist withdraws her assistance and asks the patient to move independently (Fig. 3-4).

During assistive movement, the therapist may feel that the patient's efforts to assist her are incorrect. If she feels his efforts are producing an unwanted movement pattern through activation of incorrect muscles, she must identify this for him. In this case, she instructs him to stop his attempts to assist her and concentrate again on the initiation and sequencing of her passive movement. This process is the beginning of teaching the patient to identify the muscles that he has activated and to learn to quiet or release these muscles when their activity is inappropriate.

Blocking Undesirable Movements

When the patient initiates the movement incorrectly or sequences the movement inefficiently, the therapist may select hand placements that stop the unwanted pattern. This manual technique forces the patient to initiate movement from another part of the body or with a different pattern. Many patients develop atypical movements and undesirable asymmetric compensations early in their rehabilitation. These movement substitutions persist into their recovery, even when they have regained the motor control necessary for more efficient movement. In this situation, blocking the unwanted movement pattern often forces the patient to devise new movement strategies and produce a more normal, efficient movement pattern. Since this handling technique has the potential to frustrate or confuse the patient, it is often used in combination with assisted movement. Thus, the therapist may use one hand to assist the correct initiation pattern, while her other hand stops the patient's preferred initiation pattern from occurring.

After several repetitions of the movement with any of the above handling strategies, the therapist should withdraw her assistance and ask the patient to repeat the original movement independently. This independent practice is compared with the patient's original attempts at the same movement, to determine whether there has been an improvement. When the patient's second attempt at movement is closer to the normal pattern, it indicates potential for rapid improvement in motor performance with further treatment. When the pattern has not changed, it indicates that

---

Techniques of Manual Assistance

1. Correcting alignment and postural asymmetries
2. Assisting difficult movement patterns
3. Blocking undesirable movement patterns

---

either the patient lacks the necessary muscular control to produce the movement or that secondary problems are limiting the production of the movement. From her assessment, the therapist should be able to identify which of these possibilities is the most likely explanation.

Part IV: Assessment of Relevant Impairments

In addition to assessing the patient's movement patterns, the therapist must collect information about the specific primary and secondary impairments contributing to his movement deficits and atypical/compensatory movement patterns. This includes assessment of impairments, such as loss of muscle strength, alignment, and orthopedic changes, muscle and soft tissue shortening, and abnormal muscle tone, that interfere with the production of normal movement patterns. Examples of areas of concern that might be assessed in this section include measurement of ankle joint dorsiflexion and muscle length in the gastrocnemius and hamstring muscles, determination of the amount of flexibility in the spine and rib cage, or evaluation of the passive correction in arm position that is possible when flexor spasticity has been eliminated. To ensure that the information collected is relevant to the patient's movement problems, impairments are assessed first in the areas where problems have been observed or identified during handling. This may be followed by areas where the therapist suspects a problem and desires more information. Impairments that do not appear relevant (e.g., soft tissue length in an acute patient) may safely be left untested in the initial visits.

The assessment of impairments relies on observational and manual skills that are similar to those used in the earlier stages of the assessment and during treatment. Observational skills are used to identify the alignment of body segments, to monitor the patient's reaction to tests, such as joint mobility or tissue length, that could potentially cause pain, and to look for changes in other parts of the body that may result from intervention. For example, measurements of heel cord length in sitting with knee extension may result in either knee pain or in a posterior tilting of the pelvis if the hamstrings are also tight. Observation of the patient's facial expression and body posture will tell the therapist if the movement is approaching a painful range or detect the change in pelvic position when full length of the two joint muscles has been reached. Observation is an important adjunct to all aspects of manual handling, as it gives visual information to supplement the direct contact from the hands.

Manual skills are very important for assessment of all major impairments. In testing muscle strength, length, and tone and in measuring joint alignment and mobility, the therapist must first use her hands to reestablish good body alignment and restore a stable resting position to unstable bones and joints. This establishment of normal alignment is a necessary precursor to testing of muscle strength and measurement of tone and length (Fig. 3-5). Normal alignment must be maintained during the assessment of these areas, even when this poses a considerable challenge to

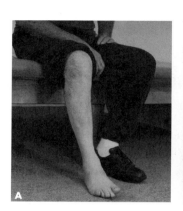
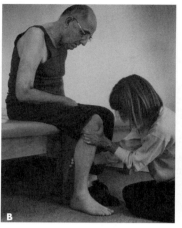
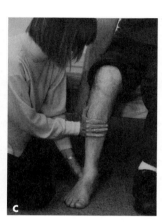

FIGURE 3-5 Correcting alignment before measuring ankle joint range of motion. (A) Uncorrected position of the leg in sitting. (B) The therapist moves the femur out of abduction and external rotation so that the hip, knee, and foot are in the same plane. (C) The therapist corrects the alignment of the heel and maintains the leg in corrected alignment.

the therapist. If alignment cannot be fully corrected during the assessment, the cause for the restrictions and the position of best correction should be identified and addressed in the early treatment goals. When normal alignment between body segments is not possible, measures of muscle strength, muscle tone, and range of motion are not reliable.

It is not possible in this space to discuss the exact procedures for assessment of all impairments that affect the movement patterns of the neurologic patient. More specific information about the effects that impairments have on the specific movements of the trunk, arm, and leg and suggestions for assessment and treatment of these impairments within the context of these movements will be addressed in the chapters of Section II.

Part V: Analysis of Information and Problem Solving

The analysis of assessment information is the last part of the assessment process. Before analysis is attempted, the therapist has assessed posture, movement control, and impairments of the trunk, arm, and leg. Since problems can often appear different when the body assumes a new position or the functional demand of the task is changed, the therapist must assess the trunk and limbs and the relationship of the trunk to the limbs in several different positions and in functional tasks, such as walking or transferring, before gaining a complete picture of the problems. When this has been completed, the therapist analyzes the information with the goals of identifying the major movement problems and relevant impairments in the trunk, arm, and leg and understanding the relationship between the problems in the trunk, arm, and leg. This analysis will be used to prioritize problems and set goals for treatment. Thus, this section of the assessment can be divided into two subsections: (1) the formation of a problem list and (2) problem solving and goal setting.

Forming a Problem List

The problem list organizes the information that has been collected during direct patient contact. It has two distinct but strongly interrelated sections: a list of movement problems and impairments and a list of functional limitations.

List of Movement Problems and Impairments The list of movement problems and impairments identifies the movement problems of the trunk, upper extremity, and lower extremity. This list contains information about the movement patterns that are performed atypically or cannot be performed, the movement deficits that affect this loss of control, and relevant impairments, such as shoulder subluxation, edema, muscle weakness, and spasticity, that also contribute to movement problems and will be addressed in treatment. In forming this list, the therapist compiles information from different positions and summarizes the important pieces of information for the trunk, arm, and leg. The list of movement problems should include all the significant factors that limit functional performance. Additional problems, such as cognitive and perceptual disturbances, lethargy, and depression, may also account for significant loss of function but are outside the realm of this book.

List of Functional Limitations The functional list itemizes the major functional limitations that decrease quality of life and interfere with independent living. Common examples of functional limitations include dependence in bed mobility, ambulation, or self-care; limitations in walking that prevent walking without a brace or cane, carrying an object in the hands while walking, or stepping up a curb without a railing; loss of upper extremity functional use for support or holding or carrying objects; or balance problems that interfere with resuming sports activities, such as golf or horseback riding. The list of functional limitations should correlate directly to both the patient's goals and concerns and with the list of movement problems and impairments. This correlation will be discussed in the following sections.

The Problem List

Functional Limitations
Movement Problems
  Trunk
    Atypical or compensatory movement patterns
    Significant movement deficits
    Relevant impairments
  Upper extremity
    Atypical or compensatory movement patterns
    Significant movement deficits
    Relevant impairments
  Lower extremity
    Atypical or compensatory patterns
    Significant movement deficits
    Relevant impairments

Problem Solving

Problem solving is the process wherein the therapist uses the information from the assessment and problem list to hypothesize how the problems of the trunk and limbs relate to each other and to the functional limitations. At the end of the problem solving process, the therapist will have identified the major functional limitations to be addressed in treatment and formulated functional goals, treatment goals, and treatment activities that relate to remediating this loss of function.

To begin the process of problem solving, the therapist should decide which of the functional limitations that she has identified will be the major focus of treatment. Each therapist will choose to address functional impairments that are important to the patient, likely to respond to treatment in a timely manner, and appropriate for her discipline and work setting. However, both the physical and occupational therapist should have collected similar information on the patient's movement problems and impairments and may ultimately select similar treatment activities, even though the goals of treatment are different for each discipline. This is true because the same problems of the trunk, arm, and leg will affect the performance of gross motor movements and skilled task performance. For example, a heavy paretic arm and asymmetric trunk will interfere equally with dressing activities in sitting (occupational therapy) and the ability to stand up from sitting with good balance (physical therapy).

When the major functional goal has been selected, the therapist should identify the problems of the trunk, arm, and leg that are contributing to this loss of function. Both movement control deficits, atypical or compensatory movement patterns, and primary and secondary impairments should be listed for the trunk, arm, and leg. The assessment process will have identified many movement problems and impairments, not all of which have a significant causal relationship to the functional limitation to be addressed in treatment. This part of the assessment helps the therapist focus on the *main* movement problems and *most significant* impairments that must be changed or ameliorated for significant changes in movement and function to be achieved. The other problems will not be totally ignored but may be addressed later in the treatment process when progress toward the treatment and functional goals has been detected.

After identifying the major movement problems and limitations that will be addressed in treatment, the therapist should begin to hypothesize how the problems of the trunk relate to the problems of the arm and leg. Since functional movement depends on both trunk and extremity movements, the problems of the trunk and the limbs should be connected during the assessment process so that treatment can link the problems of the trunk to the problems of the extremity. When the trunk, arm, and leg are treated separately, the therapist may make improvements in each of the parts without achieving a functional change. In this part of the assessment, the therapist should link the movement problems of the extremities to specific aspects of trunk control, so that treatment can reestablish the necessary pairing of trunk and limb movement that is needed for functional performance.

Establishing Goals

Goal setting is the final part of the problem solving stage of assessment. Therapy goals are divided into two categories: functional goals, and treatment goals.

Functional Goals Functional goals articulate the function or movement for which the patient will be prepared and the level of independence that will be achieved. Functional goals are identified before treatment goals. They are based on the functional limitations that the therapist has selected to emphasize. For example, for an acute care patient who is dependent in all self-care tasks, appropriate functional goals would include independent upper body dressing in sitting or transfers with minimal assistance. For the higher functioning patient, a functional goal might be walking at home without a brace or using the hemiplegic arm for weight bearing on a table. Functional goals should represent significant changes in the patient's level of independence and demonstrate the practical benefits of therapy.

Treatment Goals Treatment goals are directed toward the movement problems and impairments that are most relevant to the functional goals. Treatment goals help the therapist articulate the steps involved in meeting the functional goal. They identify the movement patterns to be reeducated and the atypical movements and primary and secondary impairments that need to be eliminated so that normal movement can be produced. To be effective, treatment of impairments must be directed toward those problems that will have the greatest impact on the functional goals of the patient. Since treatment goals are phrased in terms of problems rather than functions, they do not directly demonstrate functional improvement. Examples of treatment goals include the following examples for the acute patient described above: restore control of upper and lower body initiated trunk movements in sitting, teach compensatory one-handed dressing techniques, and reeducate sit to stand with arms supported on therapist's hips. When these treatment goals have been met, the patient will have regained some of the pieces of motor control necessary for safe performance of dressing or transfers. The patient may still need practice in specific dressing tasks or in transfers before he has achieved the functional goal. This need for practice would be articulated in another set of treatment goals.

Treatment goals are often divided further into short-term and long-term goals. *Short-term goals* address the movement problems and impairments that have the most immediate effect on the patient's inability to perform the functional goal and that the therapist believes will respond most quickly to her intervention. Short-term goals should be achievable relatively quickly, although the time required will vary from patient to patient and between treatment settings. They are based on the patient's response during the handling portion of the assessment and the therapist's past experience with the time necessary to create a response in similar types of patients. The accomplishment of a short-term goal should result in an objective change of status in one or more of the problems on the problem list, although there likely will be no change in functional level. When the initial short-term goals have been achieved, the therapist sets new goals that will move the patient closer to the long-term and functional goals.

Long-term goals take longer to accomplish and should result in a major change in a movement or secondary problem. Meeting a long-term goal will bring the patient measurably closer to accomplishing the functional goal of treatment by removing a major impediment to the desired pattern. However, even long-term goals may not accomplish the entire function. The period it takes to accomplish a long-term goal will vary tremendously, as the therapist may utilize several sets of short-term goals in meeting the long-term objective.

The following example illustrates how functional goals and short- and long-term treatment goals are related. Many hemiplegic patients experience severe shoulder pain during their rehabilitation. Because eliminating pain is an important objective to the patient but in itself may not translate into increased use of the arm, the therapist should select a function, such as "use of the hemiplegic arm in forearm weight bearing on a table," as her functional goal and address the problem of pain under her initial treatment goals. The therapist might pick a long-term treatment goal of "restoring pain-free shoulder motion to 60 degrees of forward flexion," and short-term goals of "eliminating edema in the hand, restoring mobility in the scapula in the planes of elevation/depression and abduction/adduction and practicing of passive shoulder movements to 30 degrees of flexion with internal rotation without pain." When the initial short-term goals were achieved, a new set "establishing glenohumeral external rotation to neutral, lengthening tight muscles between the scapula and trunk and humerus and scapula, and practicing of passive movements of the humerus into 30 degrees of abduction and 60 degrees of shoulder flexion" could be set. When the long-term goal was met, the therapist would be able to place the patient's arm on the table without pain and to introduce the motor compo-

---

The Problem Solving Process

Choose the MAJOR functional limitation to be addressed in treatment.

  What *main* problems in the trunk contribute to this limitation?

    Movement problems

      Movement deficits

      Atypical or compensatory patterns

    Relevant impairments

  What *main* problems in the arm contribute to this limitation?

    Movement problems

      Movement deficits

      Atypical or compensatory patterns

    Relevant impairments

  What *main* problems in the leg contribute to this limitation?

    Movement problems

      Movement deficits

      Atypical or compensatory patterns

    Relevant impairments

Goal Setting

  Relate the main *trunk* problem to the main upper extremity problem.

  Relate the main *trunk* problem to the main lower extremity problem.

  Formulate a functional goal for treatment that addresses the functional limitation you have chosen.

  Establish treatment goals to address the movement problems and impairments that are interfering with the performance of the function.

  Plan treatment activities that address the problems of the trunk, arm, and leg and prepare for the functional goal you have selected. This will be discussed further in the next chapter.

nents of forearm weight bearing. However, at this point the patient would be unable to use weight bearing for function, so that a new set of therapy goals would have to be articulated, listing the components of movement to be retrained and the significant secondary problems to be addressed during this stage of treatment to establish functional use of forearm weight bearing.

It is important to involve the patient in the process of setting therapy goals. Patient input will be derived from the first section of the assessment and from continuing conversations with the patient, his family, and other health professionals or caregivers. The therapist should select functional goals that are meaningful to the patient whenever possible, so that he can see that his goals are important and that the therapist is listening to him. It is equally important that the therapist relates the patient's inability to perform meaningful functional tasks with the specific movement problems and impairments that have been identified in the assessment. In this way, the patient understands that the treatment process has an organization and logic that may not be apparent to him and that the therapist has a plan for improving his movement patterns that will enable him to meet his functional objectives.

Realistic goal setting is based at least partially on clinical judgment and experience. The skill in goal setting is to understand the critical factors that interfere with movement control and to identify correctly the major problems interfering with the patient's ability to improve. Therapists must be able to prioritize problems for treatment, so that treatment can ignore the minor problems to achieve functional change efficiently. The ability of the therapist to choose achievable goals is increasingly important these days, for it is the means and mechanism for establishing and maintaining reimbursement for therapy.

Implementation of the Treatment Plan

As treatment begins, the therapist will collect additional information on movement problems and impairments. This additional information should clarify the information acquired in the initial assessment or the relationships between the different problems. The patient's response to treatment should also confirm that assessement and problem solving have identified the main problems affecting the patient's loss of function. When the main problems are correctly identified and treatment is directed towards these areas, the therapist should be able to see change within each treatment and an increased benefit in subsequent sessions. If a change or improvement cannot be detected in the trunk or extremities after several treatment sessions, the therapist should reassess her decisions regarding treatment priorities. The most common reason for lack of treatment progress or carryover between sessions is incorrect selection of the main problems. Whether treatment is successful or not, problem lists and problem-solving decisions must be continually updated and the patient's functional status reevaluated. In this way, treatment progress can be documented and functional status upgraded as progress is noted.

Assessments are performed during the initial patient sessions and on an ongoing basis throughout the time the patient is receiving treatment. Periodic reassessments are performed to measure progress toward the treatment goals, to document changes in functional status, and to look in depth at the problems that require further intervention. While the initial evaluation must collect information on the problems of the trunk, arm, and leg, the reevaluations may either focus on the whole body or emphasize primarily one area of the body.

4

Treatment Interventions to Maximize Functional Outcome

The goal of treatment for neurologic patients is to reestablish normal patterns of posture and movement and to develop new strategies for accomplishing functional activities. Most patients with central nervous system dysfunction will not fully recover from their impairments and will not regain completely normal movement patterns. This is true no matter what type of therapy they receive. However, there are great differences in the quality of movement, functional independence, and feelings of self-efficacy between patients who are taught to compensate for their impairments by using their uninvolved side and patients who learn to move and function with both sides of their body. Our goal in retraining normal movement is to maximize every patient's functional potential by helping him/her achieve the greatest amount of normal muscle control attainable, given the limitations imposed by their brain lesion. Treatment succeeds when the patient moves with more efficient and appropriate movements, has sufficient balance to function safely at home and in the community, accomplishes life tasks with minimal assistance and compensation, and looks and feels more like his own person again.

PARTS OF TREATMENT

To help our patients achieve their potential movement and function, treatment must be directed toward primary and secondary impairments, movement problems, and the functional limitations that contribute to disability. There are three important parts of this treatment process for neurologic patients: movement reeducation, elimination/prevention of secondary impairments, and functional training. This chapter describes these parts of treatment and briefly discusses how treatment time is allocated among the different parts. The information in this chapter is theoretical and conceptual rather than practical and serves as an introduction to our treatment approach. Specific manual treatment techniques for implementing these treatment concepts are included in the chapters in Section II.

Movement Reeducation

Reeducation or training of normal movements is one of the most important functions of neurologic treatment. The goal of this part of treatment is to increase the patient's ability to move independently in normal patterns of coordination and to use these normal movement patterns in functional activities. Movement reeducation is the part of treatment that is directed toward the primary impairments of loss of muscle strength, changes in muscle tone, and patterns of muscle activation. It is designed to minimize movement deficits and train patterns of movement that will be used to decrease functional limitations and compensations.

In neurologic patients, movement reeducation has two component parts. The first part of reeducation is directed toward training the patient to use his existing muscle strength in normal patterns of coordination and sequences of muscle activation. This type of reeducation helps the patient regain maximal functional movement from his motor recovery. When successful, it prevents or eliminates abnormal patterns of muscle activation and atypical movements and decreases compensations by replacing existing movement strategies with more appropriate patterns. Reeducation is also directed toward increasing motor control by activating muscles that cannot currently produce movement because of weakness or loss of muscle memory. This second part of reeducation is designed to enhance motor performance by strengthening weak muscles and increasing available patterns of motor control. It prepares the patient to function at a higher level than is currently possible. For patients in all stages of rehabilitation, both of these parts of reeducation are likely to be applicable, so that most treatment sessions will combine activities that strengthen existing movements and activities that produce new movements.

Movement reeducation is designed to increase muscle strength and movement control on four levels: the individual muscle level, the movement component level, the movement sequence level, and the functional movement level. Reeducation of individual muscle action is used with weak muscles of the trunk, arm, or leg to increase strength and endurance and to train concentric, eccentric, and isometric patterns of control. On the movement component level, groups of muscles in the trunk, arm, or leg are trained to work synergistically to produce movement patterns that are important for function. These patterns of muscle activation may produce simultaneous movement at more than one joint (e.g., shoulder and elbow flexion to bring the hand to the top of the head) or to stabilize joint position in one part of the body segment with movement at another (e.g., during forward reach, elbow, wrist, and forearm muscles contract isometrically to stabilize the position of the elbow and lower arm while movement occurs at the shoulder girdle). When patients have problems with abnormal patterns of muscle activation, reeducation of movement components is used to reorganize patterns of muscle firing.

At the level of the movement sequence, the therapist teaches muscles in multiple segments of the body to work together in coordinated patterns of trunk and extremity movement. Movement sequences are used primarily to change the position of the body in space (e.g., rolling or moving from supine to sitting) or to accomplish movements such as the stance and swing phases of gait that have definable beginnings and endings. Functional movement sequences combine trunk and extremity movement components to accomplish a goal. Reach patterns that combine trunk weight shifts with coordinated movements of the arm and hand are examples of the type of movement that is reeducated at this level. Reeducation of movement sequences and functional movements is only possible when the patient can perform the critical movement components in both the trunk and extremities that are used in these complex movements.

Movement reeducation should take place in normally aligned joints and body segments. This is necessary to ensure that muscles have the correct line of pull, that muscle contractions produce the desired biomechanical patterns, and that the patient does not experience joint pain during movement. When secondary problems, such as muscle tightness and joint hypomobility, are present, the therapist should begin the treatment session by treating the impairments. This is done to minimize the effects of the impairments on movement. Severe secondary impairments will probably not resolve completely within a treatment session, but the therapist should achieve the best correction possible and maintain this correction during reeducation. The treatment process for impairments is discussed later in the chapter.

In treatment, movement reeducation can be introduced with the patient in supine, sidelying, sitting, or standing. Whenever possible, movement should be trained in the position where it will be used for function, so that the patient gets the most immediate transfer of information from treatment to real life. This means that the therapist should reeducate most functional movements in sitting and standing positions because, these are the positions in which the patient will need to function. However, there are times when patient problems, such as poor endurance in the upright posture or inadequate trunk and lower extremity control, make prolonged treatment in these positions impractical or unsafe. In these cases, movement reeducation in supine or sidelying can be used to introduce the sensation of the desired movements and to activate muscles. Later in the treatment process, the therapist may need to repeat movement reeducation in the upright postures as motor control does not automatically transfer from one position to another position with a different relationship to the force of gravity. Of course, there are important functions associated with supine, and these functions must be retrained in the recumbent position.

Stages of Movement Reeducation

Movement reeducation has four stages. These stages describe the process for training new patterns of movement, increasing variability of existing movement patterns, and improving functional use of the involved side. Each successive stage of reeducation demands more active participation from the patient and correspondingly less manual assistance by the therapist. When introducing a new movement pattern in treatment, it is always best to start with the first stage, sensory education. However, the time spent in each subsequent state may vary greatly according to the patient's existing muscle strength and ability to learn what is expected, and to produce the desired movement response. The movements selected for reeducation are identified during the assessment and relate to the short-term, long-term, and functional goals that were established through problem solving.

Sensory Education

The first stage of movement reeducation is designed to teach the patient about the desired movement. In sensory education, passive movement of the body segment is used to provide sensory information about the movement and establish a kinesthetic perception of movement that will form the basis for muscle memory. Passive movement is used to teach the patient the proper initiation of the movement, the correct sequencing of muscle activation, and the completion of the movement. It also provides him with information about the correct speed of movement and the amount of force or effort that is needed during performance. The patient will need this information in the next stage of reeducation, when he will be asked to assist actively with the desired movement.

The therapist begins the process of sensory education by placing her hands on the patient's body in positions that establish correct alignment and provide control of the moving segment. For example, to reeducate the movement of elbow flexion, she first takes the wrist out of flexion and aligns the axis of the hand with that of the forearm. She uses one hand on the patient's hand and wrist to keep this distal positioning and places her other hand on the humerus above the elbow joint. To move the elbow joint, her hand in the patient's hand controls the movement, while the hand on the humerus stabilizes the proximal arm so that it does not move as the elbow is flexed.

After the therapist has established her hand positions, she directs the patient's visual attention to the part of the body that will be moved. The therapist asks the patient to focus on how the movement feels without trying to assist her. As she repeats the movement several times, the therapist gives verbal information about the movement to help the patient focus his attention on the important sensory information. For example, while flexing the elbow, the therapist would help the patient to feel that the hand initiates the movement, that the elbow muscles are active while the shoulder muscles do not contract. At the end of each repetition of the movement, the therapist pauses briefly to signal that the movement sequence has been completed and muscle activity should stop (Fig. 4-1).

As the movement is repeated, the therapist will often feel the patient's muscles begin firing to follow her movements. If the muscles are correctly assisting the movement, the goal of sensory education has been achieved, and treatment can progress to the next stage of reeducation. Sometimes the patient produces inappropriate or excessive muscle activity to assist the movement. When this happens, the process of sensory education is enlarged. The therapist must help the patient identify the way in which his motor activity was inappropriate, learn to quiet those muscles, and try a different motor strategy for producing the desired movement. If passive movement is not possible through the desired range because of tightness or poor alignment, the therapist should stop the sensory education and adjust her treatment plan to address these secondary problems.

In many patients with severe weakness or paralysis, no active muscle firing is evident during this phase of reeducation. When the patient does not spontaneously produce active muscle contractions, the therapist should ask the patient to assist

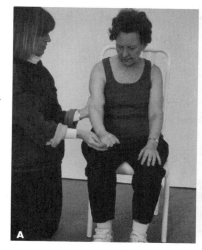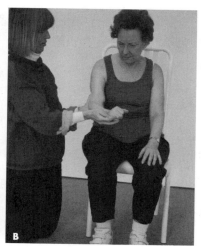

FIGURE 4-1 Sensory education of the movement of elbow flexion. (A) The therapist realigns the axes of the shoulder, elbow, forearm, wrist, and hand. (B) She maintains this alignment while moving the elbow into flexion. The patient is told to concentrate on the "feel" of the movement.

her as she repeats the movement several more times with a slower speed and smaller range. If the therapist feels no muscle contractions after the movement is repeated, this phase of treatment should be stopped. The therapist may then either start the process of sensory education again with a new movement pattern or change to a new treatment activity. For example, if no muscle activity could be elicited in the elbow flexors, the therapist could start sensory education again at the shoulder joint or move to another activity, such as forearm weight bearing, to increase muscle activity in the arm.

Assisted Practice: Muscle Activation

In the assisted practice stage of reeducation, the patient actively assists the guided movements of the therapist. This phase of movement reeducation, based on active-assistive exercise, is designed to allow the patient to practice movement in a controlled environment. The purpose of this stage is to increase muscle strength through assisted practice of concentric, isometric, and eccentric patterns of muscle firing and to increase coordination by teaching synergistic patterns of muscle activation. This stage of reeducation is complete when the patient is able to reproduce the desired movements with manual assistance from the therapist. This prepares him for the next stage of movement reeducation, independent practice, and for the first stage of functional movement reeducation.

During assisted practice, the therapist continues to use her hands to maintain correct alignment and control the range and speed of the movement. Her support limits the degrees of freedom that the patient is asked to control and makes the task easier for weak muscles by supporting partial body weight. The patient attempts to produce muscle contractions that follow along with and assist the guided movements of the therapist. To do this, he times the starting of his muscle contraction to the initiation of the movement and stops muscle activation when the therapist completes the movement. For example, the patient may actively assist movements of the arm or leg in space or work with the therapist during practice of trunk or lower extremity-initiated weight shifts (Fig. 4-2).

During the first trials of assisted movement, the therapist maintains control of all aspects of the movement. This allow the patient to continue to receive sensory information about the movement while he uses practice to increase strength and

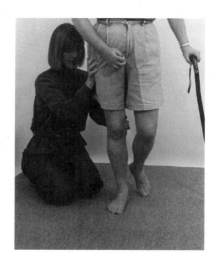

FIGURE 4-2 Assisted practice of stance phase. The therapist's hands control the position of the hip and knee and give the message to the patient to shift forward over the hemiplegic leg. The patient actively assists with the forward weight shift.

control. When the therapist senses that the patient is ready to take more control of his movements, she asks the patient to initiate the movement and control its speed and range while she supports partial body weight. The therapist also uses assisted practice to teach the patient to sustain muscle contraction in a given range (i.e., isometric contraction) and to control eccentric lengthening of the muscle. When he has learned to follow her movements in isometric and eccentric patterns of muscle activation, she lightens her control of these movements as well. Practice of these different patterns of muscle activation with the body in different positions relative to gravity varies the practice environment and encourages motor learning.

Assisted practice is also used to train synergistic patterns of muscle activation. This training expands the use of individual muscles by teaching them to work in combination with other muscle groups to produce basic movement components and movement sequences. For example, ankle dorsiflexors need to work synergistically with hip and knee flexors to lift the leg up onto a step during stair climbing. Since weak dorsiflexors are most easily strengthened in sitting, the therapist may begin her assisted practice there. When the ankle muscles consistently fire in sitting, treatment can shift to standing. The therapist asks the patient to help her flex the ankle as he lifts his foot onto the step with his hip and knee flexors and to keep the front of his foot up while he lowers his foot to the floor. A similar process is used to reeducate weak extensors of the elbow or wrist. The muscles are first taught to contract on an individual muscle level, then to contract as the arm is used in extended arm weight bearing or forward reach.

As in the sensory education phase, the therapist may feel the patient using inappropriate or excessive muscle contractions during his efforts to assist her. This may be because he is activating the wrong muscles, firing too many muscles, or incorrectly sequencing his muscle firing. His efforts may also be inappropriate if muscles are activated with excessive force or tension. When any of these problems arise, the therapist must identify the problem for the patient and help him to adjust his efforts by quieting muscles, finding the correct sequence of muscle activation, or decreasing the strength of his contraction. The therapist uses sensory education in combination with manual and verbal cues to help the patient modify his motor responses.

The therapist maintains manual contact with the patient's body during assisted practice. In this stage of reeducation, the therapist's manual cues provide the patient with critical information about how to move. When the therapist is teaching a new movement pattern, her hands use firm pressure to provide support and control the parameters of the movement. This firm pressure tells the patient that she is in charge of the movement and that he should pay attention to her messages. She lightens her pressure as the patient moves actively in the desired pattern. Light tactile contact requires that the patient control more of his body weight and allows him to initiate and control the range and speed of the movement. Manual contact with the patient's body during movement also gives the therapist information about the patient's muscle strength and control. As weak muscles grow stronger, the therapist feels less weight in her hands, and as the patient is able to produce the correct patterns of muscle activation, his body begins to move before her hands start the pattern. She reacts to this information by adjusting her manual control.

When the patient's muscle activity is consistently appropriate, and muscle strength is adequate to hold the weight of the moving segment, the patient is ready to move to the next stages of movement reeducation and begin to practice independent movement and functional movement components. Functional movement reeducation is introduced before the patient is able to move independently, so that the patient learns to associate his new movements with functional goals and begins to practice using them in functional movements with assistance from the therapist. This process is described later in the chapter.

Independent Movement

Sensory education and assisted movement are used to establish muscle memory for normal movement components and sequences and to increase muscle strength and control in the involved trunk, arm, and leg. When these sensory and motor goals have been achieved, the patient has developed a kinesthetic memory for the desired movement pattern and is able to follow the therapist's movements with appropriate muscle contractions. In the independent practice phase of reeducation, the therapist gradually decreases the amount of her physical assistance, allowing the patient to assume greater control over his new movements until he is able to reproduce the desired patterns independently. The goal of this phase of reeducation is to teach the patient to move independently with the best quality of movement possible and to perform movement components and movement sequences that are necessary for function.

The therapist can decrease her assistance by supporting less body weight, by lightening her touch to provide fewer sensory cues, or by removing one hand from contact so that the patient assumes complete control over one body segment (Fig. 4-3). To prepare for independent movement, the patient practices the movements many times and in many variations with minimal assistance from the therapist. When the quality of the patient's movements remains consistent with minimal assistance from the therapist, she removes both hands from the patient and allows him to move independently. The therapist should provide increased amounts of verbal information as the removes her manual supports to substitute for the loss of tactile and proprioceptive feedback. This verbal feedback may be used to give the patient information about how he is moving (knowledge of performance), how successful he was in producing the desired movement (knowledge of results), and how to modify his efforts to improve the quality of his independent movements.

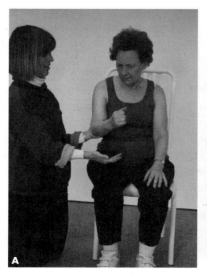 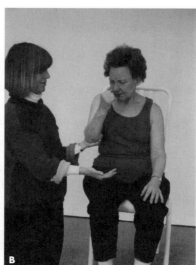

FIGURE 4-3 (A & B) Independent practice. The therapist removes her manual control of the forearm and wrist so that the patient independently controls the movement of elbow flexion.

When the therapist removes her control and asks the patient to control his own movement, the quality of movement often deteriorates. This change in movement quality may occur because the patient has difficulty maintaining correct alignment during movement, lifting body weight during movement, or controlling the speed and timing of movement when external controls are removed. Sometimes the patient is able to perform the movement independently once or twice before his control declines. In these patients, the change in movement quality is probably related to muscle fatigue. In other patients, the quality of the movement changes as soon as the therapist removes her hands. These changes probably reflect problems with motor control and insufficient motor learning. The therapist should put her hands back on the patient and return to assisted practice as soon as she feels that the patient's independent movements are not satisfactory. Muscles that are fatigued need to be rested before practice is resumed.

It is important to allow the patient opportunities for independent movement even when there are immediate changes in movement quality. Independent practice provides an opportunity for the patient to observe his own movements, to compare them with the ideal pattern introduced by the therapist, and to attempt to correct or modify his initial efforts. Moving independently also builds strength and endurance in weak muscles because the muscles are controlling more body weight. In the early stages of motor learning, the patient may be able to see that his independent movements are less than optimal, but be unable to modify them. The therapist must then help him to learn where his movement errors are occurring and give him the additional strength and control necessary to correct his movements. This is done by alternating between assisted practice and independent practice.

The stage of independent movement is completed when the patient can move independently in the desired movement pattern. The patient continues to practice this movement pattern in functional movement reeducation until he is able to incorporate his new movement into functional performance. As one movement component or movement sequence is performed independently, the therapist also identifies a new muscle group or movement pattern to be the next goal of movement reeducation. This new movement goal should relate in some way to the previous goal of movement reeducation and to the long-term and functional goals of treatment. If movement reeducation has been performed at the muscle level, the new goal of movement reeducation is often to train the muscle to work synergistically with other muscles in a movement sequence. For example, when the patient is able to control wrist extension with his elbow supported on the table, the next goal of movement reeducation may be to teach him to combine wrist extension with elbow flexion to bring his hand to his mouth or with finger flexion to grasp a cylinder.

When muscles can fire in isolation and in movement components and sequences, the therapist should identify new muscle groups to be reeducated. For example, as the patient gains independent control of ankle dorsiflexion, the therapist may choose to reeducate toe extensors. Active control of toe extension would extend the benefits of ankle joint dorsiflexion because the two muscle groups work together synergistically during swing, and control of ankle and toe muscles may allow the patient to walk without the assistance of an ankle-foot orthosis. While setting new reeducation goals, the therapist identifies any secondary impairments that are interfering with the new goal of movement reeducation and establishes a treatment plan to remove or decrease their influence.

Functional Movement Reeducation and Practice

Reeducation of functional movements is the final stage of movement reeducation. Reeducation of functional movements is used to help the patient incorporate his newly acquired movement control into functional activities, so that he uses these movements during the day when he is not in therapy. This is done by teaching the patient how to use his involved arm and leg in simple functional movements and by practicing functional movements within each treatment session. When functional reeducation is successful, the patient uses his new patterns of movement many times during the day and has a repertoire of movements that can be used to perform many tasks and functions. When it is not part of treatment, the patient may move very nicely in therapy but never apply these movements to the performance of life tasks.

While reeducation of functional movements is the end goal of movement reeducation, it is introduced in treatment before the patient can move independently so that it overlaps the other stages of movement reeducation. The therapist should start to introduce functional objects and environmental variables into the treatment session as soon as the patient is able to assist her movements with appropriate patterns of muscle activation. Whenever possible, the therapist needs to follow movement reeducation with a few minutes of functional reeducation. For example, after assisted practice of extended arm reach, the therapist could place objects on the table in various positions and use assisted practice to help the patient reach to the different objects. Or the therapist could guide the patient's arm into his shirt sleeve and help him maintain his arm in extension while he buttons his shirt cuff.

As the patient gains the ability to move independently, the therapist continues functional training through practice of simple tasks that utilize the patient's available movements. For example, when the patient can reach his arm into extension independently, he can practice putting the arm into the sleeve, reaching for the faucet or door handle, or turning on the light switch. These simple movements allow the patient to use his arm in functions before he has well-developed hand function, helping to decrease neglect and ensuring that the arm moves when the patient is away from treatment. Similarly, when the patient has mastered trunk and lower extremity movements in sitting, he should practice using these patterns in dressing or grooming.

In the stage of functional movement reeducation, the therapist also introduces specific extremity movements that are important for higher-level task performance. Once acquired, these functional movement components allow the patient to use his involved side to perform many daily living tasks without direct training from the therapist. Examples of these patterns for the upper extremity include training the hand to contour to objects (Fig. 4-4), to grasp different sizes and shapes of objects, and to combine grasp with movements of the proximal arm to lift, orient, and carry objects (Fig. 4-5). In the leg, these functional movements are designed to push gross motor and mobility skills to a higher level. Examples of these movements include training equilibrium responses in the leg and foot and increasing strength and power production in the leg through tasks such as toe walking, hopping, jumping, and kicking. Higher-level coordination requires the two sides of the body to work together in symmetric and reciprocal patterns of coordination and for the trunk and limbs to work together for balance and power. These patterns should be trained in this phase of treatment, through activities such as bilateral lifting, pushing, and pulling.

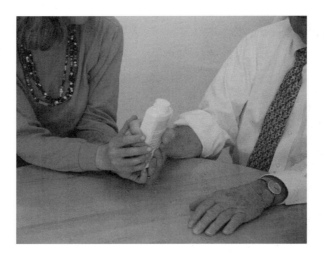

FIGURE 4-4 Training the hand to contour and grasp.

During functional movement reeducation, the therapist introduces new movements through the process of sensory education and assisted practice. For example, when training the hand to grasp cylindrical objects, such as a hairbrush, the therapist places the object in the patient's hand and guides his fingers into flexion. She asks him to help her tighten his fingers around the handle, then to release this pressure and quiet the muscle. To teach the toes to extend in a balance response in standing, the therapist places the fingers of one hand under the patient's toes. With her other hand she shifts the patient in a posterior weight shift so that his center of gravity moves back toward his heels. When the toes of his opposite foot begin to extend, she lifts the toes of his affected foot up the equivalent amount. As the patient actively assists the movement, the therapist gradually withdraws her support to allow independent practice. She then increases the complexity of the task by asking the patient to use his new functional pattern in combination with other movements. Thus, hand tasks involving grasp can be made more difficult and more functional by asking the patient to hold a jar in his involved hand while he unscrews the top with his other hand, to grasp the telephone and move it to his ear, or to hold his keys while walking across the room.

Functional reeducation and practice teach the patient how to use his new movements functionally, help him understand that new functional skills are acquired through practice and hard work, and give him permission to try to do other similar movements away from treatment. Initially, the patient will have to make a conscious

FIGURE 4-5 Training functional use of the arm in a bilateral grasp pattern. The therapist assists the patient in the task of (A) grasping, (B) lifting, and (C) repositioning the tray.

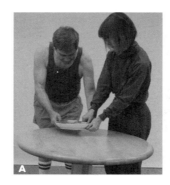 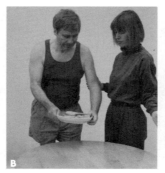 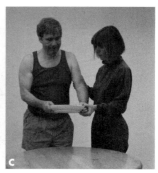

effort to remember to use his involved arm or leg in these functional patterns, and the movements will seem slower and less efficient than his compensations. However, the patient must understand the importance of this stage of reeducation and continue to practice in treatment and at home until the movements become quicker, easier, and more automatic. Otherwise, movement reeducation remains a treatment exercise, and the patient continues to rely on compensatory movements and never reaches his full potential for functional improvement.

Treatment of Relevant Secondary Impairments

Secondary impairments, such as changes in alignment, changes in joint mobility, loss of muscle and tissue length, pain, and edema, also interfere with the acquisition of movement control and functional performance. Therefore the second part of treatment is focused on the prevention and elimination of these problems. Secondary impairments begin to appear almost immediately after the brain lesion unless they are targeted for intervention from the first days of treatment. Many of the most severe problems can be prevented by prompt treatment that maintains joint alignment and mobility and muscle and soft tissue length. When these problems are already present, the therapist must set treatment goals that gradually eliminate or minimize these secondary impairments.

Neurologic patients have multiple impairments and may have different types of secondary problems in the trunk, arm, and leg of their involved side. The complexity of these impairments makes it difficult to provide a general description of the treatment process that is relevant for all of the secondary impairments described in Chapter 2. The treatment of impairments described below is designed to provide an overview of the use of movement-based techniques to influence secondary impairments. The chapters in Section II provide more detailed descriptions of techniques to manage secondary impairments of the trunk and extremities.

Whenever possible, the therapist should attempt to use movement to prevent or eliminate secondary impairments. Since the overall goal of therapy is the restoration of normal movement, using movement to address secondary impairments helps the therapist to work towards two treatment goals at once: the movement decreases the effects of the impairments and simultaneously increases the patient's movement repertoire. In our experience, selected movement activities used over a number of treatment sessions can correct most joint mobility problems and lengthen tight tissues, eliminating the need for joint mobilization and static stretching.

Although the process of meeting two goals at once sounds complicated, the therapist's knowledge of normal movement allows her to choose movement patterns that will lengthen shortened hypertonic muscles, increase joint mobility, and improve alignment. The movement patterns used to treat secondary impairments are the same movements that are taught during movement reeducation, and the handling is similar to that used in assisted movement. However, to treat secondary impairments, the therapist uses hand placements and manual messages that are different from those used during movement reeducation. These hand placements are selected to provide specific manual pressures to muscles and joints. The therapist uses her hands to influence the secondary impairments directly while the patient moves. As the movements produce the desired changes in impairment, the therapist may change her handling to use the same movements for the purposes of reeducation.

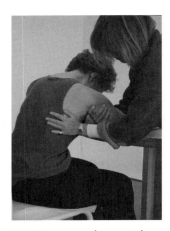

FIGURE 4-6 Lengthening tight muscles between the trunk and upper extremity through forearm weight bearing. The therapist supports the patient's hemiplegic arm on the table with one hand and uses her other hand to maintain symmetry in the trunk. The patient actively performs the trunk movements that lengthen selected muscles.

The following example illustrates how movement may be used to address secondary impairments. An asymmetric spinal position is a common trunk problem that interferes with weight acceptance on the involved hip, normal movements in the involved upper extremity, and trunk control in sitting, standing, and walking. Trunk asymmetry often results from loss of mobility in the spine, hip, and scapula and tightness in the muscles that connect the spine and ribcage to the shoulder and pelvis. To treat these impairments through movement, the therapist might place both of the patient's arms in forearm weight bearing on table and use lower trunk movements to lengthen tight muscles between the trunk and limbs and to increase mobility in the spine and ribcage. The therapist could use one of her hands to stabilize the patient's involved arm on the table, so that the movements of his trunk would lengthen the muscles between the scapula and humerus and trunk. Her other hand could be placed on the patient's spine or ribcage to guide the movements (Fig. 4-6). Pressure between her two hands would keep the spine as symmetric as possible as the body moved. A similar result could be obtained using rolling activities in supine to lengthen the shortened muscle groups and increase mobility in the spine.

To have lasting benefits, treatment of secondary impairments must be combined with a series of home exercises or activities. These activities are used to prolong or extend the benefits of therapy by providing a less specific version of the techniques used in treatment. For example, the patient described in the previous example could be given selected trunk movements in forearm weight bearing to do at home. Although his stretching at home will be less specific than during therapy, the additional movement will continue to lengthen the tight muscles and increase mobility in the spine and scapula. In cases of severe muscle contracture and loss of alignment in the hand and foot, serial orthotics with weekly corrections may be necessary to maintain the benefits of treatment and gain lasting changes in muscle length and joint range.

Although in this chapter the treatment of secondary impairments is described after movement reeducation, the order is often reversed in an actual treatment situation. Severe secondary impairments interfere with the task of movement reeducation to such an extent that treatment usually starts with movement activities to decrease the severity of these problems before new movements are reeducated. However, the whole treatment session should not be devoted to secondary impairments, because elimination of secondary problems does not translate directly into increased function. The therapist must divide her treatment time between eliminating secondary problems, reeducating movement, and doing specific functional training to maximize the patient's benefit from therapy. The exact amount of time devoted to each area of treatment will depend on the short-term, long-term, and functional goals of treatment and the severity of the patient's primary and secondary impairments.

Task-Specific Functional Training

Increasing functional independence is the ultimate goal of all rehabilitation. The final stage of treatment is devoted to training of the specific movement patterns necessary to accomplish functional tasks. The goal of this part of treatment is to give the patient the specific set of movement patterns and organized sequences of task-related behaviors that will allow him to accomplish a specific functional task.

This stage of treatment increases the range of functional behaviors and minimizes functional limitations and disability.

The patient has been prepared for functional training during movement reeducation. The stages of movement reeducation are designed to provide the patient with control of the basic movement components necessary for functional performance. When these basic movement patterns have been successfully trained, neurologic patients can learn to accomplish many functional tasks on their own, without the direct assistance of their therapist. But there are some tasks that patients are unable to reacquire on their own. This may be due to the complexity of the task or to physical limitations that interfere with normal performance. In these cases, actual task practice with the assistance or supervision of the therapist is necessary to help patients achieve specific functional goals. This task practice may involve task-specific training when the patient has the motor control necessary for normal performance or compensatory training when normal performance is not attainable.

Task-specific training is used to meet a functional goal when the patient has the movement components necessary for normal performance. Sometimes practice of the entire task is necessary to accomplish the goal. For example, to help a higher-level patient meet the goal of working out at the gymnasium, the therapist may have to accompany the patient there, select appropriate equipment for use, and go through a workout that includes getting on and off the machinery and performing the correct number of repetitions. For other functions, the patient may be able to achieve his goal by working with the therapist on a difficult segment of the task. To help a patient resume her former hobby of quilting, the therapist may only have to help her with the mechanics of using the sewing machine, needle, and thread. Given these skills, the patient may be able to proceed to fabric selection, cutting, and assembly without further assistance from the therapist.

Retraining Task Performance

The therapist should approach task-specific training by identifying the parts of the task that will be difficult or require new movement skills. If possible these movements should be practiced separately before attempting the whole task. For example, a former golfer should practice holding and swinging the golf club in therapy before trying to hit a ball. Sometimes difficulties in task performance can be identified only during trial of the task. For example, problems in the water that may interfere with swimming can only be identified by going to the pool with the patient and observing difficulties. At other times the patient identifies the problem and brings it to the therapist for a solution. A patient who wants to drive but is afraid to get into the driver's seat because it requires that he put his involved leg into the car first may request help from the therapist in learning this movement pattern.

Once the difficult movement sequences have been identified, the therapist can use assisted practice to help the patient perform the first few repetitions of the movement. The therapist can lighten and then remove her support as soon as the patient feels confident about performing the movement sequence. If the selected task has many steps and safety is an issue, practice of the difficult part of the task should be followed by supervised practice of the whole task. Thus, the patient who can swing a tennis racket should practice hitting balls thrown to him by the therapist that involve moving his body sideways, forwards, or backwards before trying it on the tennis court (Fig. 4-7).

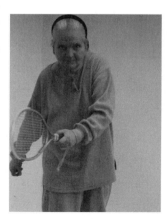

FIGURE 4-7 Training task performance. The patient practices swinging the tennis racket and hitting balls to the therapist in preparation for practice on the tennis court.

Task-specific training is generally unsuccessful when the patient lacks the movement skills necessary to accomplish the task. For example, the function of climbing a small set of stairs without a railing requires the ability to balance on one leg, produce power in the legs to propel the body up to the next step, and balance control in the trunk to maintain the body centered between the two legs. If these basic movements are not available, actual practice on stair climbing is likely to be less successful and more dangerous than devoting treatment time to training these movement components. Similarly, trying to teach a flaccid arm to bring a cup to the mouth is not likely to work if the muscles in the arm cannot contract with enough strength to lift the hand to the mouth or grasp the cup. If basic movement components are not available, the task can often be trained by teaching movement compensations to help the patient meet personal goals. The patient can learn to go up a few stairs in sitting if this will help him have access to part of his house, or he can have a railing or ramp constructed to accomplish the goal. Compensatory strategies for movement are discussed in the next section.

Training strategies for functional activities vary greatly because of the wide variety of motor, cognitive, and perceptual demands needed for the tasks of living. For functional performance without compensation, treatment begins with reeducation of the important movement components, movement sequences, and functional behaviors used to perform all phases of the task. When this has been completed, task-specific practice is the next step. Failure to achieve success at the task at this stage is often related to perceptual and cognitive limitations that are separate from motor abilities. Treatment of these cognitive and perceptual problems is beyond the scope of this book.

Teaching Appropriate Compensations

All patients with residual motor deficits must learn conpensatory strategies to accomplish the tasks of daily living. One of the main functions of therapy with neurologic patients is to teach new movement strategies for accomplishing functional needs. This compensatory training, which teaches the patient how to use what is available, is the counterpart to movement reeducation, which seeks to restore what used to be. Compensatory training is used at all stages of rehabilitation to allow the patient to meet functional goals. Its purpose is to allow the patient to regain independence using strategies that make use of his existing patterns of muscle control but that substitute for his motor deficits.

In this book we distinguish between two categories of compensation: appropriate compensations and undesirable compensations. This distinction is based on the differences in the quality of movement between the two categories and on the relationship that exists between appropriate compensations and the goals of movement reeducation. *Appropriate compensations* use movement patterns that resemble normal movements and incorporate the involved trunk, arm, and leg into the activities. The purpose of these compensations is to decrease postural asymmetries and neglect while using the potential for normal movement available on the involved side. Appropriate compensations are compatible with the goals of movement reeducation because they incorporate the patient's active movement patterns into functional performance.

Undesirable compensations use one-sided or asymmetric movements that fail to incorporate available movements of the affected trunk and limbs. These movement patterns promote asymmetries and poor alignment in the trunk and limbs, decrease weight acceptance on the involved leg, and lead to spasticity in the involved arm and leg. Undesirable compensations are "undesirable" because they lead to the development of secondary impairments, do not utilize the patient's available movement patterns, and work in opposition to the goals of movement reeducation. As the names imply, we believe the therapist should attempt to train appropriate compensations when at all possible and to replace undesirable compensations with alternatives that use the movement potential of the involved side. Undesirable compensations are eliminated in treatment through a combination of movement reeducation and training of more appropriate compensatory strategies.

Compensatory training is used in treatment in several ways. In activities of daily living, compensations are necessary to replace the action of the involved arm. To be appropriate, these compensations employ one-handed techniques in movement strategies that maintain appropriate trunk symmetry and incorporate the involved arm into the activity in the most active way possible. For example, in upper-body dressing, the hemiplegic patient may be taught the following movement strategy to put on his shirt. The patient places the shirt across his thighs so that the sleeve hangs down between his knees. He then initiates an anterior weight shift with his upper body. This causes the spine to flex and the shoulders to move forward. The movement of the trunk helps put the elbow of his affected arm in extension. As the body continues to move forward and down, the hand and arm are pushed into the sleeve. The patient may then pull the sleeve up over the shoulder and move his trunk back up to complete the dressing process (Fig. 4-8). In this example, the patient's trunk is active and appropriately symmetric, weight is supported on both hips, and the affected arm is moved in a sequential fashion that simulates the normal pattern of reaching into the sleeve. The trunk movement used to assist the dressing task is one that has already been practiced in movement reeducation. As the involved arm regains active movement, the patient practices reaching of his arm into the sleeve, eliminating the need for the compensatory trunk weight shift and incorporating active arm movements into functional performance. Similar adaptations can be used to train lower body dressing, bathing, and eating. Some examples of these compensations are included in the chapters in Section II.

Therapists should also train compensations in functional movement sequences, such as rolling, sitting up, or standing up. In these movements, compensations are necessary to substitute for loss of movement and strength in the trunk, arm, and leg. In movement sequences, compensations are used to maintain symmetry in the body and incorporate the involved trunk, arm, and leg into the activity so that they

FIGURE 4-8 An appropriate compensation for dressing. The forward movement of the trunk helps prevent trunk asymmetry and encourages elbow extension.

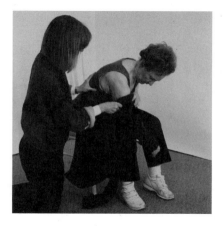

assist with the production of normal patterns of movement. The task of rolling from supine to sidelying on the uninvolved side can be used to illustrate how this type of compensation works. Rolling to the uninvolved side is difficult when the involved arm lacks sufficient strength to lift across the body as the roll is initiated. When the arm hangs back, the patient is unable to activate the flexors of his upper trunk. He is able to roll successfully only by pulling on the side of the bed. Appropriate compensatory training shows the patient how to find his involved arm in the bed, use his other hand to reach it toward the ceiling, and then initiate a flexion rotation pattern with his arm and upper body to start the roll to the side. A similar compensation may be used during sit to stand to maintain symmetry in the trunk and weight on both feet. Examples of this type of compensation are included in each of the functional chapters in Section II.

SUMMARY

This chapter has presented a model for treatment based on three different areas: movement reeducation, treatment of impairments, and task-specific functional training. These treatment parts are summarized in the box below. In most treatment settings, therapists work on all three areas of treatment with most or all of their patients. Yet for each patient, it is necessary to choose which area of treatment to emphasize and how much of each treatment session to devote to each area. This decision will depend on the level of functioning of the patient, the goals of treatment, and the intuition and skill the therapist brings to the problem-solving process.

The Parts of Treatment

Movement reeducation
  Sensory education
  Assisted practice
  Independent practice
  Functional training
Treatment of impairments
Task-specific functional training
  Retraining task performance
  Teaching appropriate compensations

5
Trunk Movements in Sitting

CONCEPTS AND PRINCIPLES

Trunk movements in sitting form the basis for postural control and functional performance in the sitting position. This chapter will describe the trunk movements that are critical for balance and function in sitting. The information in this chapter is necessary for understanding extremity movement in sitting and for the analysis of such important functional movements as sitting to standing, transfers, and supine to sitting. It will also be important for understanding the chapters on supine, rolling, and standing. In many ways, this chapter provides the best introduction to our view of functional movement, our system of movement analysis, and our model of treatment.

In sitting, the trunk moves in small ranges around midline to adjust to the movements of the extremities or in larger ranges to assume a new body position or extend the functional range of the arm or leg. When the upper extremities are active around midline, trunk movements occur as postural adjustments that maintain the body in balance over its base of support; as the arms move farther away from the center of the body, active trunk weight shifts are used to increase the range of the arms in reach. Trunk movements in sitting are also combined with lower extremity movements to transfer body weight to one leg or to change the distribution of body weight over the weightbearing lower extremities. Finally, movements of the trunk in sitting are used to move the body to a new base of support, such as occurs when forward inclination of the trunk initiates the movement of sit to stand.

Functional performance in sitting is based on the ability to maintain the trunk in a stable upright position and to generate movements that efficiently and safely position the trunk and extremities for task performance. Neurologic lesions often result in primary and secondary impairments that affect trunk control in sitting. These impairments result in an inability to move the trunk in normal patterns or to use trunk muscles to maintain or restore balance. Since sitting is such an important position for daily life, loss of trunk control in sitting leads to functional limitations and loss of independence.

Reestablishing trunk control in sitting is one of the earliest and most important goals of rehabilitation. Therapists begin to train sitting trunk movements with the acute patient. These movements help the patient regain a stable sitting position and to move his trunk safely in the patterns needed for activities of daily living. The training of trunk movements in the early stages of rehabilitation is also a crucial part of building muscle strength and tone in the muscles of the flaccid arm and of activating the weak muscles of the hip to contract during weight acceptance. Trunk movements in sitting may also be used in treatment with patients who are functioning independently in sitting, standing, and walking. With these patients, normal trunk movements are practiced to decrease atypical movements and compensation and to remedy specific movement deficits. The practice of selected trunk movements can also be used to address impairments such as muscle weakness, muscle/soft tissue restrictions, and joint hypomobility in the spine, ribcage, and hips. Higher functioning neurologic patients may have difficulty combining trunk movements with movements of the arm and leg, such as are used to reach or cross a leg. With this group of patients, practice of extremity movements with the appropriate trunk patterns is used to increase their ability to use normal patterns of coordinated movement during task performance.

TRUNK MOVEMENT COMPONENTS

The trunk is defined as the spine and the rib cage. The term *upper trunk* refers to the head, the vertebrae from C1 to T10, and the rib cage. The upper extremity is attached to the upper trunk through the clavicle and the scapula. In this book, the term *upper body* refers to the functional unit composed of the upper trunk and the upper extremity. In sitting, the *lower trunk* is composed of the vertebrae from T11 to the sacrum and the pelvis. The lower extremity attaches to the lower trunk through the pelvis. We use the term *lower body* to refer to the functional unit made up of the lower trunk and the lower extremity. It is important to recognize that the role of the pelvis is different in sitting from standing. In sitting, supine, and prone positions, the pelvis functions as part of the lower trunk.[1] In standing, the foot is the base of support and the pelvis is linked kinetically to the leg.[1]

In sitting, the body's base of support consists of the pelvis, femurs, and feet. To perform functional activities in sitting, muscle activity maintains the trunk in an erect or appropriate posture and trunk muscle tone is high enough to allow movement to occur. During periods of rest or inactivity, most people relax this erect posture and allow the spine to flex, decreasing the amount of work being done by the muscles of the trunk and lowering the state of muscle tension in the body (Fig. 5-1). When the body is in the relaxed position, the full range of trunk movements cannot

FIGURE 5-1 *(A)* Erect sitting. *(B)* Relaxed sitting.

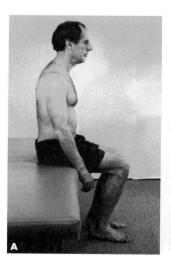
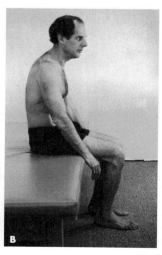

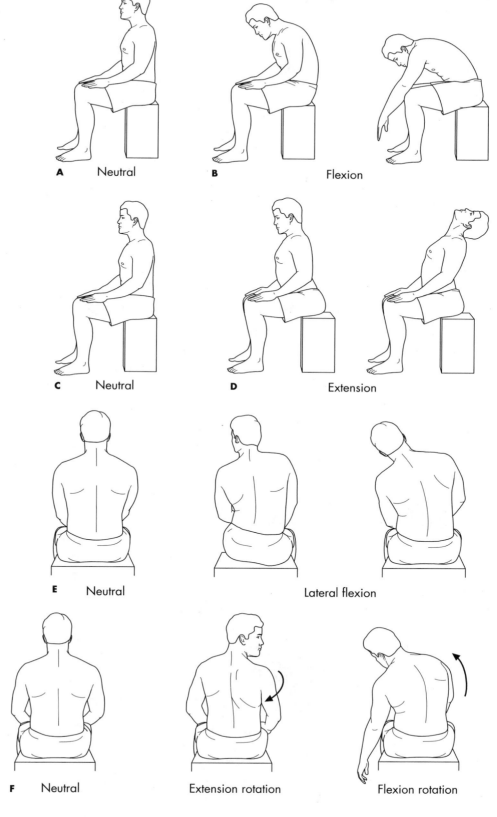

FIGURE 5-2 Planes of trunk movement in sitting. (A) Neutral. (B) Flexion. (C) Neutral. (D) Extension. (E) Lateral flexion. (F) Rotation.

A Neutral

B Flexion

C Neutral

D Extension

E Neutral   Lateral flexion

F Neutral   Extension rotation   Flexion rotation

be performed. Active and healthy people will automatically return to a more upright sitting posture before attempting movement or task performance. This automatic postural adjustment is often absent in neurologic patients, with the result that they may attempt to initiate movement with inappropriate posture and/or state of muscle readiness.

The trunk has three planes of movement in sitting: flexion/extension movements, lateral flexion movements, and rotation (Fig. 5-2). For purposes of clarity, we will define the direction of rotation as the direction in which the vertebral body is moving. These movements are the critical patterns of spinal movement that contribute to functional movement in sitting. Normal trunk movements combine these movements of the spine and rib cage with a weight shift over the base of support. Trunk movements in sitting can be initiated from either the upper trunk or the lower trunk. These two patterns of initiation result in different patterns of spinal alignment, muscular activity, and weight distribution. Both patterns are used continually for function, and both must be available for trunk control in sitting. All the movements in the section are performed from a starting position of erect sitting.

Movements Initiated from the Upper Trunk

Anterior Weight Shift

When an anterior weight shift is initiated from the upper trunk or upper body, the spine flexes forward sequentially from the head and neck (Fig. 5-3). Flexion progresses down the spine into the thoracic and lumbar vertebrae, and the hip joints move into increased flexion as the body moves forward and down (Fig. 5-3A). As the trunk flexes, the arm and hands move forward to the floor (Fig. 5-3B and C). This combination of trunk and arm movement results in scapula abduction and elevation and shoulder flexion. To return to upright from this forward flexed position, the upper trunk extends and moves back. As the upper body approaches the vertical position, extension progresses to the lower spinal segments. The movement is complete when the shoulders are upright over the hip joints.

Functional Examples

This movement is used to pick up something from the floor while sitting or to bend forward to don or tie shoes.

FIGURE 5-3 *(A–C)* Upper-trunk-initiated anterior weight shift.

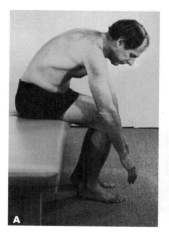
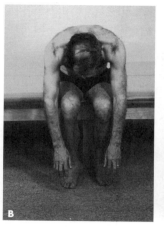
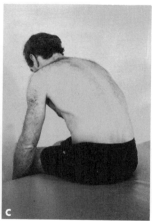

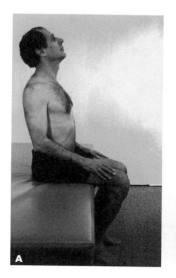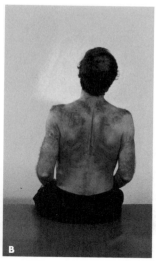

FIGURE 5-4 *(A & B)* Upper-trunk-initiated posterior weight shift.

Posterior Weight Shift

When a posterior weight shift is initiated from the upper body, the spine extends. The head and shoulders move backward until they are directly over or behind the hip joints. Extension in the spine is accompanied by an anterior tilt of the pelvis and increased flexion at the hip joints (Fig. 5-4A). In the arms, the trunk movement results in scapula adduction and depression and shoulder extension (Fig. 5-4B). The range of normal movement in this direction is small compared with the large movement available in flexion, and the pattern is less important functionally than other weight shifts in sitting.

Functional Examples

This movement is used to look up at the ceiling or position your head under the shower head for shampooing.

Lateral Weight Shift

When a lateral weight shift to the left is initiated with the upper body, the head, left shoulder, and arm move laterally and down (Fig. 5-5A). This results in lateral flexion of the spine, with the concavity on the left, and increased weight bearing on the left hip and femur. If the movement progresses far enough, the left forearm may reach the bed. The right side of the pelvis remains in contact with the support until the end range of spinal movement has been reached. At that point, it may elevate and move off the bed. In the left arm, the spinal movement is accompanied by scapula depression and downward rotation. In the right arm, the scapula elevates and upwardly rotates (Fig. 5-5B). To return to upright sitting, the shoulders move laterally back over the pelvis, so that the left shoulder moves to the left and then down.

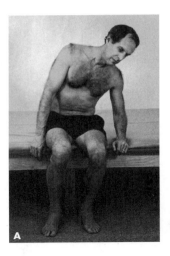 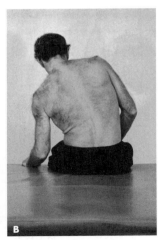

FIGURE 5-5 *(A & B)* Upper-trunk- initiated lateral weight shift.

Functional Examples

This movement is used functionally to reach sideways to the floor or to go from sitting to sidelying.

Lower Trunk-Initiated Movements

Anterior Weight Shift

When an anterior weight shift is initiated from the lower spine and pelvis, the spine extends in the cervical, thoracic, and lumbar areas and moves forward with the pelvis to produce increased hip flexion (Fig. 5-6A). Weight is transferred forward from the pelvis to the femurs and the feet as the shoulder girdle moves in front of the hip joint (Fig. 5-6B). As the body moves forward, the scapulas adduct and depress (Fig 5-6C).

Functional Examples

This sitting weight shift is used to reach forward, to move away from the back of a chair, or to stand up.

FIGURE 5-6 *(A–C)* Lower-trunk-initiated anterior weight shift.

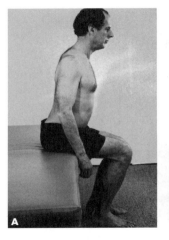 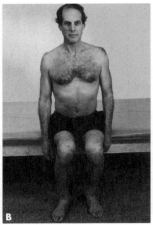 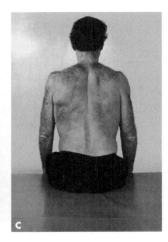

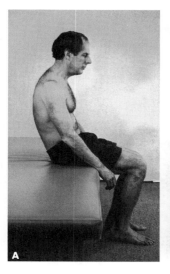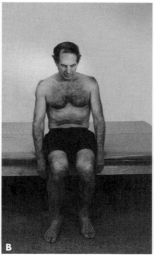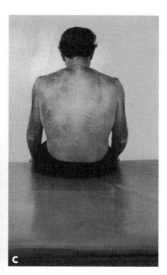

FIGURE 5-7 *(A–C)* Lower-trunk-initiated posterior weight shift.

Posterior Weight Shift

During a posterior weight shift, the pelvis and lower trunk move back and flexion occurs throughout the spine (Fig. 5-7A). This active movement of the spine shifts the center of gravity behind the hip joints, so that they are in less flexion than in erect sitting (Fig. 5-7B). As the pelvis rolls back, the upper trunk flexes, and the scapulas abduct and elevate (Fig. 5-7C).

Functional Examples

This movement pattern is used to lean back into a chair or to lift a leg to tie a shoe in sitting.

Lateral Weight Shift

When the lower trunk initiates a lateral weight shift to the left, the resulting pattern is lateral flexion of the spine with the concavity on the right and transfer of weight to the left hip (Fig. 5-8A). As the body weight is actively shifted from both sides of the pelvis and both femurs to the left hip and thigh, the right side of the pelvis lifts off the support. The left side of the rib cage moves laterally and up with the movement, resulting in increased space between the lower ribs on the left and decreased space between the ribs on the right. The left shoulder elevates and the scapula is moved into upward rotation by the lateral translation of the thoracic spine. At the same time, the left scapula moves into depression and downward rotation (Fig. 5-8B). When weight shift is complete, the left shoulder and rib cage are positioned over the left hip. At this time, the right side of the pelvis has been elevated and shifted medially, while the left side of the pelvis moves down as weight shifts to the left femur.

Functional Examples

This movement is used functionally to lift and cross one leg over another. It also occurs automatically when reaching out to one side.

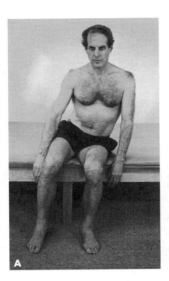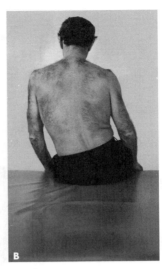

FIGURE 5-8 (A & B) Lower-trunk-initiated lateral weight shift.

Rotational Movements of the Trunk

In sitting, trunk rotation occurs during weight shifts that combine an anterior or posterior weight shift with a lateral weight shift to one side. We can visualize these movements of the body as occurring on a diagonal away from the center of the base of support. Trunk rotation is possible with the spine in either extension or flexion. Upper and lower trunk-initiated movements both result in flexion rotation and extension rotation patterns.

Flexion Rotation Patterns

Upper-Trunk-Initiated Flexion Rotation

When a weight shift on a forward diagonal to the left is initiated from the upper trunk, the movement results in spinal flexion with vertebral rotation to the left. The left hip and thigh carry more weight than the right (Fig. 5-9A). Because of the rotation that has occurred in the spine, the right rib cage and shoulder girdle move forward, and the left side of the ribs and shoulder move back. The right side of the trunk and rib cage are lengthened relative to the left side (Fig. 5-9B).

Functional Examples

This movement is used to bring both arms to the floor to tie one shoe.

Lower-Trunk-Initiated Flexion Rotation

If the lower trunk initiates a weight shift that combines posterior and lateral movement to the right, the resulting trunk position is also spinal flexion with vertebral rotation to the left. In this pattern, the right leg has more weight on it and the spine is flexed but upright (Fig. 5-10A). The rotation of the upper trunk over the pelvis causes the left shoulder and rib cage to rotate back as the right shoulder and rib

FIGURE 5-9 *(A & B)* Upper-trunk-initiated flexion rotation.

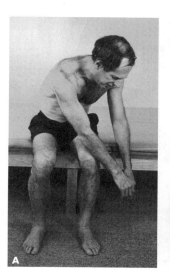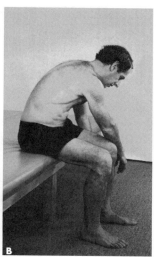

cage move forward (Fig. 5-10B). Both scapulas are abducted on the rib cage because of the flexion in the upper trunk.

Functional Examples

This movement is used as an equilibrium reaction in its extreme ranges. In smaller ranges, it is used to cross one leg over the other and bring both hands to that foot to tie the shoe.

FIGURE 5-10 *(A & B)* Lower-trunk-initiated flexion rotation.

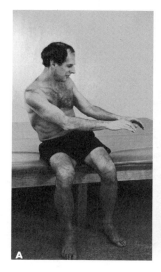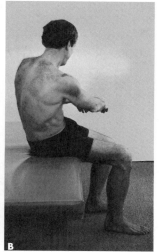

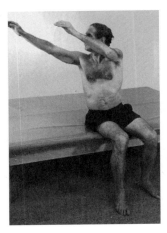

FIGURE 5-11 Upper-body-initiated extension rotation.

Extension Rotation Patterns

Upper-Trunk-Initiated Extension Rotation

When the upper trunk initiates a diagonal weight shift that combines posterior weight shift with a lateral movement to the right, the resulting trunk pattern is extension rotation to the right (Fig. 5-11). As the trunk rotates to the right, the right shoulder moves in a posterior direction behind the right hip joint, and the left shoulder girdle and arm and the left side of the ribcage move anteriorly. The pelvis remains on the supporting surface and both legs support weight.

Functional Examples

This movement is used to reach behind the body to pull your coat around or tuck in your shirt. It also occurs as an equilibrium reaction.

Lower-Trunk-Initiated Extension Rotation

The spine also moves into extension with vertebral rotation during a lower-trunk-initiated weight shift that combines anterior and lateral movements. In this rotational pattern to the left, the spine is in extension and weight is on the left leg (Fig. 5-12A). Both shoulders move forward and to the left. The forward and lateral weight shift causes anterior movement of the pelvis and listing upward of the pelvis on the right side. This makes the left side of the rib cage and spine longer than the right (Fig. 5-12B).

Functional Examples

This movement is used to use both arms together on one side of the body or to bring one arm across midline to function on the opposite side. In larger ranges, this movement pattern represents an equilibrium reaction.

Trunk Control in Sitting

Trunk control is the term used to describe the ability to move and position the trunk appropriately for balance and task performance. Trunk treatment in sitting is performed with the goal of reestablishing trunk control. For the purpose of rehabilitation, we can conceptualize trunk control in sitting as having three parts. Each of these parts must be included in movement reeducation to restore normal control in sitting.

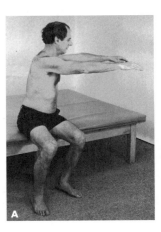
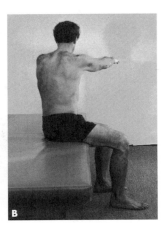

FIGURE 5-12 *(A & B)* Lower-body-initiated extension rotation.

1. Ability to perform trunk movement components. The normal trunk movements presented above are necessary for balance and function in sitting. We use these movements to perform life tasks. We must be able to perform these basic trunk movements easily and automatically for the other aspects of trunk control to be possible. For this reason, we can think of trunk movements in sitting as the movement precursors necessary for normal trunk control in sitting. Trunk treatment in sitting begins with the reeducation of these movement components and progresses to the other parts of trunk control when trunk movements can be performed normally.

2. Ability to combine trunk and extremity movements in functional sequences. During task performance in sitting, trunk movements occur in combination with movements of the arms or legs. We must be able to produce appropriate trunk movements and to coordinate movements of the trunk with those of the extremities to perform life tasks. These trunk movements are used in different ways during different tasks. For some functions, the trunk movement itself is the most critical for task performance. For example, to move from sitting to standing, the trunk must be able to initiate a lower-body anterior weight shift to allow the legs to lift the body to standing (Fig. 5-13A). In functional movements such as crossing one leg over the other to put on a shoe, the movement of the extremity is the most critical component of the task, and the trunk movements occur as background postural adjustments that facilitate the lifting of the leg and maintain the stability of the body (Fig. 5-13B). For still other activities, trunk weight shifts are used to extend the range of the arms (Fig. 5-13C). Figures 5-13D–G demonstrate the wide variety of trunk movements that are used during the task of dressing. If trunk movements can not be combined easily and automatically with movements of the arms and legs, trunk control is incomplete, and treatment must reeducate this part of trunk control.

3. Ability to combine trunk and extremity movements for balance and equilibrium. The coordination of trunk and extremity movements is equally important in balance and equilibrium. In sitting with the feet on the floor, the body's base of support is large and stable. Trunk movements and weight shifts are necessary to keep the trunk aligned over its base, but the trunk muscles do not have to work hard to maintain equilibrium because the body is not in danger of falling. The muscles of the trunk become more

FIGURE 5-13 Combined trunk and extremity movements in functional sequences. *(A)* Lower-body-initiated anterior weight shift is used to initiate the stand. *(B)* As the leg lifts and crosses, slight posterior and lateral weight shifts are necessary to maintain balance. *(C)* A lower-body-initiated anterior weight shift assists the arm in reaching the table. *(Figure Continues)*

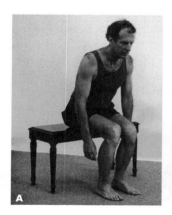
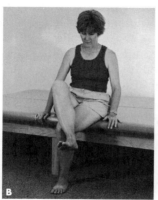
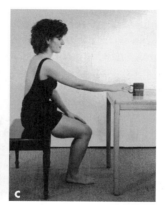

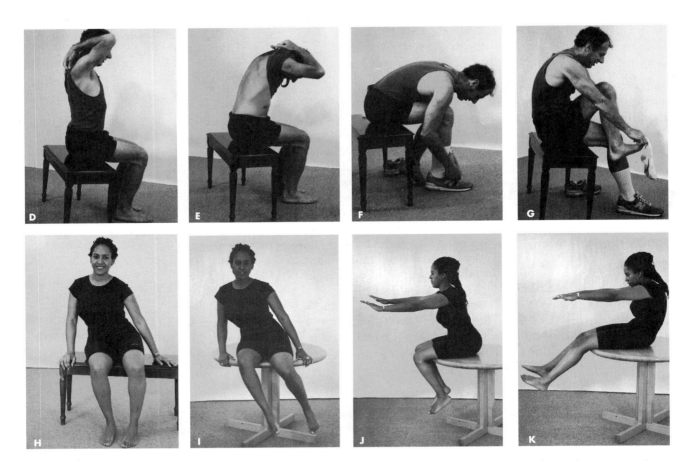

FIGURE 5-13 *(Continued)* *(D–G)* Trunk movements during dressing and the different roles that trunk movements play in a functional task: *(D)* Upper-trunk-initiated posterior. *(E)* Upper-trunk-initiated anterior. *(F)* Upper-trunk-initiated anterior, larger weight shift. *(G)* Lower-trunk-initiated posterior. *(H)* Trunk movement with the feet on the floor. The body position is relatively stable. *(I)* When the feet are not supported, the base of support is less stable, and the trunk is correspondingly more active. Note the movement of the lower leg to the left to counterbalance the trunk weight shift to the right. *(J & K)* Equilibrium responses in the arms and legs provide additional stability when trunk muscle activity alone is not enough to keep the body from falling.

active when the base of support becomes smaller e.g., when the feet are not in contact with the floor or when the trunk moves through a bigger range so that it balances closer to the edge of its original base) (Fig. 5-13H & I). As the the position of the body becomes more precarious, the muscles of the trunk work harder. Eventually the task of maintaining stability becomes too difficult for the trunk muscles alone, and the muscles of the arms and/or legs become active to provide additional stability to the trunk. The ability of the trunk muscles to work harder against gravity and to combine with movements of the extremities to keep the body from falling is the equilibrium demand of trunk control (Fig. 5-13J & K). If the trunk cannot work hard enough to move the body through a large weight shift or work together with the arms and legs to balance on a small base of support, this aspect of trunk control is incomplete and should be reeducated.

The therapist must systematically train the three parts of trunk control in sitting. In the treatment section of this chapter, we describe specific activities to reeducate trunk movements, prepare the trunk and limbs to work together in functional activities, and increase strength and control in the trunk and extremities to improve balance and equilibrium. The movements described above are summarized in Table 5-1.

TABLE 5-1 Summary of Movements

UPPER-TRUNK-INITIATED MOVEMENTS			
MOVEMENT	SPINE	SCAPULA	PELVIS/HIP
Anterior	Flexion	Abduction Elevation	Pelvis moves forward, more hip flexion
Posterior	Extension	Adduction	Less hip flexion
Lateral			
WB	Lateral flexion, concavity	Depression	Not much movement
NWB	Lateral flexion, concavity	Downward rotation Elevation	Pelvis stays on support

UPPER-TRUNK-INITIATED ROTATION	
Flexion rotation	
Direction of weight shift LE WB	Anterior and lateral Weight on side to which body is rotating
Trunk rotation	Rotation back of side to which body is rotating
Extension Rotation	
Direction of weight shift LE WB	Posterior and lateral Pelvis stays on support, weight on both legs
Trunk rotation	Rotation back on side to which rotating

LOWER-TRUNK-INITIATED MOVEMENTS			
MOVEMENT	SPINE	SCAPULA	PELVIS/HIP
Anterior	Extension	Adduction Depression	Anterior tilt, more hip flexion
Posterior	Flexion	Adduction Elevation	Posterior tilt, less hip flexion
Lateral			
WB	Lateral flexion, convexity	Elevation Upper rotation	Pelvis lists down Increased weight
NWB	Lateral flexion, concavity	Depression Downward rotation	Pelvis lists up Less weight on leg

LOWER-TRUNK-INITIATED ROTATION	
Flexion rotation	
Direction of weight shift LE WB	Posterior and lateral Increased weight on side opposite to rotation
Spinal pattern	Rotation forward of WB side
Extension Rotation	
Direction of weight shift LE WB	Anterior and lateral Increased WB on side to which rotating
Spinal pattern	Rotation backward, WB side of trunk

Abbreviations: LE, lower extremity; NWB, non-weight bearing; WB, weight bearing.

SIGNIFICANT IMPAIRMENTS THAT INTERFERE WITH PERFORMANCE

Muscle Weakness in the Trunk

Trunk muscle weakness/paralysis has a significant effect on the neurologic patient's ability to move and function safely in sitting. Loss of muscle control in the trunk affects sitting posture, automatic postural and balance responses, and functional movement patterns. Most neurologic patients in the early stages of rehabilitation demonstrate weakness or paralysis in the muscles of the trunk on the involved side. This hemiplegic pattern of trunk weakness makes the center of the body asymmetric and unstable, as the trunk muscles on the hemiplegic side of the body cannot be active to maintain alignment in the spine and rib cage against the force of gravity or to perform movements over the base of support.

When most of the trunk and extremity muscles on one side of the body are weak, the patient's involved side will not be able to maintain an erect posture or sit without support. Patients with this pattern of muscle weakness use their uninvolved trunk and arm for stability and develop asymmetric patterns of posture and trunk movement (Fig. 5-14A). In less severe strokes or injuries, some, but not all, of the trunk muscles on the involved side have adequate strength to be used for stability. In these patients, the use of available muscles in excessive or inappropriate patterns may also contribute to postural deviations and atypical movement patterns. In sitting, trunk posture and movement are also influenced by muscle weakness in the shoulder girdle and hip. These problems are discussed in separate sections below.

Muscle weakness/paralysis is addressed through movement reeducation. After assessing the trunk to determine the pattern of weakness and resulting problems with posture and movement, the therapist selects hand placements and handling techniques that allow her to control the patient while teaching him to perform upper-trunk- and lower-trunk-initiated movements. When the patient has very little movement control in the trunk, the therapist usually faces the patient and supports the hemiplegic arm. This allows her to use the hemiplegic arm to help control the position of the upper trunk and keep it aligned over the pelvis. The therapist uses this grip during treatment on the mat and during functional training of transfers or activities of daily living (Fig. 5-14E). The patient will use this movement pattern functionally to transfer to the mat and to dress and bathe. The therapist may have difficulty controlling the trunk and hemiplegic arm in sitting, since the severe weakness makes the arm and trunk heavy and difficult to control. In this situation, forearm weight bearing can be used to support the heavy arm, freeing the therapist's hands for maintaining trunk alignment and retraining the correct patterns of trunk movement (Fig. 5-14F). This technique is described in Chapter 7. In facilities where co-treatment is possible, having one therapist support the hemiplegic arm while the second therapist assists the trunk weight shifts also simplifies the task of reeducation.

When the patient begins to regain strength in the muscles of the trunk, treatment of the trunk in sitting is easier. The patient is now able to sit without use of his uninvolved arm and to perform some trunk movements without assistance or loss of balance. At this point, the therapist changes her handling techniques so that the patient learns to use his trunk more actively or through bigger ranges. The therapist may move to more distal hand placements on the arm and/or leg to facilitate the trunk movements (Fig. 5-14G). She may position the patient on a high plinth to

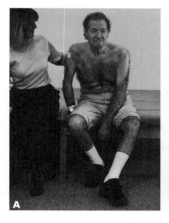
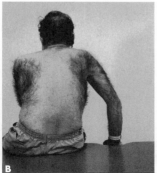
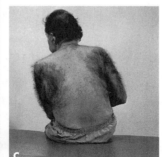
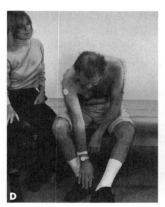
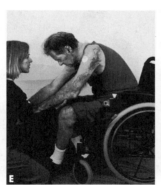
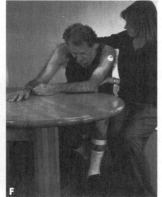
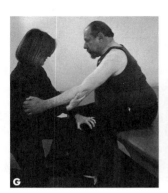
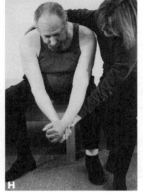
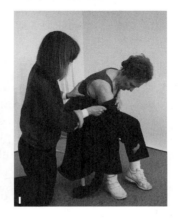

FIGURE 5-14 *(A)* Left hemiplegia with severe muscle weakness in the trunk, arm, and leg. The patient has shifted his trunk over his right hip and uses his right arm for balance. *(B)* From the back, the use of the right arm to stabilize the trunk is very obvious. Note how the left side of the pelvis does not appear to be in contact with the bed. *(C)* When he lifts his right hand off the mat, the trunk lists to the hemiplegic side. *(D)* During an upper-trunk-initiated anterior weight shift, the hemiplegic side does not participate symmetrically in the movement. *(E)* The therapist supports the patient's arms to maintain symmetry in the upper trunk and assists his performance of an upper-trunk-initiated anterior weight shift. *(F)* The therapist has placed the patient in forearm weight bearing. The table supports the weight of the hemiplegic trunk and arm and makes it easier to align the upper trunk over the pelvis. *(G)* The therapist is supporting the hemiplegic arms and leg while the patient actively controls the weight shift in the trunk. *(H)* The patient supports his hemiplegic arm with his right hand and reaches to the floor in an upper-trunk-initiated anterior weight shift. The therapist is providing only light support of the trunk and hemiplegic arm. *(I)* Practice donning a sweater using an upper-trunk-initiated anterior weight shift to the hemiplegic right arm at the shoulder.

work on trunk movements, making his base of support smaller so that the trunk must be more active to maintain balance. Trunk control in sitting can also be improved by having the patient attempt to move independently (Fig. 5-14H). The therapist may also combine trunk movement reeducation with daily living activities such as dressing and bathing, so that the patient learns to associate the trunk movements with specific life tasks (Fig. 5-14I). The patient's ability to use his trunk actively in sitting will improve through these treatment activities.

Loss of Alignment and Stability in the Upper Extremity

Loss of alignment and stability in the upper extremity also affects the postural alignment of the trunk and the performance of trunk movements. Changes in upper extremity position are frequently associated with flaccid paralysis of the upper extremity, hypertonicity, and unbalanced muscled return. These alignment changes primarily affect the stability of the upper trunk and the position of the thoracic spine and rib cage. The flaccid arm pulls the upper trunk forward or laterally, creating excessive flexion in the thoracic spine or a lateral flexion in the spine with the involved arm on the concave side of the curve. When the trunk moves, the arm dangles without control, affecting upper trunk control and alignment (Fig. 5-15A & B). Flexor spasticity in the arm is associated with elevation of the scapula and rotation backward of the hemiplegic rib cage (Fig. 5-15C & D). The asymmetric trunk postures associated with both flaccidity and spasticity in the arm interfere with normal performance of some critical trunk movement components.

When the weight and position of the arm exert a significant influence on alignment of the upper trunk, the therapist must correct the position of the scapula and arm before reeducating trunk movements. In flaccid patients, the excessive weight of the hemiplegic arm pulls on the trunk and interferes with movement. To prepare the trunk for movement in these patients, the therapist corrects the position of the scapula and glenohumeral joint and supports the weight of the arm on her body. The therapist maintains this manual support of the arm while retraining trunk movements (Fig. 5-15E). However, performance of trunk movements in sitting will always be strongly influenced by weakness in the hemiplegic arm. Therefore, the therapist should include activities to activate and strengthen shoulder girdle and arm muscles in weight bearing and non-weight bearing patterns to increase control of the upper trunk and prepare the arm and trunk to work together.

When spasticity or muscle shortening maintain the upper extremity in an abnormally flexed position, the therapist may not be able to easily correct the position of the patient's trunk and arm to support it on her body. In these patients, specific treatment techniques to lengthen the shortened muscles and restore mobility and alignment to the shoulder girdle may be necessary before the arm can be extended and supported on the therapist's body. The therapist can use activities such as scapula mobilization in sitting or forearm weight bearing to reduce the hypertonicity in the arm and lengthen tight muscles. The therapist then maintains her control of the arm during treatment of the trunk to ensure that muscle tone in the arm does not increase excessively as the trunk moves (Fig. 5-15F & G). Techniques for incorporating the hemiplegic arm into treatment of the trunk are described in this chapter. Information on reducing flexor hypertonicity in the arm are included in Chapters 6, 7, and 10.

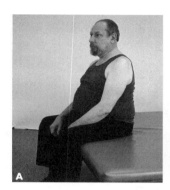

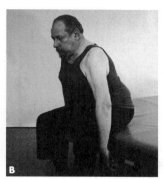

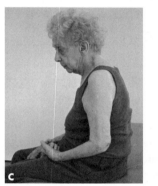

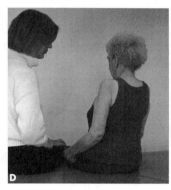

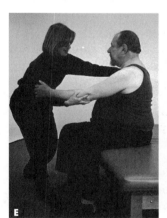

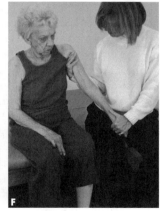

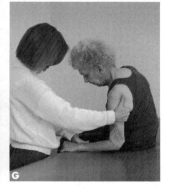

FIGURE 5-15 *(A & B)* The hemiplegic right arm is weak and subluxed. During trunk movements the arm dangles by the side, pulling the right upper trunk forward. *(C & D)* Flexor hypertonicity in the hemiplegic left arm is associated with elevation of the scapula and rotation backward of the rib cage on the hemiplegic side. The difference in height between the two shoulders makes the left side of the trunk appear longer than the right. *(E)* The therapist has corrected the position of the shoulder joint and is supporting the hemiplegic arm against her body while retraining trunk movements. *(F)* The therapist uses scapula mobilization in sitting to decrease hypertonicity in the shoulder, elbow, and wrist. *(G)* She continues to control the position of the arm as the patient performs an upper-body-initiated lateral weight lift.

Loss of Trunk Alignment with Soft Tissue/Joint Restrictions

As has been mentioned above, problems with muscle weakness and/or abnormal muscle tone in the trunk, arm, and leg lead to abnormal alignment in the spine and rib cage, shoulder girdle, and pelvis/hip. These changes in trunk posture are important because they create an abnormal starting position for movement in sitting, interfere with efficient muscle activation and weight transfer, and limit the movement patterns that can be safely executed. Several common trunk postures are associated with hemiplegia:

1. *Excessive upper trunk flexion.* This pattern is common in acute hemiplegia, where it is associated with a flaccid arm (Fig. 5-16A).
2. *Excessive lumbar extension/anterior pelvic tilt.* This trunk pattern occurs most commonly in patients with unbalanced recovery in the trunk and hypertonicity in the hemiplegic leg (Fig. 5-16B).
3. *Lateral flexion with shortening on involved side.* This pattern is common in acute hemiplegia but may persist throughout rehabilitation. It is associated with weakness/paralysis in the hemiplegic arm and leg. Muscle weakness in the arm pulls the upper trunk forward and down, while weakness in the leg interferes with weight bearing on the leg (Fig. 5-16C).
4. *Lateral flexion with lengthening on the involved side.* In this pattern, the trunk is laterally flexed with the concavity on the uninvolved side. The hemiplegic shoulder appears higher, the hemiplegic side of the rib cage appears longer, and the pelvis is angled toward the hemiplegic side with the appearance of increased weight bearing on that hip (Fig. 5-16D).
5. *Rotation backward on the hemiplegic side.* This pattern is not present in the acute phase. It develops over time and is associated with hypertonicity in the arm and leg (Fig. 5-16E).

Each of these postural changes affects the performance of selected movement patterns and is associated with predictable patterns of atypical movement and compensation. For example, excessive trunk flexion blocks movements in the anterior/posterior plane that require trunk extension. Lateral movements are also difficult because the posterior tilting of the pelvis and position of the rib cage prevent changes in spine or weight transfer at the hip. Similarly, when the trunk is laterally flexed toward the hemiplegic side the patient will perform anterior/posterior movements in an asymmetric position and will be unable to initiate lower-trunk-initiated lateral weight shifts to the involved side.

Secondary impairments in muscle and tissue length and selective loss of joint mobility are associated with changes in resting alignment in the trunk. Restrictions in muscle tissue length and joint mobility may develop from problems associated with muscle weakness or problems associated with atypical patterns of muscle activation and incomplete motor recovery. These secondary impairments develop over time and become increasingly severe if the abnormal trunk posture does not improve as the patient progresses through rehabilitation. In the early stages of rehabilitation, normal tissue extensibility and joint mobility are available even though the body is in an atypical posture. But when atypical alignment in the trunk continues for longer periods and becomes part of the patient's preferred

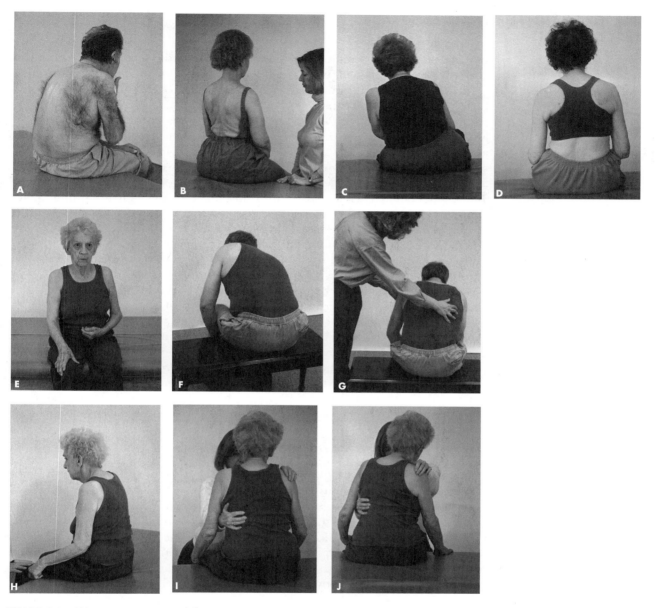

FIGURE 5-16 *(A)* Excessive upper trunk flexion. *(B)* Excessive lumbar extension. *(C)* Trunk lateral flexion with shortening on the hemiplegic right side. Note the rotation forward of the right upper trunk and shoulder. *(D)* Trunk lateral flexion with the convexity on the hemiplegic right side. *(E)* Left hemiplegia. The left side of the trunk is rotated backward. *(F)* The patient's hemiplegic left side is rotated backward during an upper-body-initiated anterior weight shift. *(G)* The therapist corrects alignment in the trunk and maintains the correction while the patient performs the movement more symmetrically. *(H–J)* Left hemiplegia: *(H)* In relaxed sitting the hemiplegic side is rotated backward relative to the right side. *(I)* The therapist selects hand placements to restore symmetry to the trunk, *(J)* The therapist's hands guide the patient into extension rotation to the right side; this movement brings the hemiplegic rib cage farther forward, lengthening tight tissues and increasing mobility in the spine and rib cage. The result of this treatment activity should be a more symmetric trunk position.

movement patterns, alignment changes gradually lead to contractures of muscle and soft tissue and loss of joint mobility in the spine, hip, and shoulder girdle. In sitting, changes in joint mobility in the spine and rib cage, hip, and scapulothoracic joints limit performance of trunk movements. The range and quality of trunk movements are also altered by shortening and contracture in the muscles and tissues that connect the pelvis to the hip/leg and the trunk to the scapula and arm.

Since normal movements in the trunk are based on normal trunk posture, alignment, and mobility, the therapist will have to correct the position of the trunk and maintain her corrections during movement reeducation in sitting. When alignment problems in the trunk are due to muscle weakness and there is no loss of range of motion, the therapist should restore normal alignment and maintain this corrected position while reeducating movement (Fig. 5-16F & G). However, severe joint stiffness in the spine, rib cage, and pelvis/hip is difficult to treat successfully in sitting, because it is not possible to fully correct trunk posture. With these severe problems, the therapist should correct alignment as much as possible and maintain this corrected trunk position while beginning movement reeducation. The therapist can use movements of the trunk to increase mobility in the spine and ribcage and lengthen tight muscles. For example, extension rotation to the uninvolved side could be used to correct the ribcage position in a patient with rotation backwards on his hemiplegic side (Fig. 5-16H–J). Forearm weight bearing in sitting and supine activities are also very effective in increasing length and mobility in the trunk, pelvis, and rib cage. These treatment activities are described more completely in later chapters.

Loss of Lower Extremity/Hip Control in Weight Bearing

The ability to support body weight on both legs is an important aspect of postural stability and movement control in sitting. Trunk movements in sitting are accompanied by constantly changing muscle activity in the weight bearing lower extremities. This muscle activity is used to maintain the legs in position to function as an appropriate and stable base of support, to increase muscle contraction to adjust to the demands of increased body weight, and to fire leg muscles to assist trunk movements. In sitting, trunk movements result in both symmetric lower extremity weight bearing patterns, where body weight is distributed equally on both legs, and asymmetric weight bearing, where more weight is taken on one leg and the body mass is aligned over one leg and foot. Symmetric weight bearing on both legs in sitting occurs during anterior/posterior movements and is an important precursor to function in sit to stand and in standing; lateral weight shift onto one leg is important for the transition from sitting to supine and for reaching movements of the arm. Thus, loss of control of weight bearing on one lower extremity has an immediate effect on the body's ability to balance and move in sitting and important related effects on function in other positions.

Neurologic patients frequently have difficulty shifting body weight onto their involved leg and actively controlling this leg to support body weight. These problems occur primarily because of muscle weakness in the lower trunk and leg. Muscle weakness in the leg causes the leg to fall into abduction in sitting. If muscle activity in the leg does not stabilize the hip and foot during lateral

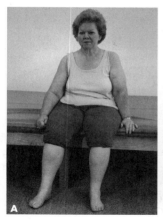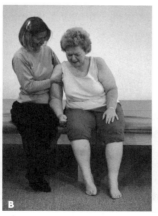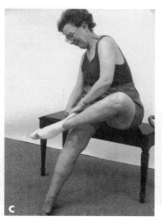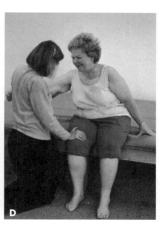

FIGURE 5-17 *(A)* The hemiplegic right leg is excessively abducted in sitting, with no weight on the foot. *(B)* When the patient attempts a lower-trunk-initiated lateral weight shift to the right, the right foot adducts. The hemiplegic leg is not active during this weight shift. *(C)* Extensor hypertonicity in the right leg interferes with weightbearing on the hemiplegic leg. The patient has moved her upper trunk laterally to the right to allow herself to balance in this position. *(D)* The therapist's right hand is correcting the abduction of the femur and stabilizing the foot on the floor, while her left hand supports the hemiplegic arm and helps the patient shift over her right hip.

weight shifts to the hemiplegic side, the foot will slide into adduction as the trunk moves laterally (Fig. 5-17A & B). Problems with weight bearing on the hemiplegic leg also exist because of muscle tightness in the pelvis, hip, or lower leg or hypertonicity that causes knee extension and plantarflexion in the involved leg and restricts pelvic and hip motion (Fig. 5-17C). Tactile and proprioceptive deficits that make it difficult for the patient to trust his involved leg for weight bearing may also contribute to loss of weight bearing on the hemiplegic side. When the hemiplegic leg cannot accept or support body weight, anterior/posterior and lateral weight shifts will be affected. In some patients, loss of control of weight bearing on one leg is the major cause of atypical performance of trunk movements in sitting. In other patients, atypical performance results from a combination of problems with control of the trunk and problems with control of the leg.

Reestablishing weight bearing control of the leg in sitting is an important goal of treatment. The patient with poor hip control will not regain normal trunk movements until he can shift weight onto his involved leg and support weight on that side. Training the patterns of lower extremity weight bearing can be done as part of the treatment of trunk movements in sitting, using hand placements that control pelvic/femur position (Fig. 5–17D). When problems in the leg are severe, it may be necessary to treat the leg to correct alignment and prepare for weight bearing before adding trunk movements. Detailed information about weight bearing problems in the leg and treatment activities to improve this control is presented in Chapter 8. Weight bearing control of the leg can also be trained during forearm weight bearing activities in sitting and standing, during the task of sit to stand, and in supine.

Poor Trunk Control During Task Performance

The trunk movements described in this chapter are functionally significant because they are used for balance and task performance in sitting. To be functional in sitting, the neurologic patient must be able to both move his trunk in all the normal patterns and combine these trunk movements functionally with those of the arms and legs. Many patients have lost control of the normal movements of the trunk and are either unable to perform tasks safely in sitting or can function only by using atypical movement strategies. Other patients, who have regained control of trunk movements, fail to utilize them appropriately during task performance. While it is not surprising that the patient who has no control of trunk movements on the exercise mat does not use normal trunk patterns during task performance, learned compensatory strategies often persist after trunk control has improved. Compensations persist when the patient either cannot move his trunk with his extremities or when he fails to see the connection between the treatment "exercises" and real life. To avoid this problem, the therapist must make every effort to relate trunk movements to function so that as soon as the patient regains control of some trunk movements, he practices these patterns in specific tasks of everyday life.

ATYPICAL TRUNK MOVEMENTS IN SITTING

The impairments discussed above are associated with predictable patterns of atypical movement. The most common atypical movements are described below. These atypical movement patterns are identified during the assessment. The therapist then selects hand placements that allow her to maintain appropriate trunk alignment and block the use of these movements, while reeducating the normal trunk patterns.

Asymmetric Performance of Anterior/Posterior Movements

Anterior/posterior movements are performed with symmetry in the trunk, because the two sides of the body do the same movement at the same time. When the two sides of the body are asymmetric during these movements, the resulting movement pattern is atypical and undesirable. Asymmetries during anterior/posterior movements are common during both upper-body- and lower-body-initiated weight shifts. These asymmetries occur in two different patterns.

Lateral Flexion Asymmetry

Lateral flexion asymmetry is present when the spine is C-curved with the concavity on the hemiplegic side during upper-body- or lower-trunk-initiated anterior or posterior movements. In this type of movement deviation, the greatest asymmetry is between the length of the two sides of the trunk (Fig. 5-18A). The reverse of this pattern is also common. In this group of patients the trunk is laterally flexed with the convexity on the hemiplegic side, so that the hemiplegic side is inappropriately long (Fig. 5-18B).

Rotational Asymmetry

Rotational asymmetry is the second movement deviation that is commonly observed during anterior/posterior movements. In this pattern, the spine appears to rotate during the movement, so that the hemiplegic side stays back as the body moves forward (Fig. 5-18C & D). Rotational asymmetry with the hemiplegic side rotating farther forward than the uninvolved side is also observed.

Atypical Performance of Lateral Movements

During upper-body- and lower-trunk-initiated lateral weight shifts, the two sides of the body should not be symmetric. Lateral flexion of the spine and compatible changes in the heights of the two shoulders and length of the two sides of the rib cage and appropriate weight bearing patterns in the legs are critical for normal performance of these movement patterns. Atypical movements occur during lateral weight shifts when the appropriate pattern of trunk lateral flexion is not produced or when the weight bearing response in the hemiplegic leg is abnormal. Several different movement deviations can occur during upper-trunk- and lower-body-initiated lateral movements.

An *inappropriate straight spine* is present when the spine does not laterally flex during a lateral weight shift initiated by either the upper or lower trunk. In this type of atypical movement, the body moves laterally, but the spine remains straight and there is no difference is position between the two sides of the rib cage. During upper-trunk-initiated patterns, the pelvis often lifts off the bed inappropriately as the straight spine moves laterally (Fig. 5-18E & F).

Inappropriate rotation of the hemiplegic side often occurs during lateral weight shifts to either side. In this atypical movement, the lateral weight shift is performed as a rotational rather than a straight place movement. The hemiplegic side may rotate either forward or backward during lateral movements. Many times, the hemiplegic side will rotate backward when the body is moving toward the hemiplegic side and forward during movements to the opposite side. The movements are atypical because of the backward or forward movement of the hemiplegic upper trunk; the spinal lateral flexion often occurs appropriately during these rotational weight shifts (Fig. 5-18G–I).

Excessive lateral movement of the upper trunk, a very common atypical movement, occurs mostly during lower-trunk-initiated lateral weight shifts. In this movement pattern, the patient does not initiate the movement from his pelvis but instead moves his head and shoulders laterally over one hip. At first glance, the movement pattern appears normal. The patient's head and upper trunk line up over one side of the pelvis, and the opposite side of the pelvis may elevate off the bed by the time the movement is complete. However, careful assessment of the trunk reveals that the resulting position of the spine, rib cage, and shoulder girdles are incorrect. When the patient has used a lateral movement of the upper trunk to initiate the weight shift, the shoulder on the weight bearing side ends up lower than on the non-weight bearing side. It is also positioned lateral to the weight bearing hip. The spine does not laterally flex in this movement pattern (Fig. 5-18J & K).

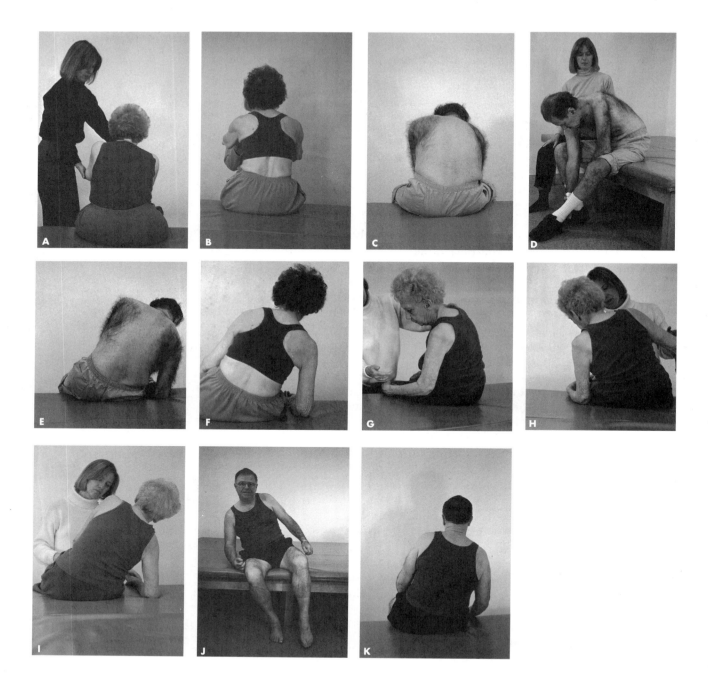

FIGURE 5-18 *(A)* Right hemiplegia with trunk shortening on the hemiplegic side. The therapist is supporting the patient's hands while the patient performs a lower-body-initiated anterior weight shift. Note the lateral flexion in the spine and the difference in height between the two shoulders. The pelvis appears level, telling us that the asymmetry is higher up in the spine. *(B)* Lateral flexion asymmetry in the trunk with the convexity on the hemiplegic right side during an upper-trunk-initiated anterior weight shift. Note how the pelvis appears tilted to the right in this patient. *(C & D)* Rotational assymmetry, left hemiplegia. *(C)* The patient is performing an upper-trunk-initiated anterior weight shift. Note that the left shoulder girdle, rib cage, and pelvis have not moved as far forward or down as those on the right. *(D)* From the side angle, the backward rotation of the left side of the body is very obvious. *(E)* Lack of lateral flexion in the spine during an upper-body-initiated lateral weight shift to the uninvolved side. The patient is able to move independently to his uninvolved side. Note how the trunk is in flexion without lateral flexion. The left pelvis is off the bed, and the two sides of the rib cage appear to be the same length. *(F)* The patient is performing an upper-body-initiated weight shift to her hemiplegic side. Her trunk is in more extension than the patient in the previous figure, but the lack of side bending in the trunk is equivalent. *(G)* Left hemiplegia. As the patient moves her hemiplegic shoulder girdle laterally, the upper trunk and ribcage are beginning to rotate backward. The therapist's hand on the right shoulder gives a visual marker for the backward movement of the left shoulder. *(H)* As she reaches her hemiplegic arm to the bed, the trunk is appropriately shortened on the left side but inappropriately rotated backward on the left as well. *(I)* When she performs the same movement on the right side, the hemiplegic shoulder and upper trunk rotate forward. *(J)* The patient has moved his upper trunk excessively to the right rather than initiating the movement from his pelvis. As a result, his hemiplegic right shoulder is lower than the left and his weight bearing side is not correctly lengthened. Although he appears to have shifted weight onto his right leg, the right foot is not planted on the floor and has moved medially as his trunk leans to the right. *(K)* From the back, the lateral movement of the upper trunk without lateral flexion in the spine is apparent. Note how the left side of the pelvis is elevated, even though the spinal pattern of initiation is incorrect.

ASSESSMENT GUIDELINES

Assessment of the trunk in sitting should include an assessment of the patient's posture and control of movement and an assessment of the problems that influence his movement control. The questions listed below are intended to provide a framework for trunk assessment. More general information about the assessment process and goal setting is included in Chapter 3.

I. Describe the position of the trunk at rest. Include the position of the spine and rib cage and note weight distribution and position of the legs. Does the patient change this position before moving?

II. Describe what happens when you ask the patient to perform the normal trunk movements. Identify which movements are normal, which movements are performed abnormally, and which movements cannot be performed.

What asymmetries and/or problems do you observe during these movements?

What impairments are contributing to these problems?

III. Describe the changes in movement patterns that occur when you put your hands on the patient to change alignment and assist movements. Where do you put your hands to make these changes? What movements improve when you put your hands on the patient to correct alignment?

What problems and movements do not respond to handling? How will you treat these problems and their underlying impairments to improve trunk posture and movement control further?

THERAPY GOALS

Functional Goals

The retraining of trunk movements in sitting is necessary to help the patient meet the following functional goals:

1. To be able to maintain a secure sitting position and to perform the trunk movements that are critical for function.

2. To be able to use normal trunk movements automatically to maintain or restore balance.

3. To be able to combine trunk and extremity movements for task performance in sitting and during the transitional movements of sit to stand and sitting to/from supine.

Treatment Goals and Techniques

To meet the functional goals outlined above, treatment of the trunk in sitting must include both techniques of movement reeducation and techniques to address the impairments that are interfering with movement. The treatment techniques described in this section are designed to demonstrate how the therapist uses her hands to correct specific problems and meet specified treatment goals. Because of spatial constraints, it is impossible to demonstrate how each of these treatment techniques is used to produce every trunk movement. However, we have tried to demonstrate several movements with each technique and to include enough information to allow the reader to produce other movements without difficulty. Similar treatment goals and techniques are included in all subsequent chapters of the book, helping the reader to see how trunk problems in sitting relate to the movement problems in other positions and how treatment in other positions can be used to increase trunk movement control in sitting.

Treatment Goal: To reeducate normal trunk movements in sitting.

In the section below, we describe a variety of treatment techniques for reeducating trunk movements in sitting. These handling techniques are designed to allow the therapist to correct the position of the hemiplegic side, restore symmetry to the trunk, and maintain appropriate trunk alignment during the performance of trunk movements. They are also designed to allow the therapist to teach the patient the normal patterns of initiation and weight shift and prevent the use of undesirable postural asymmetries and atypical movements. The therapist should decide which hand placement and treatment techniques to use on the basis of the patient's impairments and the movement patterns she chooses to reeducate. The process we use to determine where to place our hands to control the trunk is illustrated immediately after the treatment techniques.

Treatment Technique: Reeducating trunk movements using a rib cage or rib cage/pelvis grip. Hand placements on the patient's trunk or trunk and pelvis provide the therapist with the most direct control of the patient's trunk movements. The therapist may place both hands on the patient's trunk, both hands on the pelvis, or use uneven hand placements, with one hand on the pelvis and the other hand on the opposite rib cage. These hand placements are most useful for reeducating lower-trunk-initiated weight shifts, since the therapist's hands are placed directly over the part of the patient's body that should be moving. They may also be used for training upper-trunk-initiated movements, although they do not provide control of the upper trunk or support for the hemiplegic arm (Fig. 5-19A–L).

Treatment Technique: Support of the hemiplegic arm during trunk movements. This treatment technique is used for patients with a shoulder subluxation and for patients with poor control of upper trunk extension. It is designed to give the therapist control of the trunk through the arms (Fig. 5-20A–K). Support of the upper extremities is also a useful technique with patients who have excessive upper trunk flexion and difficulty with trunk extension, with or without shoulder subluxation. When the weight of the upper trunk and arms makes it difficult for the therapist to use the technique shown above, an alternate version may be useful (Fig. 5-20L–P).

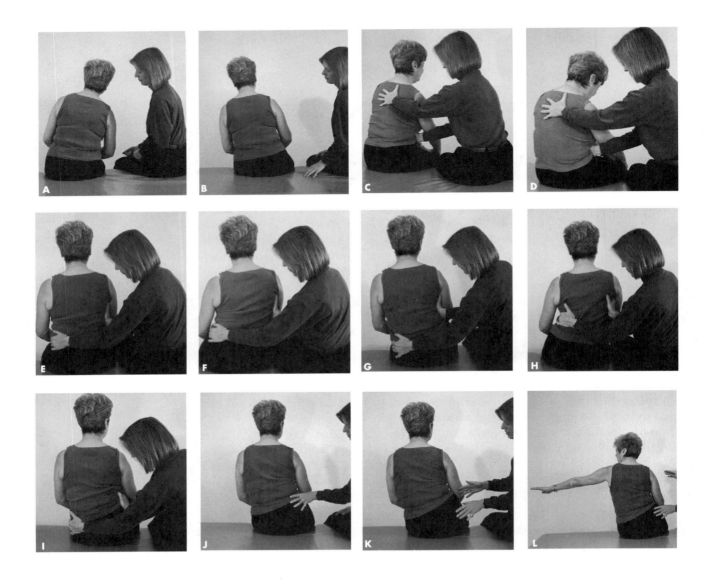

FIGURE 5-19 *(A & B)* Right hemiplegia. The patient performs lower-trunk-initiated lateral movements using an atypical movement pattern of excessive upper trunk sway. Her trunk pattern does not show appropriate lateral flexion to either side. She also has difficulty with anterior/posterior movements. *(C)* To reeducate lower-trunk-initiated anterior/posterior movements, the therapist places her hands on the front and back of the trunk. She presses both hands lightly into the patient's trunk, so that the trunk is supported front and back between her hands. *(D)* To produce a posterior weight shift, the therapist uses her right hand on the front of the rib cage to move the lower trunk and pelvis back. Her left hand supports the back of the trunk. As the therapist moves the lower trunk back, the pressure from her left hand prevents excessive backward movement of the upper trunk and encourages upper trunk flexion by delivering a forward and downward pressure to the thoracic spine. For an anterior movement, the therapist reverses the position of her hands. Her right hand moves to the front of the chest and her left hand is placed over the lumbar spine. The therapist gives a forward message with her left hand to start the movement. Her right hand prevents excessive trunk flexion by providing light upward support to the upper trunk. *(E)* The therapist selects a rib cage/pelvis grip to control the trunk during lower-trunk-initiated lateral movements. She places her right hand over the rib cage on the patient's right trunk. Her left hand is placed on the left side of the patient's pelvis so that her thumb lies along the pelvic crest and her fingertips are near the anterior superior iliac spine (ASIS). The therapist presses both hands lightly into the patient's trunk, so that the trunk is stabilized between her hands. *(F)* During a lateral weight shift to the hemiplegic side, the therapist's hands move the middle of the trunk to the right. Her left hand lifts the left side of the patient's pelvis up and moves the lower trunk and pelvis to the right, while her right hand lifts the right side of the rib cage up and holds it over the right hip. As the patient completes the weight shift to her right hip, the therapist's left hand delivers a diagonal pressure from the top of the left pelvis down into the right hip to increase the sensation of weight bearing. *(G)* The therapist keeps her hands in the same position for the weight shift to the left. In this figure, both hands are moving the trunk laterally over the left hip. The therapist's right hand is starting the movement by moving the right side of the rib cage to the left. As the trunk begins to move, her right hand tucks the right ribs and delivers a diagonal message downward through the spine into the left hip. The therapist's left hand moves the left side of the pelvis down and delivers a message down into the left hip joint. *(H)* An alternate hand placement. The therapist has both her hands on the rib cage. This grip works well to increase lateral flexion in the spine and rib cage when the patient is able to perform the pelvic movements without assistance. *(I)* A second alternate hand placement using both sides of the pelvis to train the weight shift. This hand placement provides maximal input to the pelvic motion but offers no control of the trunk. This pelvic grip also can be used during anterior/posterior movements. *(J–L)* This treatment series demonstrates a progression from the handling techniques used in the previous figures. *(J)* The therapist first lightens her control to begin practice with less assistance. The therapist assists the pelvic motion, while the patient controls the movement of her trunk. *(K)* The patient performs the movement independently. The therapist's hands are close by during independent practice. She may place them back on the trunk/pelvis if the quality of the movement deteriorates. *(L)* The patient practices combining the weight shift with reaching movements of her left arm. This sequence could also be demonstrated with all other trunk movements.

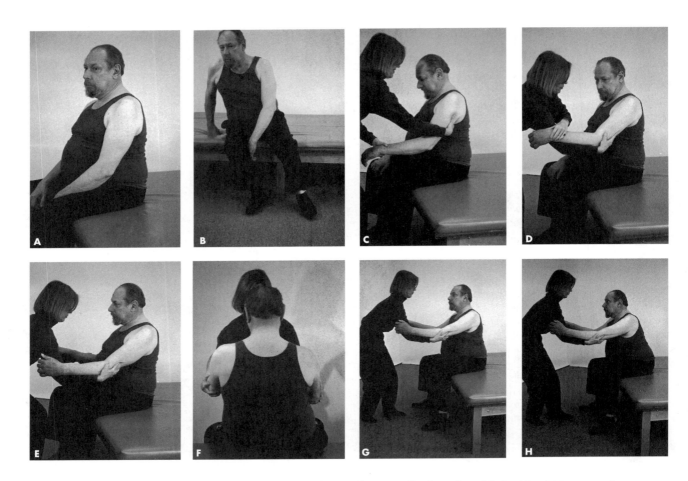

FIGURE 5-20 *(A)* At rest, the patient has an inferior subluxation of his hemiplegic left shoulder. *(B)* During trunk movements, the left arm dangles without control by the side of the body. The weight of the flaccid arm pulls the shoulder joint and scapula out of alignment, increasing the instability of the shoulder joint. Note how the heavy left arm has pulled the upper trunk forward on the left side. The therapist will support the hemiplegic arm on her body during treatment of the trunk. This hand placement is designed to protect the shoulder joint from tractioning and pain and to increase trunk symmetry by taking the weight of the hemiplegic arm off the trunk. *(C)* The therapist lifts the hemiplegic arm, using an axillary/hand grip. Her hand in the patient's axilla lifts the humerus up into the fossa and takes the shoulder joint out of internal rotation by rotating the humerus to neutral. Her hand placement at the wrist aligns the distal arm with the shoulder. Both arms support the weight of the arm and reach it forward. The therapist should avoid lifting the arm into more than 60 to 70 degrees of forward flexion, because her hands cannot ensure appropriate scapula rotation. *(D)* The therapist cradles the patient's forearm against her forearm, sliding her hand from the axilla to the distal humerus and elbow. Her other hand retains control of the patient's wrist and hand. *(E)* The patient's hemiplegic hand is placed against the therapist's arm. She now can control the patient's hemiplegic arm with her right arm and hand. The patient places his uninvolved right arm in a similar posture on the therapist's other arm, and she places her left hand against his left forearm/elbow. *(F)* The therapist stabilizes the patient's upper trunk between her two hands, by tucking the patient's arms close to the sides of his trunk. *(G)* To prepare for trunk movements, the therapist adjusts her body position relative to the patient's trunk. In this figure, the therapist is preparing for a lower-trunk-initiated anterior weight shift. She places her feet in step-stance position, so that she can shift her weight backwards to her right foot as the patient moves toward her. *(H)* The therapist asks for the lower-trunk-initiated anterior weight shift by bringing the patient's upper body toward her. Her hands on the patient's arm lift up slightly as she brings them toward her to keep the trunk in extension. Note how the therapist shifts her weight to her right leg as the patient moves, so that the distance between her body and the patient's body remains constant. If she did not shift backward, the patient would end up too close to her body. Similarly, to reeducate lower-trunk-initiated lateral weight shifts with this grip, the therapist shifts her weight to her right leg as the patient moves to his left. *(Figure continues.)*

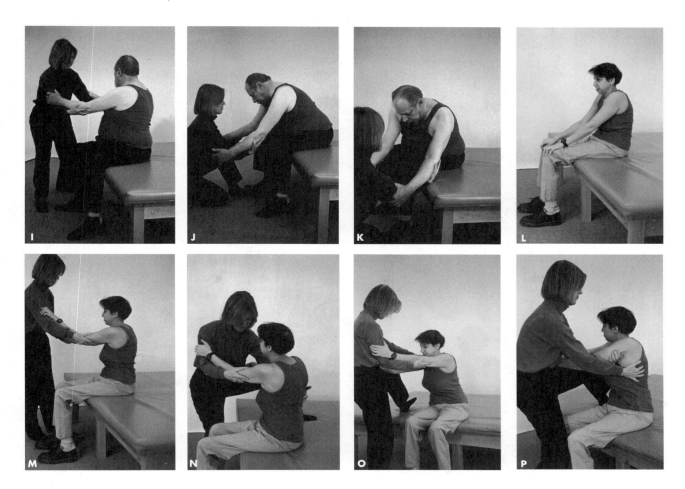

FIGURE 5-20 (Continued) (I) The therapist maintains this trunk grip while reeducating other trunk movements. Here, she is teaching extension rotation to the right. Her right hand rotates the patient's left trunk and arm forward. At the same time, she gives a message with her left hand to the patient's arm and trunk to move backwards. The therapist steps her feet to her left during this movement. This is done to keep her feet under her trunk and arms during the movement. Note how the therapist faces the patient directly, with her upper body position a mirror image of his. (J) To facilitate an upper-trunk-initiated anterior weight shift, the therapist has to lower her body closer to the floor. The therapist starts in half kneeling with the left leg forward. As the patient moves forward and down, she shifts her weight backwards and sits down over her right foot. To shift the patient back to sitting, she extends her right hip and shifts forward to her flexed left leg. (K) The therapist assists the patient in upper-trunk-initiated flexion rotation. Note how she has moved her legs to her right before starting the trunk flexion. (L) Before treatment, the patient sits with her trunk in flexion. (M) The therapist supports the hemiplegic left arm on her right arm as shown previously. (N) The patient rotates her trunk to the right. The therapist places her left foot on the mat near the patient's right leg and places her left hand on the patient's upper trunk/rib cage. The patient rests her right hand on the therapist's left thigh. By bringing her leg to the mat, the therapist is able to use her legs to support more of the weight of the patient's upper body, decreasing the load on her arms. (O) The therapist asks the patient to shift toward her. This diagonal weight shift increases extension in the spine. Note how the therapist has clearly shifted her weight backwards onto her right foot as the patient moves forward. The patient practices shifting back and letting her trunk flex, then coming forward again with trunk extension. The therapist could then rotate the patient's trunk to the left, bring her right leg to the mat, and repeat the movements. (P) An alternate hand placement. The therapist has placed the patient's hemiplegic arm across her thigh. She is supporting the glenohumeral joint with her left hand. Her right hand is rotating the rib cage forward and helping the trunk extend. This hand placement makes the job of supporting the weight of the arms and trunk the easiest.

Treatment Technique: Reeducating trunk movements using an upper trunk/rib cage grip. The upper trunk/rib cage grip provides the therapist with control of the patient's upper trunk and rib cage. It can also be used to correct rotational and lateral flexion asymmetries in the trunk. Since there is no direct control over the pelvis with this grip, the therapist's ability to influence the pelvis or leg is minimal (Fig. 5-21).

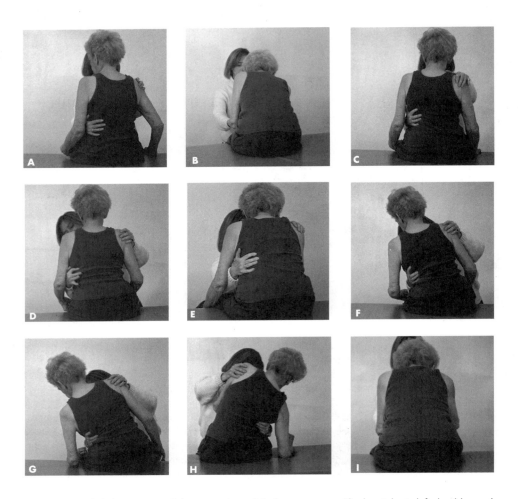

FIGURE 5-21 *(A)* The position of the patient's trunk before treatment. The hemiplegic left shoulder and the left side of the rib cage are rotated behind the right side. The therapist's hands are in position but have not yet corrected the patient's alignment. *(B)* The patient is performing an upper-trunk-initiated anterior weight shift. The left side remains rotated back during this weight shift. *(C)* The therapist first uses her hands to correct the rotation backward of the left side. The therapist's right hand rotates the hemiplegic side of the rib cage forward, as her left hand brings the right side of the upper trunk back. The therapist's two hands exert equal but opposite pressures and move the same distance at the same speed. The result is a more symmetric trunk position. *(Figure caption continues)*

FIGURE 5-21 *(Continued)* *(D)* The therapist maintains the correction in the trunk while assisting the patient in trunk movements. Here the patient is performing a lower-trunk-initiated anterior weight shift. The therapist is using her hands to encourage trunk extension during the movement. Her left hand is lifting the front of the patient's right shoulder up and back and adducting the scapula as the trunk moves forward. The fingers of her right hand push down lightly on the back of the rib cage to tell the lumbar spine to extend. To assist the weight shift back, the therapist will use the heel of her right hand against the front of the rib cage to move the spine out of flexion. At the same time, she will provide a message to the right scapula to abduct and the upper trunk to flex. *(E)* During an upper-trunk-initiated anterior weight shift, the therapist's hand placements stay the same, but the message of the hands is different. Here, both hands are keeping the trunk in flexion and guiding the body forward. The compatible pressures from the therapist's hands maintain symmetry in the trunk and prevent rotation backward of the hemiplegic side. *(F & G)* The therapist is assisting an upper-trunk-initiated weight shift to the left. The therapist uses her right hand to tuck the patient's hemiplegic rib cage by delivering a downward and inward pressure to the ribs. Her left hand is guiding the patient's shoulder girdle to her left. As the patient completes the movement, the downward and inward message of the therapist's right hand is clearly visible. The therapist will use her left hand to start the movement back up. Her right hand can lift the patient's hemiplegic side if necessary. *(H)* Upper trunk movements to the opposite side are easiest if the therapist changes her hand placements. Her right hand now controls the movements of the upper trunk and her left hand guides the appropriate rib cage movement. *(I)* After treatment, the patient moves independently. Note the symmetry of the shoulders and rib cage that has resulted from the treatment.

Treatment Technique: Control of the hemiplegic side with an axillary/rib cage grip. This hand placement gives the therapist the best control over the hemiplegic side (Fig. 5-22).

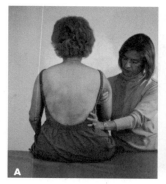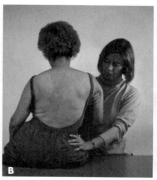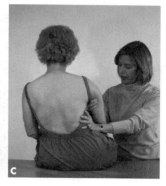

FIGURE 5-22 *(A)* The therapist faces the patient and places her right hand under the patient's hemiplegic arm to lift and support the hemiplegic shoulder. She places her left hand on the hemiplegic rib cage or pelvis. *(B)* During a lower-trunk-initiated lateral weight shift to the hemiplegic side, the therapist lifts the hemiplegic shoulder with her right hand and depresses the hemiplegic side of the pelvis with her left hand. Note how the therapist's two hands have moved farther apart. The wrinkles on the left side of the trunk, indicate that the hemiplegic side of the trunk has appropriately lengthened. *(C)* The patient is shifting to her uninvolved hip. The therapist's left hand is tucking the right rib cage and moving the trunk to the left. As the weight shift progresses, the therapist will deliver a diagonal message through the rib cage into the left hip to increase the pelvic weight shift.

Treatment Technique: Cotreatment. Therapists often find it difficult to maintain appropriate alignment during trunk movements. This is especially true in acute care, where many patients are weak and floppy on their hemiplegic side. It is also a problem when the patient has acquired an atypical movement pattern that the therapist must try to eliminate while training a new pattern of movement. Cotreatment by two therapists provides two sets of hands to support the weight of the trunk, prevents the use of atypical movements, and reeducates normal movements. When two therapists work together, the messages of their hands must be compatible. This happens most easily when one therapist makes her correction while the second therapist watches and then places her hands on for further correction (Fig. 5-23).

Additional suggestions for improving trunk movements:

Forearm weight bearing
Supine treatment
Standing treatment

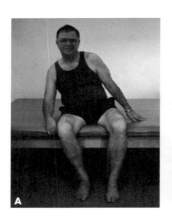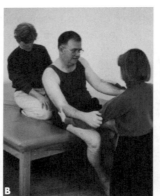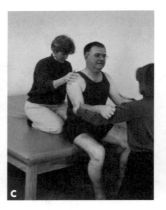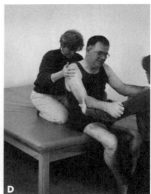

FIGURE 5-23 *(A)* Before treatment, the patient shows excessive upper body lateral movement during lower-trunk-initiated weight shifts to his hemiplegic side. *(B)* The first therapist supports both arms against her hips. She is attempting to use her control on the arms and upper trunk to stop the excessive upper trunk movement. The patient's movement is still atypical because he is not initiating the movement from his lower trunk. The second therapist is observing. *(C)* The second therapist puts her hands on the patient's trunk. Her first input increases the amount of extension in the trunk. This increases muscle activity in the trunk and will make it easier for the patient to initiate from his lower trunk. *(D)* The two therapists work together to control the lateral weight shift. The second therapist's hands on the patient's trunk and shoulder are stopping the excessive lateral movement of the upper trunk and helping the patient initiate the movement from the lower trunk. The result is a more normal movement. The two therapists' hands have to give compatible messages and move the patient at the same rate and distance for their handling to make sense to the patient. This kind of treatment can be very effective but is difficult to do correctly.

Problem Solving to Determine Optimal Hand Placements

Selecting the proper hand placements and delivering the appropriate messages with the hands are probably the most difficult aspects of movement reeducation. In the section below, we describe the process for deciding where the therapist should put her hands and how to use them. We have selected two patients with very different trunk problems to illustrate the problem-solving process (Fig. 5-24). In the course of problem solving to correct trunk alignment, the therapist selects the same hand placements for both patients. However, her hands are giving quite different messages to each patient despite their being in the same place. Readers should refer back to the assessment guidelines for a more complete description of trunk assessment in sitting.

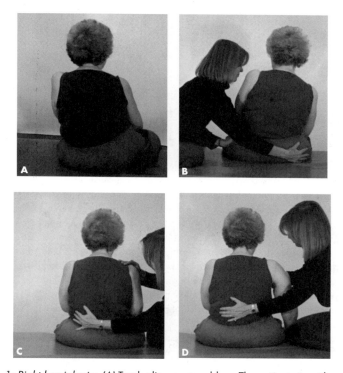

FIGURE 5-24 *(A–D) Patient no. 1: Right hemiplegia. (A)* Trunk alignment problem: The patient sits with most of her weight on her left hip. The trunk is laterally flexed, with the concavity on the right. The right pelvis is elevated. The right shoulder appears lower and farther forward than the left. *(B)* Correction of the pelvic position makes the asymmetry in the trunk more pronounced. The therapist has shifted the patient's weight toward the right, which dropped the right side of the pelvis and made the pelvis level. This has resulted in more trunk lateral flexion. *(C)* The therapist maintains the pelvis in a level position while bringing the right shoulder girdle up and back. This adducts the scapula and increases extension in the thoracic spine. This correction combined with the correction of pelvic position are both necessary to make the trunk more symmetric. *(D)* The therapist selects an axillary trunk grip for movement reeducation of the trunk. Her control of the hemiplegic shoulder girdle is used to increase upper trunk extension and scapula adduction/upward rotation. Her control of the lower trunk is needed to maintain weight on the hemiplegic hip and increase lower trunk extension. *(Figure continues.)*

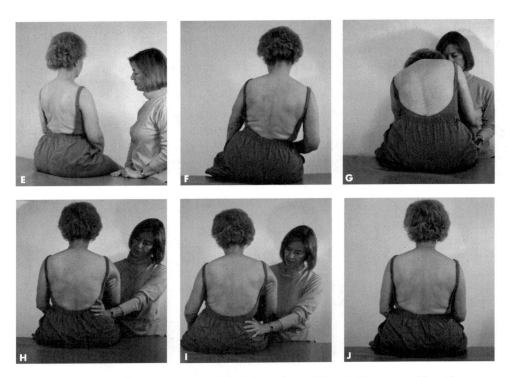

FIGURE 5-24 *(Continued)* *(E–J) Patient no. 2: Right hemiplegia. (E)* Trunk alignment problem: The patient sits with excessive trunk extension. Her pelvis is in an anterior tilt, and both scapulas are adducted. *(F)* During lower-trunk-initiated lateral weight shift to the right, the trunk remains extended and the right shoulder and rib cage rotate backwards. The spine appears straight rather than laterally flexed during this weight shift. *(G)* During an upper-trunk-initiated anterior weight shift, the excessive lumbar extension and rotation backward of the right upper trunk are also apparent. Spinal flexion occurs only in the thoracic spine. *(H)* The therapist uses her hands to introduce flexion in the spine and rotate the right shoulder and rib cage forward. Her hand on the lower trunk and pelvis tilts the pelvis backward to neutral. *(I)* The therapist uses her hands to keep the spine in slight flexion and prevent rotation backward to the rib cage during a lower-trunk-initiated lateral weight shift to the right. Her control of the shoulder maintains the scapula in abduction and the upper trunk in slight flexion. Her hand on the lower trunk is taking the pelvis from an anterior tilt to neutral while rotating the right side of the ribcage forward. She will use the same messages while practicing other trunk movements. *(J)* Following treatment, the patient sits with less trunk extension. Excessive trunk extension is not desirable because it limits active movement patterns in sitting and standing; it also interferes with the use of abdominal muscles, hip extensors in the legs, and scapula muscles in the arms.

Treatment Goal: Reeducate compatible trunk and arm movements. As soon as the patient is able to sit independently and assist with upper- and lower-trunk-initiated movements, the therapist should try to reeducate trunk movements in combination with movements of the hemiplegic arm. This is done to improve arm function in sitting and to increase the automatic use of normal trunk movements during functional performance.

Treatment Technique: Use of an axillary/hand grip to support the hemiplegic arm and coordinate arm movements with trunk weight shifts (Fig. 5-25). The therapist should prepare for this treatment technique using the arm treatment techniques described in Chapter 6 and the treatment techniques described in Figure 5-20A–O.

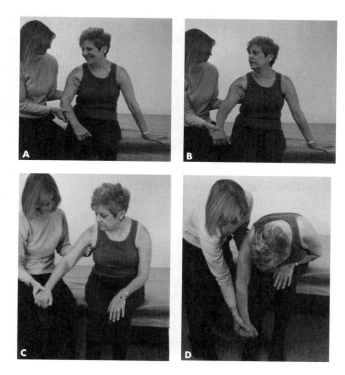

FIGURE 5-25 Right hemiplegia. *(A)* The therapist sits close to the patient's hemiplegic side. She places her right hand in the axilla to support the hemiplegic shoulder from underneath. The therapist lifts up under the arm until she is supporting some of the weight of the shoulder girdle. She also flexes her wrist to externally rotate the glenohumeral joint to neutral. *(B)* The therapist places her left hand under the hemiplegic wrist/hand to support the distal arm. The pressure of this hand extends the elbow and holds the forearm in pronation. If the muscle tone in the arm is hypertonic, the therapist will feel resistance to elbow extension, forearm pronation, or shoulder external rotation. The tension in the muscles should be reduced before proceeding with movement reeducation. Readers should refer to Chapter 6 for techniques to decrease flexor hypertonicity. *(C & D)* The therapist controls the hemiplegic arm in extension and asks the patient to reach with her arm. She maintains control of the arm as the patient performs an upper-body-initiated anterior weight shift. *(Figure continues.)*

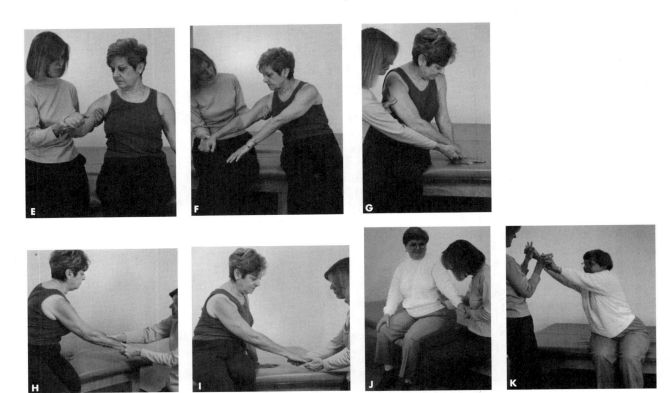

FIGURE 5-25 (Continued) (E & F) The therapist lifts the arm up in preparation for reaching to the side. The patient rotates her trunk to the right and reaches both arms to the therapist. Note how the patient shifts weight to her right hip as she reaches her arms to the side. The therapist should provide verbal information to the patient about the appropriate trunk movement, so that the arm and trunk patterns are compatible. (G) The therapist has guided the hemiplegic arm to the patient's left, with appropriate trunk rotation and weight shift to the left. In this treatment series, rotational movements of the trunk were combined with arm movements, because the patient has good control of straight plane movements. (H) The therapist has asked for more trunk rotation and a bigger weight shift. In this figure, the therapist has changed the activity by letting the patient weight bear on her left arm while reaching with her right. The therapist has also changed her control of the hemiplegic arm from the axilla to the forearm. The therapist is able to remove her control of the shoulder when the patient has more active control of shoulder and elbow movements. (I) The therapist is now holding only the hemiplegic hand, indicating that the patient is controlling both her trunk movements and the position of her arm during this weight shift. Note that the hemiplegic hand, which was fisted in the previous figures, is now open and relaxed. This reduction in hypertonicity has occurred because of the lengthening of tight muscles and activation of muscles in normal patterns in the trunk and arm. (J) A variation of the treatment technique. The therapist is holding the hemiplegic hand with her hand in a handshake grip, using her other hand to facilitate weight shifts at the pelvis. The handshake grip can be used when the fingers of the hemiplegic hand are open and relaxed. (K) An alternate hand placement. The therapist holds both of the patient's hands. The patient holds her arms up in extended arm reach with only light support from the therapist. The therapist asks her to reach both hands to her, producing an extension rotation weight shift in the trunk. The therapist will change the position of her body and the patient's arms to ask for other trunk movements. Refer to Chapter 6, Figure 6-29A–H, for more information about this technique.

Treatment Goal: Reeducate compatible trunk and leg movements.

Treatment Technique: When the hemiplegic leg is not appropriately active in weight-bearing, the foot moves on the floor during lower-trunk-initiated weight shifts. The therapist should stabilize the hemiplegic leg on the floor to increase weight bearing on the hemiplegic hip and foot (Fig. 5-26).

Treatment Technique: Additional techniques for improving weight bearing control of the hemiplegic leg are described in detail in Chapter 8.

FIGURE 5-26 *(A)* Before treatment, the patient sits with most of her weight on her left hip. The hemiplegic right leg is abducted and externally rotated. *(B)* The therapist has taken the femur out of abduction and external rotation so that the hip, knee, and foot are in a line. She exerts a downward pressure from the knee into the foot to stabilize the foot on the floor. Here the patient is shifting onto her hemiplegic hip so that weight is shifted toward the outside of her right foot. The therapist has also brought the hemiplegic arm into shoulder flexion/abduction. This increases the amount of trunk extension and improves the quality of the weight shift. These techniques are described in more detail in Chapter 8. *(C)* Lower-trunk-initiated lateral weight shifts can also be controlled completely from the legs, when the patient is able to perform the trunk movements with minimal assistance. This technique is used to increase activity in the hemiplegic leg and weight transfer over the foot in sitting. The patient has her feet on a box because the plinth is too high to allow her feet to touch the floor. This treatment technique requires that the feet be firmly supported. The therapist faces the patient and places both hands over the tops of the knees. *(D)* To assist the weight shift to the left, the therapist slightly adducts and internally rotates the right femur and externally rotates the patient's left femur. Both hands deliver downward pressure into the feet to keep them firmly on the support. *(E)* The therapist is helping the patient shift weight onto the hemiplegic leg. The therapist is placing the hemiplegic femur in adduction and external rotation and delivering a downward message from the right knee into the foot. The patient must have some ability to perform these weight shifts for this technique to work.

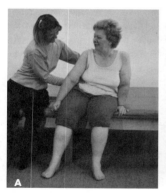
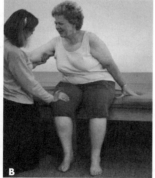

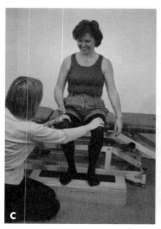
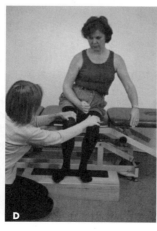
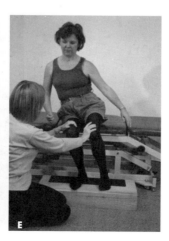

Treatment Goal: Activating equilibrium responses in the trunk and extremities.

Treatment Technique: Higher levels of trunk control and equilibrium responses in the hemiplegic side are trained on high plinth. On the high plinth, the feet are not part of the body's base of support but are free to move and respond to weight shifts of the trunk. In training equilibrium, the therapist is trying to push the level of trunk muscle strength and control to the highest possible level and to produce automatic extremity movements to assist the balance of the trunk. The therapist uses light hands and minimal sensory cues to produce the desired trunk and extremity movements. This type of treatment is called facilitation because it produces flowing, effortless movement patterns with minimal assistance from the therapist. The patient must work very hard with her trunk and extremities to stay balanced during these movements (Fig. 5-27).

FIGURE 5-27 *(A)* The patient before treatment on the plinth, right hemiplegia. *(B)* The therapist uses both the patient's arms to produce the trunk movements. When her control is on the arms, she is looking primarily for a response in the lower trunk and legs. *(C)* The therapist asks for a lower-trunk-initiated anterior weight shift. The patient responds with trunk extension and increased knee flexion. *(D)* The therapist shifts the patient backwards. Trunk flexors become more active, and the knees extend to counteract the backward movement of the trunk. *(E)* Extension rotation to the right is initiated from the lower trunk. The patient has increased weight on her right hip and appropriate adduction of her right lower leg and abduction of her left lower leg. Note how the therapist has very light contact with the patient's hands, indicating that the patient is actively controlling her position with her trunk muscles. *(F)* The therapist can also use both legs to activate the trunk and increase equilibrium responses in the arms. Here the therapist has flexed both legs and shifted the trunk backwards. She is looking for increased flexion in the upper trunk and forward movement of the arms to counterbalance the trunk. Trunk flexors are clearly active, but the arms are not being recruited for equilibrium. *(G)* The therapist is using the legs to assist a lower-trunk-initiated lateral weight shift to the right. The patient's trunk pattern is appropriate, and her hemiplegic and uninvolved arms are responding appropriately with slight abduction. *(H)* The therapist is now using the hemiplegic arm and leg to produce the trunk movements. This type of control allows her to assist the response in the hemiplegic extremities. Here the therapist is controlling the trunk weight shift through the patient's right leg. Her control on the hemiplegic arm is increasing the lateral flexion in the right side of the trunk and assisting the abduction of the arm. *(I & J)* The therapist is now using only the hemiplegic arm to facilitate equilibrium reactions in the trunk and other extremities. To use an arm to shift control to the trunk, the therapist must give a message along the arm into the trunk that tells the trunk which direction to move and which muscles to activate. These two pictures demonstrate very nicely how rotation of the trunk occurs at the end of lateral movements. *(I)* The patient shifted her weight completely to the left hip so that the right hip has left the plinth. The legs have responded to the weight shift by moving to the right, and the left arm is abducted. *(J)* As the therapist continues to shift the body to the left, the patient's upper trunk begins to rotate to the right. This allows the patient to use trunk flexors to help hold her upright. This type of treatment is very difficult for the therapist to perform. The patient must work her trunk muscles very hard to avoid loss of balance. *(K)* At the end of treatment, the patient's hemiplegic hand and arm are totally relaxed. Although the hemiplegic arm appeared stiff during part of the treatment, the patient had been using appropriate muscle activity or the hand and arm would be tight after treatment.

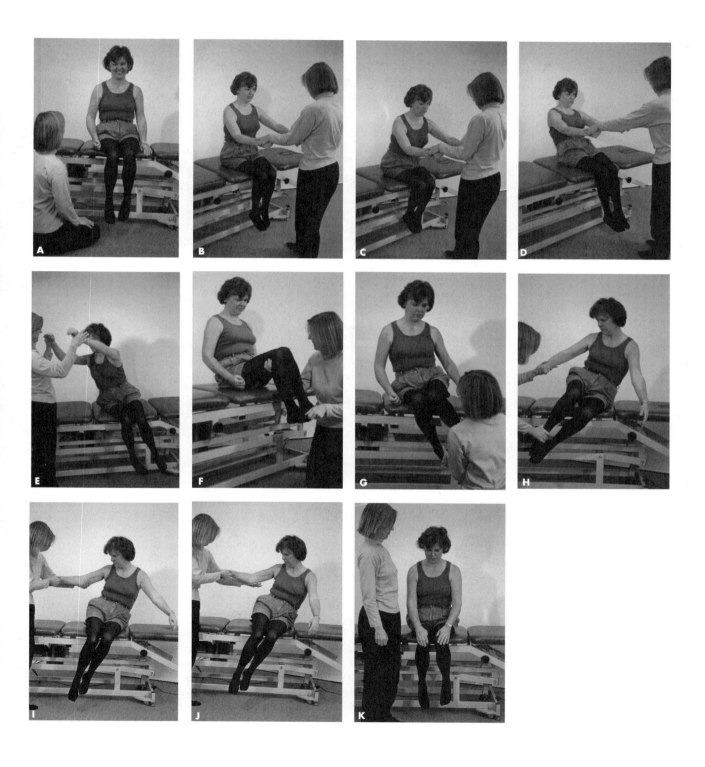

Treatment Goal: Increase independent functioning in sitting.

Treatment Technique: Independent practice of trunk movements with clasped hands. Independent practice of trunk movements will help the patient increase strength and control in his trunk. When the hemiplegic arm is weak or subluxed, the patient should hold this arm with his uninvolved arm during practice (Fig. 5-28).

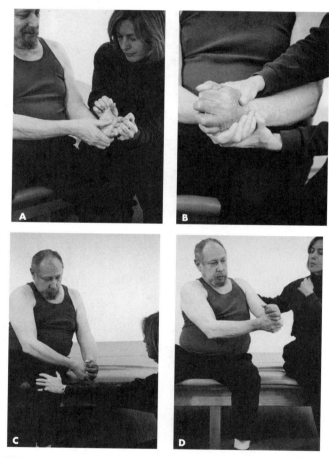

FIGURE 5-28 The patient is shown how to grasp his hemiplegic hand. He places his thumb in the palm while supporting the ulnar side of the hand with his fingers. *(B)* When he closes his left hand, the hemiplegic hand is held securely with the thumb up, the wrist extended, and the forearm in neutral rotation. *(C)* The patient practices an upper-body-initiated flexion rotation to the hemiplegic side. The therapist is supporting the hemiplegic leg in weight bearing but is not assisting the movement of the trunk or arms. *(D)* Practice of extension rotation to the hemiplegic side. The patient will use this arm grip to practice other trunk weight shifts. This treatment technique is often part of the patient's home program.

Treatment Technique: Combining trunk and extremity movements in functional tasks. This treatment activity gives the patient practice combining normal movement components of the hemiplegic arm with appropriate trunk movements during functional performance in sitting. It should begin once the patient can perform all trunk movements in sitting without assistance and has control of arm movements in space. Practice of trunk and arm movements should be included in treatment to ensure that the patient develops normal functional movement sequences (Fig 5-29).

Additional suggestions:

Upper extremity movements in sitting
Lower extremity movements in sitting

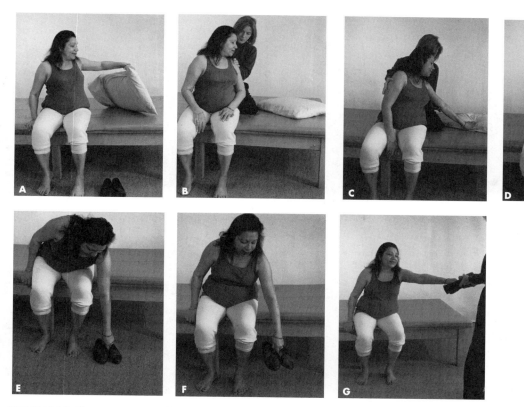

FIGURE 5-29 The patient is using her hemiplegic left arm to reach behind her body. Although she has accomplished the movement independently, the movement patterns in her trunk and arm are inefficient. The patient has not shifted her weight onto her left hip. She has substituted scapula elevation and humeral abduction for appropriate shoulder external rotation. *(B)* The therapist is preparing for an appropriate reach pattern by establishing the correct pattern of trunk rotation. She is guiding the patient's left shoulder back, while shifting weight onto the hemiplegic hip. *(C)* With this pattern of trunk rotation, the patient practices reaching for the pillow with external rotation at the shoulder. *(D)* The therapist helps the patient maintain her shoulder joint in external rotation and move the trunk and arm together to bring the pillow to the edge of the bed. Compare the quality of movement in this figure to the patient's movements in Figure 5-29 A. *(E–G)* Independent practice of trunk and arm movements in treatment. The patient performs these movements with normal trunk and arm components. This practice helps the therapist identify movement patterns that are difficult or performed with atypical movements. She will treat these movement patterns with hands-on practice.

REFERENCE

1. Kapandji A: Physiology of the Joints. Vol. 1: Upper Limb. 5th Ed. Churchill Livingstone, New York, 1982

6

Upper Extremity Movements

CONCEPTS AND PRINCIPLES

In daily life, we use our arms to perform a wide variety of tasks and functional movements. For the purpose of movement analysis, these functional movements of the arm (and leg) can be divided into two categories: movements in space and weightbearing movements. Functional performance in the arm is most closely associated with the ability to move in space. Arm movements in space are complex movements that rely on well coordinated and calibrated movements of the shoulder, elbow, forearm, and wrist to position the hand efficiently for function. In this chapter, we describe the movement components in the arm that are most important for functional movements in space. Since the arm is used in so many different patterns, we have simplified this information by directing it toward the major movement problems of the neurologic patient. Fine motor coordination and grasp patterns are not presented in this book. Weightbearing movements of the arm are discussed separately in Chapter 7.

The simplest patterns of arm movement are reach patterns. Reaching movements are used to position the hand at arm's length from the body. During reach, extension at the elbow and wrist joints stabilizes all the segments of the arm into one functional unit, and movement occurs at the shoulder joint. More complex arm movements require coordinated sequences of movement at multiple joints. For example, to bring the hand from a resting position on the knee to the top of the head, we combine movements of elbow flexion with forearm supination to initiate the movement, followed by shoulder flexion to lift the hand to the desired height, and then wrist flexion to bring the fingers to the head. For movements such as this to progress smoothly and efficiently, the exact range of movement at each of the joints must be precisely controlled and the sequence of joint movement planned correctly. Upper extremity movements become even more complex when we add a unilateral hand function like brushing the hair or a bilateral function, such as hair braiding, to the movement pattern described previously. Yet, despite the apparent infinite complexity of arm movements, it is possible to identify basic movement components for the arm that form the basis for many functional movements. These movement components are presented later in the chapter.

Loss of arm function is one of the most common long-term effects of neurologic pathology and one of the biggest contributors to disability. Most neurologic patients regain enough strength and control in their affected leg to stand and walk.

Unfortunately, the arm often does not achieve an equivalent amount of functional return. This loss of controlled movement in the involved arm has a devastating effect on functional use of the hemiplegic extremity and also on bilateral upper extremity coordination, which forms the basis for task performance. While some functional movements and tasks can be relearned with one-handed compensations, many cannot. Thus, loss of movement control in the involved arm and hand has a direct effect on independence and quality of life.

Movement problems in the hemiplegic arm result from several different impairments. Acute neurologic lesions are associated with primary loss of muscle strength, hypotonia, or flaccid paralysis, and changes in the patterns of muscle activation. As the patient progresses through rehabilitation, secondary impairments that also affect movement may begin to develop in the hemiplegic side. Incomplete motor return in the arm is a common problem that results in significant movement deficits, especially in the distal muscles of the forearm, wrist, and hand. In addition, hypertonicity, loss of alignment, soft tissue shortening, and pain become more prevalent in the months after stroke. These primary and secondary impairments result in persistent movement deficits, inefficient or atypical patterns of movement, and loss of function.

Treatment of the hemiplegic upper extremity is an extremely important part of rehabilitation. From the patient's perspective, regaining movement and function in the involved arm is one of the major goals of rehabilitation. The arm should be treated from the earliest days of rehabilitation to maximize recovery in the arm and to give the patient hope of regaining function. For the therapist, arm treatment is important because of its role in function and because of the influence that the arm has on functional movements of the trunk and leg in sitting, standing, and walking. In the acute stage, treatment of the arm prevents the development of secondary impairments, strengthens weak muscles of the upper trunk and arm, prevents the development of secondary impairments, and teaches the patient to incorporate the arm into task performance so that patterns of learned neglect are not established. Later in rehabilitation, arm treatment must address secondary impairments, such as problems with alignment and tissue length, as well as reeducate movement and function. Our clinical experience has demonstrated that improvements in upper extremity movement and function are possible for many years after a stroke or neurologic injury. For this reason, we believe that treatment of the involved arm should be part of all rehabilitation programs.

MOVEMENT COMPONENTS

The upper extremity is attached to the trunk at the sternoclavicular joint and through muscular attachments at the scapulothoracic joint. The shoulder complex comprises three bones: the scapula, the humerus, and the clavicle. Each of these boney segments have well-defined planes of movement. For normal shoulder movement to occur, the three bones of the shoulder must move together in the correct relationships to each other. In the section below, we review the planes of movement for each boney segment and describe the composite movements that are important for function.

Scapula Movements

The scapula has mobility in three planes: elevation/depression, abduction/adduction, and upward/downward rotation. These planes are illustrated in Figure 6-1.

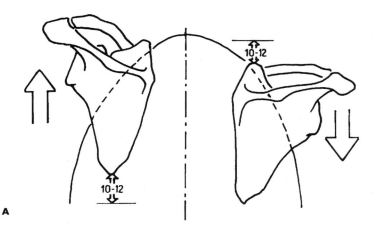

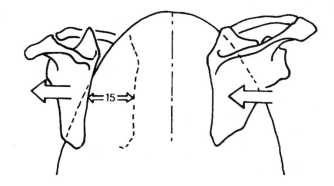

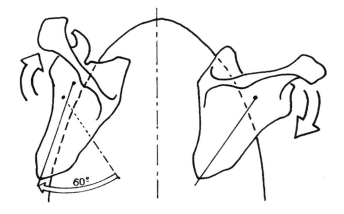

FIGURE 6-1 Normal scapular movements. (*A*) Elevation/depression. (*B*) Abduction/adduction. (*C*) Upward/downward rotation. (From Kapandji[2] with permission.)

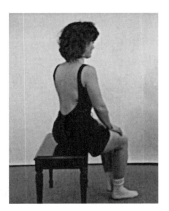

FIGURE 6-2 Starting position for functional arm movements in sitting.

Humeral Movements

The humerus also has three planes of movement: flexion/extension, abduction/adduction, and internal/external rotation.

Clavicular Movements

There are three planes of movement in the clavicle as well: elevation/depression, protraction/retraction, and rotation.

The movements of the scapula, humerus, and clavicle occur in coordinated sequences during functional movements of the arm. These movement sequences were first identified by Codman,[1,7] who labeled them "rhythms" of the shoulder girdle. In daily life, Codman's shoulder girdle rhythm can be observed most easily during reaching with an extended elbow. The movement components used in extended arm reach are described below. In all these movement patterns, the hand moves first to initiate the arm movement.

Forward Reach

The range of forward reach is potentially 180 degrees of movement. This arc moves the hand from the side of the body to full overhead elevation. When the arm is at rest by the side of the body, the humerus hangs in neutral rotation and the forearm is in neutral rotation or slight pronation with the hand resting along the femur. In sitting, the hand often rests on the thigh or on an arm of the chair, so that the elbow is slightly flexed and the forearm is pronated. This position is the natural starting point for functional arm movements in sitting (Fig. 6-2).

The position of neutral rotation at the shoulder joint is generally maintained as the hand moves forward to reach. While it is possible to raise the hand overhead with either internal rotation or external rotation at the shoulder, the hand is most efficiently positioned for function in front of the body, if the humerus is maintained in neutral rotation or slight external rotation and the forearm in neutral position so that the thumb faces up. For the shoulder joint to be the fulcrum of the movement, the wrist and elbow joints must be extended. Elbow extension fixes the humerus and forearm into one functional unit. Similarly, wrist extension stabilizes the position of the hand in line with the forearm.

It is helpful to divide the arc of forward flexion into four stages of movement. These stages roughly correspond to distinct phases of movement, but we have also chosen them because they have different functional roles. Since these movements are taking place with the elbow in extension, the starting position of the arm is by the side of the body.

0 to 60 Degrees of Forward Flexion

In the 0 to 60 degrees of forward flexion, initial phase of movement, the hand moves forward and up away from the thigh. As the hand and forearm move forward, the shoulder joint gradually moves into flexion. When the distal end of the humerus moves forward, the humeral head moves back in the fossa. This humeral movement is accompanied by a posterior rotation of the clavicle. While the scapula muscles are active to stabilize the scapula on the rib cage during this phase of the

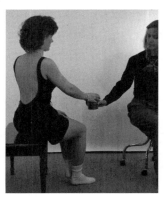

FIGURE 6-3 Forward flexion, stage I: 0 to 60 degrees of forward flexion.

movement, the scapula does not move with the humerus until approximately 60 degrees of flexion has been reached (Figs. 6-2 and 6-3). This initial arc of humeral movement without scapular rotation is one of the most important ranges for arm function. It is used for reaching for objects on a table or counter and for tasks like pushing a shopping cart or opening a door.

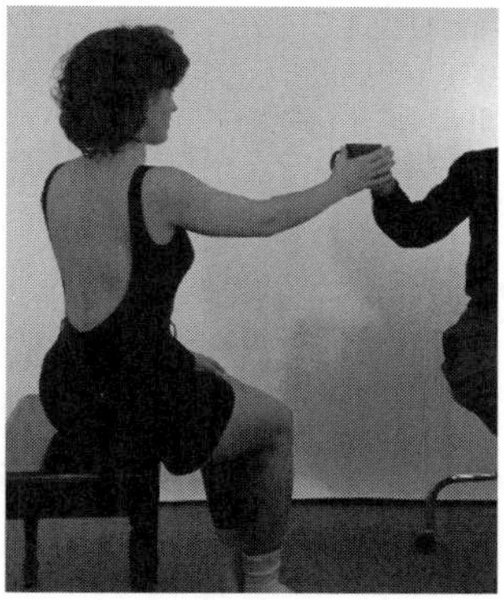

60 to 90 Degrees of Forward Flexion

When the humerus has moved through approximately 60 degrees of flexion, the scapula begins to rotate upwardly with the movement of the humerus. The ratio of humeral to scapular movement was found by Codman[1] to be 2:1, so that for every two degrees of humeral movement the scapula moves one degree. While modern investigations have disputed Codman's ratio, examination of normal movement demonstrates that scapular rotation does begin to occur sometime during this arc of movement. During this phase of movement, the clavicle continues axial rotation (Fig. 6-4). This range of movement is where many reaching tasks take place in sitting and standing. Examples include turning on a light switch or reaching for a book on the bookshelf.

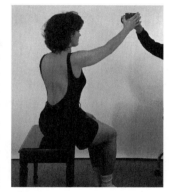

FIGURE 6-4 Forward flexion, stage II: 60 to 90 degrees of flexion.

90 to 120 Degrees of Forward Flexion

As the hand moves above the height of the shoulder, the distal humerus is positioned above the glenohumeral joint for the first time. At this point in the movement, the humeral head must move down in the fossa to allow further elevation to occur. External rotation to neutral is thought to assist this downward movement of the humeral head by keeping the bicipital tuberosity clear of the coracoid process. Upward rotation of the scapula moves the superior angle close to the spine, allowing the glenoid fossa to face superiorly. As the hand moves higher, continued scapular rotation is necessary to keep the humeral head in contact with the fossa. At the same time, the clavicle rotates on its axis in a posterior direction (Fig. 6-5). This range of movement is used to comb your hair, put on a pullover shirt, or to reach for something on a shelf above your desk. It brings the hand above the height of the shoulder.

FIGURE 6-5 Forward flexion, stage III: 90 to 120 degrees of flexion.

120 to 180 Degrees of Forward Flexion

At 120 degrees of forward flexion, the arc of scapula rotation and humeral movement is essentially complete. Most functional tasks for the arm will take place at or below 120 degrees of elevation. Further elevation of the arm requires accessory lengthening in the spine and rib cage. The final degrees of elevation are obtained by lengthening of the rib cage, extension of the lumbar spine, and a superior glide of the upwardly rotated scapula (Fig. 6-6). This range of movement brings the hand to its maximal height over head. It is used to reach for very high objects or to stretch your trunk and arms.

Shoulder Protraction

During forward reach, the length of the arm can be increased through the movement of shoulder girdle protraction. To perform this movement, the humerus must be in forward flexion in a range of 60 to 90 degrees of elevation, with the scapula in upward rotation. To protract the arm, the hand moves farther forward away from the trunk.

FIGURE 6-6 Forward flexion, stage IV: 120 to 180 degrees of flexion.

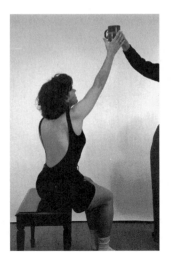

FIGURE 6-7 Shoulder protraction.

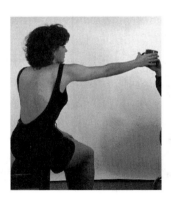

This causes the scapula to glide around the rib cage into abduction while maintaining its upwardly rotated position. If the hand reaches forward as far as it can, the scapula glides around the rib cage and the rib cage rotates forward simultaneously. This movement is called protraction (Fig. 6-7). During the forward glide of the scapula, the lateral end of the clavicle moves anteriorly. Retraction is the movement of the scapula backwards on the rib cage. This pattern is used when the arm is not long enough to bring the hand into the desired position. This might occur during a game of catch or when reaching for something on the very back of the supermarket shelf.

Abducted Reach

Reaching movements also occur in the plane of partial or complete horizontal abduction. During abducted reach, the shoulder joint is more externally rotated than in the forward reach. External rotation at the shoulder and forearm supination is increased during shoulder abduction to keep the hand oriented for grasp with the thumb facing up. When the arm moves from the side of the body into abduction, the components of scapulohumeral rhythm are similar to those described for forward reach. However, the scapula is more adducted during this reach pattern, and the thoracic spine has more extension (Fig. 6-8).

Functional Example

This movement pattern is used to reach for objects to the side of the body.

FIGURE 6-8 Abducted reach.

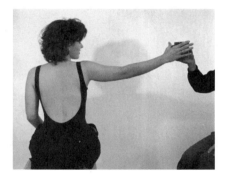

Backward Reach

The arm reaches backward during tasks that require hand placement behind the body. As the hand reaches backward, the distal humerus moves behind the shoulder joint into hyperextension. Humeral hyperextension is characterized by an anterior movement of the humeral head in the fossa. It is accompanied by scapula downward rotation and forward movement of the clavicle (Fig. 6-9).

Functional Example

Shoulder hyperextension is used to bring the hand behind the body to pitch a softball or tuck in the back of your shirt.

Reaching Away From Midline

To move the humerus from forward flexion to abducted reach by the side of the body, another pattern of scapula/humeral rhythm is employed. As the arm moves in the plane of horizontal abduction it is accompanied by adduction of the scapula and external rotation of the humerus to position the hand for function. The head of the humerus moves anteriorly in the fossa as the distal humerus moves to the side. During horizontal abduction, the rotational component of the scapula does not change because the arm stays at a constant level of elevation (Fig. 6-10).

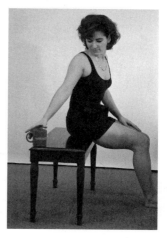
FIGURE 6-9 Backward reach.

Functional Example

These movement patterns are used to change the position of the hand relative to the body midline. They are used in tasks such as washing dishes in the sink and stacking them in the drain board. This is a very important movement pattern of the arm for function.

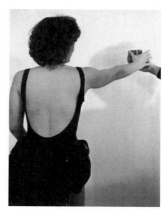
FIGURE 6-10 Reaching away from the midline.

Reaching Across Midline

The arm and hand can also be moved across the midline of the body to achieve about 30 degrees of horizontal adduction. During this movement, the scapula moves into abduction and the clavicle moves forward. Horizontal adduction of the humerus is blocked by the body until partial flexion of the shoulder has occurred to move the arm ahead of the rib cage. Therefore this pattern of arm function is used when the arm is flexed greater than 60 degrees (Fig. 6-11A). Movements of the arm across midline are often combined with trunk rotation to the same side. Trunk rotation extends the range of the reaching arm by allowing scapula abduction to supplement humeral adduction (Fig. 6-11B).

Functional Example

Movements across midline are very common for lifting and positioning large objects, such as trays, that require both hands to lift and carry. They are also used during eating to use the fork on the salad plate.

FIGURE 6-11 Reaching across the midline. (*A*) Crossing the midline using horizontal adduction of the humerus. (*B*) Reaching across the midline with rotation of the trunk.

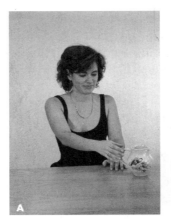
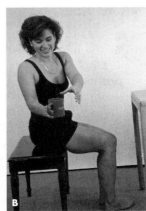

Complex Patterns of the Upper Extremity

In the previous section, the patterns of shoulder girdle rhythm were presented as they occur during extended arm reach. With the exception of reach, most functional movements of the arm combine shoulder movements with elbow flexion. This type of movement is more complex, since the movement of several different joints must be correctly planned and sequenced. Functionally, elbow flexion is used to raise the height of the hand or to bring it closer to the body. These elbow movements decrease the range of shoulder movement that is required to keep the hand in an optimal position by placing a second fulcrum of the movement at the elbow and decreasing the length of the lever acting at the shoulder. In this section we will examine how elbow flexion combines with scapular and humeral movements to position the hand for function.

Elbow Flexion/Extension

The elbow joint is described as a hinge joint, with its plane of movement in flexion and extension. Full flexion of the elbow moves the bones of the forearm from along the side of the leg until it touches the humerus, an arc of 145 degrees. To initiate elbow flexion, the wrist extends to bring the hand and carpal bones in line with the radius and ulna. The position of the forearm may vary from supination, mid-position, and pronation, depending on the orientation of the hand that is desired. When elbow flexion is combined with forearm supination, the palm touches the shoulder, while pronation orients the palm away from the body. Several important movements that combine elbow flexion with shoulder movement are described in the next section.

Reach Combining Shoulder and Elbow Flexion

The combination of elbow flexion with shoulder flexion is used to bring the hand forward to reach in a range close to the body. To reach forward using this pattern, the elbow first flexes to 90 degrees with the wrist extended. This brings the hand from its position of rest on the leg to the approximate height where it will function. In the next phase of the movement, the humerus moves forward into flexion and the elbow simultaneously extends, so that the hand moves forward without

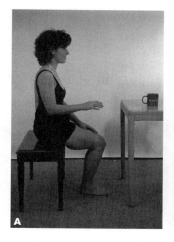
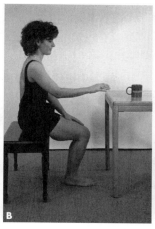
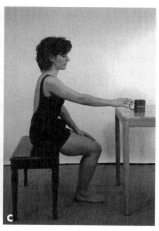

FIGURE 6-12 *(A–C)* Reach combining shoulder and elbow flexion.

moving higher. The amount of shoulder flexion and elbow extension required depends on how long the arm must be for the hand to reach its intended target (Fig. 6-12).

Elevation Combining Shoulder and Elbow Flexion

To bring the hand to the top of the head for grooming or to the mouth for eating or drinking, greater than 90 degrees of elbow flexion and greater than 60 degrees of shoulder flexion is necessary. This type of movement is initiated with elbow flexion to around 90 degrees. It continues from there with simultaneous elbow and shoulder flexion. The exact combination of shoulder and elbow flexion will depend on the demands of the task for height of the hand and length of the arm. When the shoulder flexes more than 60 degrees, scapular rotation accompanies humeral flexion/abduction in accordance with scapulohumeral rhythm (Fig. 6-13).

Elbow Flexion with Shoulder Extension

Movements combining humeral extension or hyperextension with elbow flexion are used to bring the hand closer to the anterior surface of the body from the forward position described above. To maintain the hand at a constant height, the elbow flexion increases as the position of the shoulder joint changes from flexion to neutral and into extension (Fig. 6-14).

FIGURE 6-13 *(A & B)* Elevation combining shoulder and elbow flexion. The scapula must upwardly rotate to allow the hand to reach the top of the head.

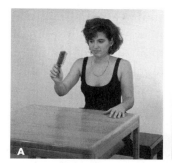
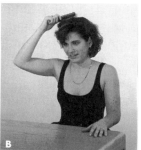

FIGURE 6-14 *(A & B)* Elbow flexion with shoulder extension is used to bring the hand closer to the body.

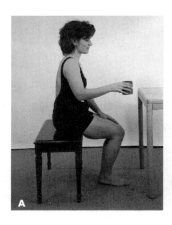 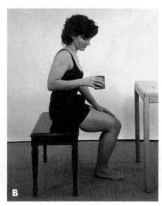

Elbow Flexion with Shoulder Internal/External Rotation

When the elbow is flexed to 90 degrees, rotation at the glenohumeral joint is used to move the hand around the midline of the body. Neutral rotation at the shoulder keeps the hand parallel with the line of the body, facing forward. As the shoulder internally rotates, the hand comes across midline, so that the forearm and hand approach the front of the chest or opposite side of the body (Fig. 6-15A). External rotation at the shoulder moves the hand away from the midline towards its own side of the body (Fig. 6-15B). These movements are very important for positioning the hand for grooming and dressing activities and for function at a table.

Functional Performance

Arm movements are generally performed with the goal of positioning the hand for function. Thus, most arm movements are initiated by movement of the hand and forearm. These distal movements are used to orient the hand for the task, so that the thumb and fingers are in position for grasp or manipulation. The correct orientation of the hand is obtained through distal movements that combine forearm rotation and wrist flexion/extension. Orientation of the hand for function occurs early in the movement sequence, so that the hand is ready to be used as soon as the targeted object is reached.

Rotational movements of the forearm are used to orient the hand. This orientation establishes the position in which the palm and fingers will approach the object and determines the pattern of grasp that is available. Pronation of the forearm is

FIGURE 6-15 Elbow flexion with shoulder internal/external rotation. *(A)* As the shoulder internally rotates, the hand comes across the midline, so that the forearm and hand approach the front of the chest or opposite side of the body. *(B)* External rotation at the shoulder moves the hand away from the midline toward its own side of the body.

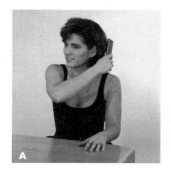 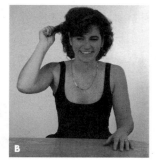

FIGURE 6-16 Pronation of the forearm. *(A)* With an overhand grasp. *(B)* Neutral forearm rotation allows thumb and fingers to directly approach the handle.

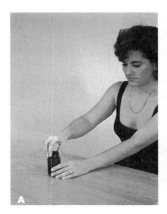
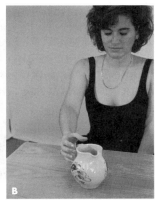

used to position the hand for grasp over the top of the object (Fig. 6-16A). Mid-position of forearm rotation places the thumb on top and is used for a sideways approach to the object (Fig. 6-16B). Supination of the forearm places the palm up during approach and is used to lift from under an object. During functional performance, forearm rotation is often used to change the orientation of the hand. For example, to open a book, the grasp pattern remains stable, but the forearm rotates from pronation to supination (Fig. 6-17).

Movements at the wrist joint determine the position of the hand relative to the forearm. Wrist extension is used to bring the hand in line with the distal radius and ulna, so that the hand and forearm move together as a unit. Wrist extension that maintains the hand in line with the forearm is a very important part of the initial arm movements that position the hand for the task. Once the hand has reached its desired position, wrist extension may or may not be maintained. Wrist extension is important for hand functions that require a flat open hand and for a strong palmar grasp. Wrist flexion is used to bring the fingers closer to the object for grasp and for fine manipulative finger movements and grasp patterns.

When the distal orientation of the hand has been achieved through movements of the forearm and wrist, the hand is moved into position for task performance with the patterns of shoulder and elbow movement described in the previous sections.

FIGURE 6-17 Using rotation to change the orientation of the hand. *(A–D)* To open a book, the grasp pattern remains stable, but the forearm rotates from pronation to supination.

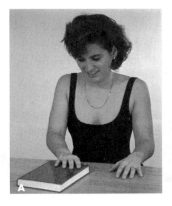
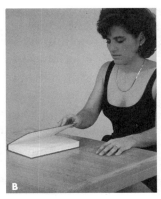
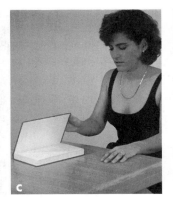
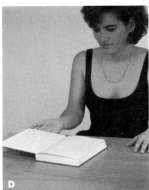

By orienting the hand first, the shoulder and elbow movements that most efficiently target the object can be used to approach the task. After the desired hand position has been achieved, the position of the arm and hand must be stabilized through muscle activity of the shoulder and elbow while the hand performs. When grasp is complete, or the task finished, shoulder and elbow movements return the hand to the body for further performance or rest.

SIGNIFICANT IMPAIRMENTS THAT INTERFERE WITH PERFORMANCE

Muscle Weakness in the Arm

Muscle weakness and paralysis are the major causes of loss of movement, atypical movement, and functional limitation in the hemiplegic arm. There are several common patterns of muscle weakness in the hemiplegic arm.

Total Paralysis or Severe Weakness in All Muscle Groups

Total paralysis/weakness, the most extreme example of the problem, is usually found in the early days after stroke, although in rare cases it persists throughout rehabilitation. In this group of patients, the hemiplegic arm cannot move without assistance because none of the arm muscles are strong enough to produce movement. In most patients, total paralysis in the arm is followed by gradual recovery of motor function.

Moderate Weakness in All Arm Muscle Groups

Moderate weakness in all arm muscles is often found immediately after stroke. It may develop later in rehabilitation as the patient recovers muscle strength in previously paralyzed muscles. In this group of patients, proximal and distal muscle groups of the arm are equally affected, and all arm muscles have less than normal muscle strength. When all the muscles in the arm are weak, active range of motion in the arm is less than normal, and the muscles fatigue quickly. Patients with overall weakness produce arm movements similar to normal movement patterns in their initiation and sequencing. Their arms remain limited functionally because they are unable to move the arm up above shoulder height or to keep the arm up while grasping with the hand (Fig. 6-18A–D). These problems may gradually resolve with a treatment program designed to increase strength and endurance in the arm, and patients with this recovery pattern have the potential for good function in the arm and hand.

Distal Weakness

Distal weakness occurs when recovery of muscle strength begins at the shoulder girdle and progresses down the arm. In this recovery pattern, shoulder and elbow muscles have sufficient strength to produce movement, but weakness in the forearm, wrist, and hand muscles interferes with functional use of the hemiplegic arm (Fig. 6-18E–G). Some patients with this weakness pattern eventually regain movement control in the distal muscles of the arm.

Unbalanced Muscle Strength

Unbalanced muscle strength in the hemiplegic arm exists when some proximal and distal arm muscles recover strength and control, while other proximal and distal muscle groups remain severely weak or paralyzed. Typically, patients with this recovery pattern regain strength in the muscles that control shoulder elevation, humeral abduction, and internal rotation, and elbow, wrist, and finger flexion. However, they do not regain control of shoulder flexion and external rotation, or extension of the elbow, wrist, and fingers. All patients with unbalanced muscle strength have deficits in some critical arm movements. These movement deficits may profoundly affect the patient's ability to produce functional arm movements or merely interfere with skilled, efficient task performance. For example, patients who have severe weakness in elbow and wrist extensors are usually unable to use the hemiplegic arm functionally, while a loss of humeral external rotation affects the positioning of the hand for grasp but does not limit function as completely (Fig. 6-18H).

Atypical arm movements frequently develop as a way of compensating for muscle paralysis and unbalanced muscle strength. For example, many patients learn to lift up their hemiplegic arm by elevating the scapula, abducting the humerus, and flexing the elbow (Fig. 6-18I & J). This atypical movement pattern is associated with recovery of shoulder muscles and weakness/paralysis of muscles in the forearm, wrist, and hand. The patient uses an improper pattern of initiation because the muscles in the lower arm are paralyzed or too weak to initiate a normal reach. If the therapist carefully evaluates muscle control in the lower arm, she frequently finds that the patient can contract elbow, forearm, and wrist muscles with assistance. This indicates the potential for more normal movements if muscle strength in these groups can be increased (Fig. 6-18K). The motivated patient may be able to use atypical movements to accomplish simple functions like lifting the arm onto the table or bringing the hand over an object to prepare for grasp (Fig. 6-18L). However, most atypical movement patterns are too abnormal or inefficient to be of use in life tasks.

Muscle weakness in the arm is treated by a program of movement reeducation that includes retraining proximal and distal movement patterns and functional task-oriented movements. The goal of treatment is to increase strength and control in weak muscles, to teach these muscles to be active synergistically with other muscle groups in functional movements, and to encourage further motor recovery in paralyzed muscles. When most arm muscles are weak or paralyzed, the therapist must control the proximal and distal arm during movement reeducation. The therapist's hands preserve normal mechanical relationships between the segments of the arm and between the arm and trunk and make it easier to teach normal initiation, sequencing, and completion of functional movements. The therapist should train extended arm reach and complex patterns of reach that combine shoulder and elbow flexion (Fig. 6-18M). The arm should be elevated above 60 degrees of shoulder elevation for at least part of each treatment session to reeducate the muscles of scapula rotation. The therapist should also introduce movements of forearm rotation, wrist flexion/extension, and finger and thumb movements, even if the patient is unable to assist these movements. As distal muscle strength improves, the therapist can add objects to movement reeducation to prepare the hand for grasp, release, and manipulation. Objects can also be used to increase overall arm strength and to allow independent practice of arm movements. For example, traditional cane exercises can be used to reinforce the patterns of arm movement prac-

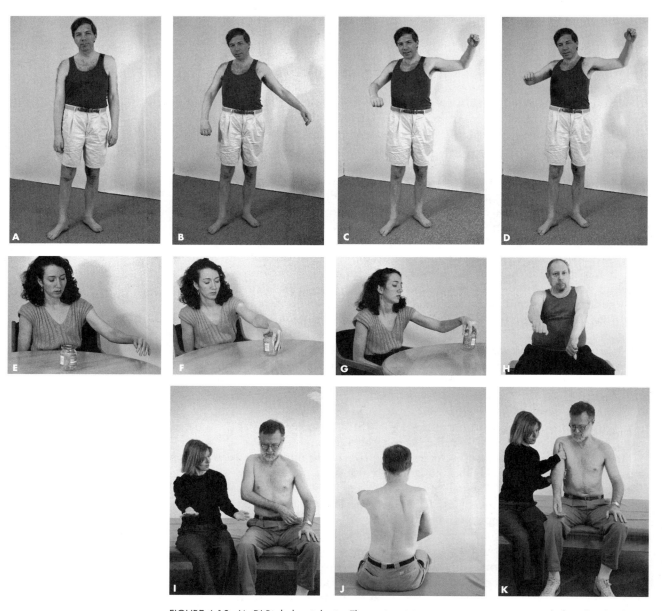

FIGURE 6-18 *(A–D)* Right hemiplegia. The patient initiates movements appropriately from his distal arm, but he is unable to lift the hemiplegic arm above shoulder height because of muscle weakness in all major muscle groups of the right arm. *(E–G)* The patient has suffcient muscle strength in her proximal arm to bring the hemiplegic hand to the jar, but weakness in the wrist and fingers interferes with normal grasp. *(H)* Loss of control of shoulder external rotation in the hemiplegic arm. This movement deficit causes the thumb to face down during forward reach, interfering with efficient approach and grasp. *(I)* The therapist asks the patient to reach his hemiplegic arm forward with an extended elbow. He responds with shoulder elevation and elbow flexion. *(J)* The back view of his arm movement pattern showing elevation and apparent upward rotation of the scapula. These muscles are active because they are the strongest muscles in the arm. *(K)* When the therapist stabilizes the position of the shoulder joint and humerus, the patient is able to extend his elbow. This indicates the presence of weak elbow extensors. *(Figure continues.)*

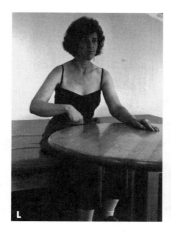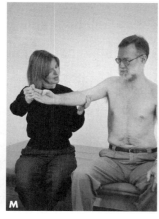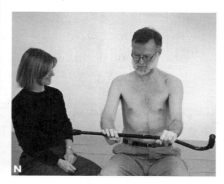

FIGURE 6-18 (*Continued*) (*L*) The patient is using an atypical movement to bring her arm from her lap to the table. (*M*) The therapist's hands control the position of the proximal and distal arm during movement reeducation of reach. (*N*) With both hands on the cane, the patient can practice extended arm reach patterns independently.

ticed in treatment, building strength and automatic movements. When these exercises are part of the patient's home program, muscle strength will increase more rapidly than through treatment alone (Fig. 6-18N). These abilities can also be increased through selected use of functional tasks, crafts, and sports activities.

When muscle weakness is a major arm problem, it is also very important for the therapist to incorporate the hemiplegic arm into treatment of the trunk and leg. To do this, the therapist may support the hemiplegic arm against her body, place the arm in weightbearing, or reeducate movements of the arm with the trunk and/or leg. Incorporating the hemiplegic arm into as many treatment activities as possible helps teach the weak muscles of the shoulder girdle to work against gravity and helps prevent the development of subluxation and flexor hypertonicity. Specific techniques for supporting the arm during trunk and leg treatment are included in all the treatment sections of the book.

Loss of Trunk Control

In normal functional movement, the arm moves on a normally aligned trunk, and arm movements are automatically coordinated with trunk movements. Trunk movements in sitting and standing are necessary to compensate for the distracting force that the moving arm places on the center of the body and to increase the range of the arm as it moves and functions. The muscles of the hemiplegic side of the trunk are often affected by primary and secondary impairments. These impairments result in a loss of normal trunk alignment and a loss of control of trunk movements, both of which interfere with efficient use of the arms for function.

Loss of Trunk Alignment

Loss of normal trunk alignment and changes in trunk posture have a major effect on the position of the hemiplegic shoulder and arm. The resting position of the scapula and clavicle are influenced by changes in alignment in the spine and rib cage. In neurologic patients, several typical patterns in the trunk have a major influence on position of the shoulder. These changes in spinal position may be fairly symmetric between the two sides of the body or may affect only one side of the trunk and one scapula.

Excessive Flexion in the Thoracic Spine

Excessive flexion in the thoracic spine will cause increased scapula abduction and an arm that rests in front of the body (Fig. 6-19A).

Excessive Extension in the Spine

Excessive extension in the spine and rotation backwards of the hemiplegic rib cage cause the scapula to rest closer to the spine in a position of adduction and the arm to posture in shoulder abduction and internal rotation or shoulder hyperextension (Fig. 6-19B).

Lateral Trunk Flexion

Lateral trunk flexion with the concavity on the hemiplegic side results in scapula downward rotation (Fig. 6-19C).

When the involved side of the trunk is the longer side, the involved scapula is elevated (Fig. 6-19D). In many patients, the position of the trunk on the hemiplegic side combines trunk flexion with lateral flexion, so that the involved scapula is both abducted and downwardly rotated. These changes in scapula position are important

FIGURE 6-19 *(A)* Excessive trunk flexion is associated with scapula abduction. *(B)* Excessive trunk extension is associated with scapula adduction. *(C)* Trunk lateral flexion with the concavity of the curve on the hemiplegic side causes downward rotation of the hemiplegic scapula. *(D)* Lateral trunk flexion with the convexity on the hemiplegic left side causes elevation of the hemiplegic scapula. *(E)* The patient is unable to maintain his trunk in a stable position during movements of the hemiplegic arm. The hemiplegic side of the trunk flares laterally and rotates backard as he lifts the right arm. Note how the patient has most of his weight on his uninvolved leg during this bilateral symmetric arm movement.

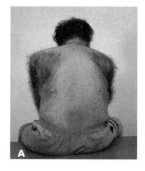
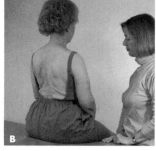
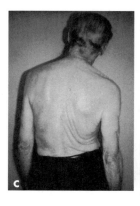
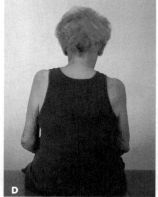
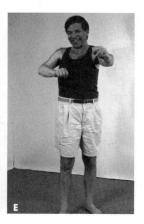

because they result in glenohumeral joint subluxation, disrupt scapulo/humeral rhythm, and contribute to atypical patterns of arm movement. To correct these atypical scapula positions, the therapist must first correct the position of the trunk.

Loss of Trunk Movement Control

Loss of trunk movement control is a second major trunk problem that interferes with efficient arm movements. During task performance, the trunk must be able to maintain a stable upright position and to produce weight shifts that counterbalance the movements of the arm and assist in task performance. Many hemiplegic patients are unable to perform some or all of the trunk movements necessary for function in sitting and standing or to combine trunk and arm movements. In acute patients, trunk control is not adequate to allow the trunk to remain stable without use of the uninvolved arm for balance. These patients tend to move the arms close to the body and avoid reaching movements that require active trunk weight shifts. For these patients, reeducation of trunk movements in sitting is necessary to prepare for functional arm movements of the hemiplegic arm and improved use of the uninvolved arm. Later in rehabilitation, many patients are able to move their trunks in sitting but have difficulty maintaining the trunk in a stable position during arm movements or coordinating weight shifts with arm movements (Fig. 6-19F). This compensation allows them to sit securely, but blocks many functional movements of either arm. As the patient learns to sit unsupported and to perform trunk movements in sitting, trunk balance improves. However, the patient may lack the ability to coordinate trunk responses with arm movements or to initiate a trunk weight shift to extend the range of arm function. With these patients, reeducation of movements that coordinate trunk and arm movements is necessary to improve functional performance and dynamic balance.

Since changes in trunk alignment and loss of trunk movement control interfere with arm function in the upright positions, they have to be addressed as part of the rehabilitation of the hemiplegic arm. Specific techniques for treating trunk problems in sitting and standing are described in Chapters 5 and 9. Treatment techniques that support the hemiplegic arm in forward flexion during reeducation of trunk movements or that combine upper extremity weightbearing with trunk treatment are the most beneficial to the hemiplegic arm.

Subluxation (Loss of Alignment at the Shoulder)

The integrity of the glenohumeral joint is maintained by the position of the scapula on the rib cage and tension in the joint capsule and the tendons and ligaments connecting the various bones of the arm to each other and to the trunk.[3,6] The resting position of the scapula and angulation of the glenoid fossa with its cartilaginous lip provide an inferior support for the humeral head. The humerus remains seated in the glenoid fossa despite the downward forces generated by the weight of the arm because of this inferior support and the support provided by the capsule and muscular attachments. Studies by Basmajian[4] and others have failed to demonstrate any active muscular contributions to the stability of the shoulder girdle at rest (Fig. 6-20).

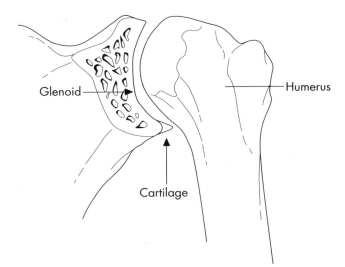

FIGURE 6-20 Normal resting position of the scapula.

In many neurologic patients, the hemiplegic scapula does not rest in the normal position on the rib cage. This change in the orientation of the scapula results in changes in the alignment and integrity of the shoulder joint and of the lower arm. Changes in shoulder girdle alignment and subluxation are caused by impairments that affect the trunk, shoulder girdle, and arm. The most important of these are changes in muscle tone or tension and muscle weakness or paralysis. In the flaccid patient, the weak/paralyzed muscles of the trunk and shoulder girdle do not have sufficient strength or background muscle tone to resist the distracting force that the weight of the arm places on the scapula and shoulder joint. The weight of the paretic arm pulls the scapula into a position of downward rotation and abduction. The weight of the arm probably also contributes to the lateral and forward flexion that develops in the hemiplegic side of the trunk. As the position of the hemiplegic scapula and trunk change, the stability of the glenohumeral joint is compromised. The shoulder girdle may also assume abnormal positions in patients when hypertonicity and inappropriate or unbalanced muscle firing are present in the upper extremity. In these patients, unopposed muscle firing pulls the scapula/humerus into an abnormal position. Both weakness/low tone and hypertonicity/unbalanced muscle firing can lead to subluxation or permanent changes in shoulder joint integrity.

There are three major patterns of shoulder joint subluxation: inferior, anterior, and superior. Each of these secondary impairments is associated with a particular pattern of muscle tone, muscle strength, and motor recovery.

Inferior Subluxation

Inferior subluxation, the most common type of shoulder subluxation, is found in patients with severe muscle weakness and low tone and usually develops in acute hemiplegia. In flaccid hemiplegia, the weight of the arm pulls the scapula into downward rotation. When the scapula downwardly rotates, the slope of the glenoid fossa becomes more vertical. This change removes the inferior support from under the humeral head, allowing the humerus to slip below the lip of the glenoid fossa (Fig. 6-21). The weight of the arm stretches the joint capsule and the tendons con-

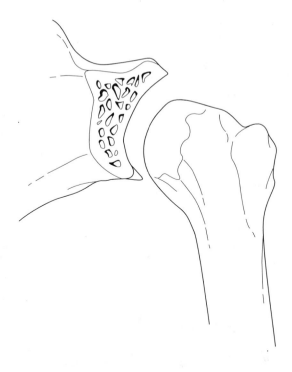

necting the humerus to the scapula. These tissues are non-elastic, and with prolonged traction they passively lengthen. This allows the humerus to move below the level of the glenoid fossa.

The inferior position of the humerus can be observed and the amount of separation quantified by finding the superior boney markers for the top of the shoulder joint and the boney prominence of the bicipital tuberosity inferior and slightly anterior to these markers (Fig. 6-22A & B). The distance between the top of the shoulder and the humerus is the amount of subluxation. The bicipital tuberosity lies anterior to the acromium because of internal rotation of the humerus that occurs with the inferior subluxation. Internal rotation appears to develop for several reasons, including trunk flexion, which causes the arm to rest across the body, the increased weight of the thumb side of the arm, and early unopposed activity in the pectoral muscles.

Before the therapist can introduce active or passive movements of the shoulder joint, she must reduce the inferior subluxation and restore normal joint mechanics to the shoulder girdle. To do this, the therapist must first correct the trunk position to restore symmetry to the spine, rib cage, and pelvis. This allows the therapist to identify the true resting position of the scapula and to reposition the scapula on a correctly aligned rib cage. Next, the therapist upwardly rotates the scapula to neutral and lifts the humerus superiorly into the glenoid fossa. Finally, the therapist rotates the humerus from internal rotation into slight external rotation, so that the arm hangs naturally by the side of the trunk. When these steps are done correctly, the separation between the bones is removed and the normal contouring of the shoulder girdle returns (Fig. 6-22C & D). The therapist must maintain this corrected joint position during all arm treatment activities, until the muscles of the trunk and scapula become appropriately active to hold the scapula in the correct position.

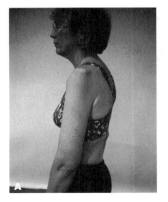

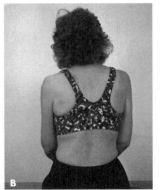

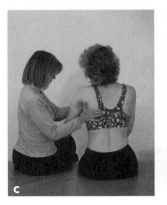

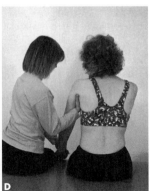

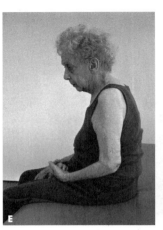

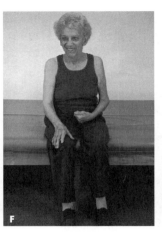

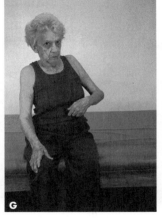

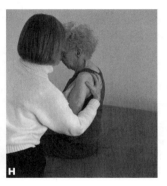

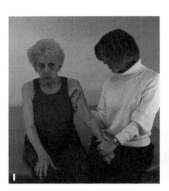

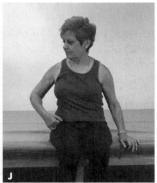

FIGURE 6-22 *(A)* Inferior subluxation. From the side, the boney markers of the spine of the scapula and clavicle are clearly visible, as is the contour of the humerus. *(B)* From the back, the downward rotation of the scapula can be identified. *(C)* The therapist corrects the subluxation by upwardly rotating the scapula to neutral, lifting the humerus up into the fossa, and externally rotating the shoulder joint to neutral. This control restores the normal contouring of the left shoulder. *(D)* The therapist maintains her control of the shoulder while reeducating arm movements. *(E & F)* Anterior subluxation. *(E)* From the side, the forward position of the proximal humerus and hyperextension of the distal humerus are evident. *(F)* The rotation backward of the rib cage on the hemiplegic side is evident from the front. *(G)* When the patient attempts to reach her arm forward, the shoulder elevates, the elbow flexes, and the ribs flare and rotate backwards on the hemiplegic side. *(H)* Reduction of anterior subluxation. The therapist is moving the scapula into depression and upward rotation while moving the humeral head back in the fossa. *(I)* The therapist is lengthening the tight elbow flexors. She uses her right hand to maintain the shoulder joint in normal alignment and her left hand to extend the elbow. The bands of muscle tightness in the upper and lower arm are clearly visible. *(J)* Superior subluxation. The humerus is locked in a position of abduction and internal rotation.

Anterior Subluxation

Anterior subluxation occurs when the humeral head separates from the glenoid fossa in an anterior direction and the distal end of the humerus moves posteriorly into hyperextension. This subluxation pattern is associated with hypertonicity and unbalanced muscle return in the shoulder girdle, trunk, and leg. Anterior subluxation is usually found in combination with a trunk pattern of rotation backward of the hemiplegic side and anterior pelvic tilt and extensor hypertonicity in the hemiplegic leg. The humerus appears to sublux anteriorly when the downwardly rotated scapula is pulled into elevation with a forward tilt and the humerus is pulled into hyperextension and internal rotation. Muscles that influence the scapula and humeral position in anterior subluxation, include upper trapezius and levator, latissimus, pectoralis major and minor, and biceps. As the humeral head moves forward of the glenoid fossa, it places increased tension on the long head of the biceps, causing the elbow flexion and the forearm supination. In this way, the abnormal position of the shoulder joint causes increased hypertonicity in the elbow and lower arm (Fig. 6-22 E–G). Anterior subluxation prevents the shoulder joint from moving into forward flexion and external rotation. When a patient with this type of subluxation attempts to reach an arm forward, the scapula elevates, the elbow flexes, and the trunk and shoulder girdle rotate backwards.

To reduce an anterior subluxation, the therapist corrects trunk alignment, takes the humerus out of internal rotation and hyperextension, depresses and upwardly rotates the scapula, and glides the humeral head back into the fossa (Fig. 6-22H). When this subluxation has persisted for a long period, the muscles connecting the trunk, scapula, and arm develop severe hypertonicity and muscle shortening. The therapist must decrease abnormal muscle tension in the scapula elevators and pectoral and biceps muscles to influence this subluxation. Once hypertonicity is decreased, it may be necessary to lengthen shortened muscles to restore normal resting alignment to the arm, forearm, wrist, and hand (Fig. 6-22I).

Superior Subluxation

Superior subluxation occurs when the head of the humerus becomes tightly lodged under the coracoid process in a position of elevation and internal rotation. In this position, the humerus is locked and cannot move freely in the glenohumeral joint. This means that every movement of the humerus is accompanied by simultaneous movement of the scapula, regardless of whether this is appropriate to the range and pattern being produced. In the neurologic patient, superior subluxation is associated with muscle cocontraction and hypertonicity. It appears to develop when the scapula is abducted and elevated, the humerus internally rotated and abducted away from the rib cage, and the forearm adducted across the body with flexion at the elbow and usually supination of the forearm (Fig. 6-22J).

Superior subluxation is associated with inappropriate muscle firing in the middle deltoid, pectoral muscles, and biceps. Because mobility of the humeral head in the glenoid fossa and disassociated movement between the humerus and scapula are necessary for normal arm movements, superior subluxation of the humeral head must be reduced before normal shoulder movements can be produced or reeducated. This process begins with stopping the unbalanced muscle firing and cocontraction and restoring normal alignment to the trunk and scapula. When these problems have been decreased or eliminated, the humeral head can be manually taken out of internal rotation and moved down in the fossa.

Whenever the hemiplegic shoulder is subluxed, the therapist must correct the position of the trunk, scapula, and shoulder joint before attempting to reeducate movements. Since subluxation at the shoulder joint results in changes in muscle length-tension relationships and alters the line of muscle pull, the patient will be unable to produce normal shoulder movements until joint position is returned to normal. Treatment techniques such as shoulder mobilization and forearm weightbearing can be used to return the scapula to its normal orientation on the rib cage, allowing the therapist to reseat the humerus. (see also Chs. 7 and 10) The therapist must maintain alignment of the shoulder joint and provide normal scapula humeral rhythm during movement reeducation to activate normal patterns of shoulder movement. As the patient learns to move the arm using normal patterns of coordination, subluxation and the related problems of hypertonicity and soft tissue shortening will gradually decrease.

Changes in Distal Alignment

Alignment changes below the shoulder joint are also common. These changes also have a great effect on movement and function in the hemiplegic arm. Neurologic patients have changes in distal alignment because of the changes of alignment at the shoulder girdle and because of the influences of gravity and unbalanced muscle pull on the structures of the forearm, wrist, and hand. Changes in alignment in the distal arm are significant for two reasons. First, these changes interfere with normal movement patterns in the distal arm and hand. Second, changes in distal alignment alter the normal mechanical relationship between the hand and shoulder joint, interfering with the patterns of movement that can be produced at the shoulder. Alignment problems in the lower arm and hand include excessive elbow flexion, changes in forearm rotation that are incompatible with shoulder position, wrist flexion, and fisting or flattening of the hand.

Distal alignment problems can be observed in patients with hypotonicity and weakness and in patients with hypertonicity and unbalanced muscle strength. In patients with low tone and weakness/paralysis, the hemiplegic arm rests in internal rotation, with passive extension of the elbow, and forearm pronation. This pattern appears to develop because of the position of the trunk and shoulder joint, the greater amount of muscle bulk on the front and top of the arm, and the greater weight of the thenar side of the hand (Fig. 6-23A). The weight of the hand on the forearm pulls the wrist into flexion and often causes the carpal bones and the hand to pronate on the forearm. In addition, the low-tone hand quickly develops flattening of the palmar arches with extension of the fingers. These alignment changes are accompanied by loss of tissue mobility in both the flexors and extensors of the forearm, wrist, and hand, and joint stiffness that interferes with forearm rotation, wrist extension, flexion of the fingers, and rounding of the palm.

In patients with hypertonicity in the arm, the resting position of the elbow is in flexion, with either pronation or supination of the forearm and flexion of the wrist (Fig. 6-23B). Elbow flexion develops because of the changes in scapula and glenohumeral joint alignment, discussed in the previous sections, and unbalanced muscle return in the arm. Strong tension in the biceps muscle rotates the forearm from pronation into neutral or supination. As the elbow flexes, the forearm bones become more horizontal. This places the wrist in flexion, since gravity pulls the hand down, and muscle activity in the wrist extensors would be necessary to maintain the hand in line with the forearm. Wrist flexion is quickly associated with short-

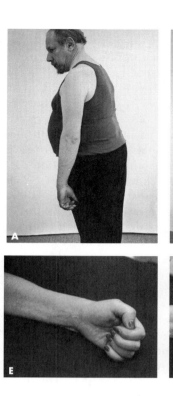
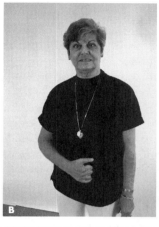
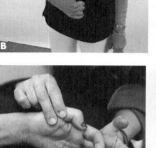
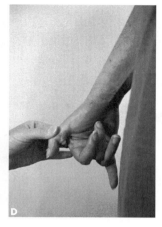
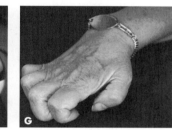
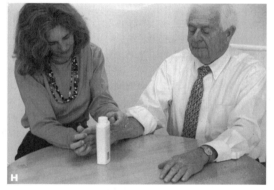

FIGURE 6-23 *(A)* Low tone hemiplegia. The hemiplegic arm hangs in internal rotation, elbow extension, forearm pronation, and wrist flexion. *(B)* Flexor hypertonicity in the arm is associated with elbow flexion and supination of the forearm. *(C & D)* Wrist and finger flexion and shortening of the flexor tendons above and below the wrist. *(E)* The fisted hand. *(F)* The finger flexor tendons have shortened in the palm, causing resistance to finger extension. *(G)* The claw hand. Muscle shortening of the intrinsic finger flexors and extensors leads to this pattern of hand deformity. *(H)* Practice opening the hand in preparation for grasp and release.

ening of the extrinsic wrist and finger flexor tendons. The tendons shorten first above the wrist joint, causing an excessive tendodesis response in the fingers when the position of the wrist is moved from flexion to neutral or slight extension (Fig. 6-23C & D). Later, finger flexor tendons also shorten in the hand, gradually pulling the fingers into flexion until the hand is fisted and resists opening (Fig. 6-23E & F). Wrist and finger flexor muscles frequently develop hypertonicity or are active before the extensors, which also contributes to the flexed posture of the wrist and hand. In some patients, the extrinsic finger extensor tendons shorten along with the extrinsic flexors. This leads to a claw hand deformity, in which the metacarpal phalangeal joints of the fingers are hyperextended and the interphalangeal joints are flexed (Fig. 6-23G).

When distal alignment of the arm is abnormal, normal movement patterns of both the proximal and distal arm are compromised. Wrist flexion makes it difficult to raise the arm without internal rotation and elevation at the shoulder. Similarly, if the elbow cannot be actively extended because of abnormal activity in the biceps, an atypical movement using abduction and internal rotation of the shoulder to lift the hand up, followed by forward rotation of the upper trunk, is necessary to accomplish reach.

Distal alignment problems and the associated changes in muscle length and joint mobility are largely preventable with appropriate arm treatment. In all cases in which distal arm alignment is abnormal, the distal problems must be addressed along with the proximal for normal patterns of arm movement to be possible. This may involve lengthening tight muscles, reestablishing normal mechanical relationships, and reeducating distal movement patterns. Distal arm treatment should reeducate the components of the forearm, wrist, and hand necessary for normal reach and grasp, as well as practice the movement components necessary for higher-level hand skills (Fig. 6-23H).

Abnormal Muscle Tone

Abnormal tone is a source of frustration to both patient and therapist. Although it may not be the primary cause for the inability to perform normal movements,[5] abnormal tone in the arm is associated with abnormal limb position and abnormal amounts of stiffness in the arm at rest and during movement. Most hemiplegic patients are concerned about problems related to abnormal muscle tone in their arm. The hypotonic arm is heavy and floppy. It pulls on the trunk and interferes with balance. When the arm is hypertonic, it feels stiff and assumes an unnatural and uncosmetic posture. It is difficult to get the arm to straighten during dressing or the hand to open to be washed. Therapists are also concerned about abnormal muscle tone, because changes in the tension of muscles lead to changes in alignment and muscle length and interfere with reeducation of normal movement. Therapists treating neurologic patients must be able to change hypertonicity quickly in preparation for movement reeducation. They also need treatment techniques that allow them to build strength and control in hypotonic muscles without causing the arm to become stiff or spastic. In most cases, the patient's movements will not have normal qualities of speed, timing, and effort until muscle tone is brought into the range where it is high enough to resist the pull of gravity but low enough to allow movement.

In the acute stage, most stroke patients have hypotonia in the involved trunk and limbs. Some hemiplegic arms remain low tone, while others develop hypertonicity. Hypertonicity in the muscles of the arm develops over a period of weeks or months. Its appearance is noted first when the arm assumes a flexed posture during difficult activities, as a reflex that accompanies yawning, or by unnatural curling of the fingers at bedside. The change from hypotonic to hypertonic muscle tone is marked by fluctuations from one extreme to the other for some time. During this period, the arm may assume a flexor pattern during some daily activities, but relax while the patient rests in the wheelchair or lies in bed. Gradually, the flexor pattern of the arm comes to predominate, and there is resistance to passive elbow or finger extension. Extensor hypertonicity in the arm is much less common than flexor hypertonicity. In these patients, the hemiplegic elbow locks in extension, and the fingers may be stiff and straight and resist bending.

Several situations seem to contribute to the development of hypertonicity in the hemiplegic arm. These factors are listed separately below.

Abnormal Alignment

The development of increased tension in the biceps muscle and elbow flexor spasticity is related to anterior subluxation of the head of the humerus. This mechanism is discussed above, in the section on subluxation. When anterior subluxation is the cause of elbow joint flexion, the tension in the biceps muscle is decreased when the head of the humerus is moved back into the glenoid fossa and the resting alignment of the scapula restored to normal orientation on the thorax (Fig. 6-24A–C). For these changes to be permanent, treatment must return the scapula to a normal resting alignment on the rib cage and activate the muscle and movement patterns in the trunk and arm necessary to maintain this alignment.

Poor Trunk Stability

Flexor posturing of the arm is frequently first observed during the patient's initial attempts at standing and walking. These involuntary changes in arm posture are also observed when the patient performs functional activities, such as dressing or bathing, that challenge his balance. In these situations, weakness in the involved leg and poor control of trunk movements in sitting and standing create an unstable balance situation for the patient. The flexor muscles of the arm appear to be activated as part of an automatic response. When this is true, the patient is unconsciously recruiting muscle activity in the hemiplegic upper trunk and arm to react to this instability. Flexor posturing of the arm is uncosmetic. It also prevents functional use of the arm.

In acute hemiplegia, hypertonicity in the arm that is occurring as a balance reaction is immediately diminished when the therapist provides more stability to the patient's hemiplegic trunk and leg or assists his balance (Fig. 6-24D & E). However, the posturing of the arm will persist until the patient gains sufficient trunk and lower extremity control to feel safe and stable in these situations. If the patient's balance and walking pattern remain unstable, the posturing of the arm becomes part of the patient's movement repertoire. Over time, the flexed arm posture is permanently maintained by severe hypertonicity and soft tissue contracture.

Volitional Muscle Activation

Excessive flexor muscle activity and atypical flexion of the arm are also evident during the patient's efforts to move his arm either to command or during attempts to perform a function. The arm flexes because the patient is activating the muscles that he has available for movement in the best way that he knows how. Volitional movement patterns increase flexor hypertonicity in the arm; when the patient has unbalanced muscle strength, he fires his available muscles in the wrong sequence or he fires them with excessive effort and cocontraction (Fig. 6-24F & G). These "spastic" or "synergistic" movements can rarely be used for function. Frequently, the patient has difficulty "turning off" the muscles once they have been activated, so that he learns to avoid trying to move his arm for fear that it will stay in a flexed position. The abnormal flexed posture of the arm during movement will change when the patient learns to initiate and sequence normal patterns of muscle firing and to control the intensity and duration of muscle contraction. These skills are learned through movement reeducation of functional arm movements.

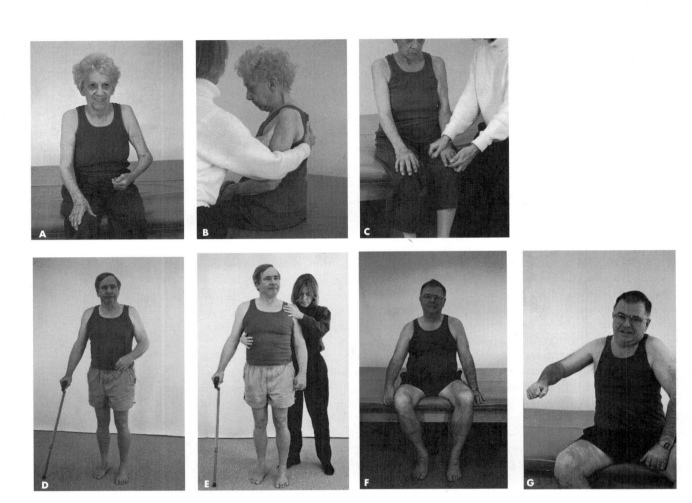

FIGURE 6-24 *(A)* Before treatment, the hemiplegic arm is hypertonic, with an anterior subluxation. *(B)* The therapist changes the position of the scapula and glenohumeral joint to move the humerus back into the glenoid fossa. *(C)* This results in an immediate reduction of hypertonicity in the hemiplegic arm. *(D & E)* Flexor posturing of the hemiplegic arm caused by poor balance. *(D)* The patient's hemiplegic arm flexes in standing. Although his trunk posture is fairly symmetric, the position of his cane tells us that he is avoiding supporting full weight on his hemiplegic leg. *(E)* The therapist has shifted more weight onto the hemiplegic leg and is lightly stabilizing the trunk. The patient's arm relaxes and hangs in extension by his side. Note how the position of his cane is more upright. *(F & G)* Increased muscle tone during volitional arm movements. *(F)* Before movement, the hemiplegic right arm rests in extension by the side of the body. *(G)* The patient lifts his arm using his available pattern of muscle control. The excessive effort used to produce this movement is evident from the patient's facial expression. *(Figure continues on p.161)*

Soft Tissue Shortening

Hypertonic muscles that have been maintained in shortened positions for weeks or months lose extensibility. These muscles gradually develop soft tissue shortening/contracture that prevents the muscle from being brought to its full length even when the resistance from hypertonicity has been reduced. Hypertonicity is often difficult to distinguish from soft tissue shortening and contracture, because both problems maintain the arm in a flexed position that resists extension. The therapist should suspect soft tissue restriction whenever treatment to decrease hypertonicity does not result in full muscle length. The experienced therapist learns to distinguish between the feel of hypertonicity and tissue restriction.

Treatment of Hypertonicity

Hypertonicity is associated with resistance to passive stretch. Hypertonic muscles are lengthened by correcting alignment, stabilizing the proximal end of the muscle, and gradually lengthening the distal end. Proximal muscles are lengthened first, beginning at the shoulder girdle and progressing to the elbow, wrist, and fingers. The selected muscle is lengthened to the maximal length available without resistance and held in this lengthened position until the recoil tension subsides and the muscle shows no further resistance to passive lengthening. At this time, the muscle is lengthened further to its full length. Sometimes the release of hypertonicity is gradual, so that the muscle lengthens a little bit, stops, and then lengthens a little more. Other times, the tension in the muscle gives way completely, allowing the muscle to be brought to its full length without further resistance. Hypertonicity caused by inappropriate muscle activation can also be decreased by asking for active movement in the spastic muscle and/or its antagonist muscle. Hypertonic muscles that have developed secondary problems of length will require stretching over multiple treatment sessions before full muscle length has been restored.

Permanent changes in muscle tone are not possible until the underlying causes of hypertonicity have been addressed. When the posturing of the arm results from poor trunk and leg control, the hemiplegic arm will continue to flex until the trunk is more stable and symmetric and the hemiplegic leg is able to support weight and move easily. On the other hand, if the cause of upper extremity hypertonicity is poor alignment of the scapula and shoulder joint, treatment of the shoulder to restore normal mechanical relationships and lengthen shortened muscles will result in relatively quick improvements in arm position. If hypertonicity in the arm is due to excessive muscle activation or inappropriate coactivation of muscle during active movements, treatment must stress quieting unwanted muscle activity and reeducation of the correct sequences of muscle firing. The wide number of possible explanations of hypertonicity probably explains the inconsistent results that antispasticity medications, such as baclofen, have for most stroke patients and the transient results from treatment that only stretches spastic muscles without addressing the underlying movement problems. In our experience, it is possible to reduce hypertonicity dramatically and sometimes to eliminate it. These changes occur through treatment that addresses the appropriate underlying causes for the hypertonicity and provides the patient with new patterns of movement and coordination that replace undesirable patterns of muscle activation.

Pain

Pain in the hemiplegic shoulder, arm, and hand is a common problem in patients with many types of neurologic pathology. Arm pain may be directly related to primary and secondary impairments (e.g., the muscle pain that comes with flaccid hemiplegia and inferior subluxation or is a result of trauma to muscles and joints caused by accident or therapy). The type, location, frequency, and intensity of pain vary widely among patients. Every patient with a painful arm must be thoroughly assessed to identify the type of pain and its causes before treatment is started. The more common types of arm pain are discussed below.

Pain Related to Changes in Joint Alignment and Mobility

The most common cause of shoulder pain in hemiplegia is poor joint mechanics at the shoulder joint. There are two reasons for this disruption of normal joint mechanics:

1. Scapula and glenohumeral joint positions are abnormal, with inferior subluxation. When the humerus is inferiorly subluxed, passive movements of the humerus are not accompanied by appropriate scapula rotation. Joint pain will occur at about 90 degrees of forward flexion, when the capsule is pinched between the acromium and the humerus.

2. Hypertonicity and muscle shortening prevent the scapula from moving on the rib cage in accordance with scapulohumeral rhythm. If muscle restrictions block scapula rotation from accompanying humeral movements, shoulder pain occurs when the humerus impinges on the acromium at around 90 degrees of forward flexion.

Shoulder pain is localized to the shoulder joint and is described by the patient as being "sharp" or "stabbing." It resolves when the humerus is lowered below the height where scapulohumeral rhythm is necessary (i.e., below 90 degrees of flexion). The cause of this pain is removed by reseating the humerus in the fossa and/or freeing the scapula to rotate correctly. Once these goals have been accomplished, the arm should be able to be moved above 90 degrees of flexion without pain.

Pain Related to Changes in Muscle Tone and Length

Muscle and/or soft tissue pain occurs when shortened structures are lengthened too quickly or stretched beyond their comfortable resting length. Muscles and soft tissues in the hemiplegic arm shorten when changes in alignment alter the resting length of muscles and when spasticity or involuntary muscle contraction cause active shortening. Over time, the affected tissues lose elasticity; skin, muscle, and fascia become thick and resistant to active or passive lengthening. In the arm, the problem is complicated by the fact that this tightness is often found in muscles that cross two joints and connect multiple segments of the arm (e.g., biceps and wrist flexors) or that connect the arm to the trunk (e.g., latissimus and pectoral muscles). The therapist's attempts to restore normal alignment to the trunk, shoulder girdle, and arm may cause these muscles to be lengthened at their origins and insertions simultaneously. Stretching both ends of the muscle often provokes muscle pain in the muscles placed on stretch. Since multiple muscle groups in the arm are often tight, treatment to restore normal alignment may also result in stretch of tight muscles from the trunk down the length of the arm. Muscle pain often also occurs during treatment when multiple tight muscles are all placed on stretch at the same time.

Pain in muscles and tissues that are being stretched is experienced over the length of the stretched areas. The patient will rub his hand over a muscle or group of muscles to identify where he hurts. The pain is described as a pulling or stretching sensation, which can vary in intensity from "a good stretch" to a feeling of "tearing" or "burning". During treatment, the pain decreases or resolves when the amount of stretch-induced tension on the muscle is decreased or the number of tight muscles being simultaneously lengthened is reduced. This generally allows the therapist to continue arm treatment without causing further discomfort. If the therapist ignores the patient's pain and does not decrease the amount of stretch, the patient may develop chronic myalgia, which makes any change in tissue length painful. Restoring normal alignment and lengthening tight tissues are important parts of the process of retraining movement patterns. However, the therapist must develop sufficient manual skill to identify when the tissues are on stretch and the amount of stretch she is imposing on the different segments of the body. Selective pain-free stretching combined with movement reeducation will result in gains in tissue length without pain.

Pain Associated with Changes in Sensation

Many patients experience diminished sensation or problems with sensory interpretation in the hemiplegic arm as one of their primary impairments. Pain occurs in patients with sensory impairments when either sensory messages are not perceived during treatment until severe pain is produced or when sensory messages from multiple sensory systems overload the processing capabilities of the nervous system and are perceived as painful. Arm pain related to sensory impairment is most common in the acute care stage of treatment and in patients with severe weakness and hypotonia.

When pain related to poor sensory processing occurs during a treatment session, the patient may not be able to describe the pain or locate where exactly he is uncomfortable. It often occurs unexpectedly in the middle of a treatment session, leaving the therapist puzzled over what suddenly went wrong. The patient's description of his pain is often vague or confusing. Descriptions such as "It just doesn't feel good" or "I don't like what you're doing" are common. The patient is usually unable to localize this type of pain, often pointing to multiple places on the arm.

Whenever sensory impairments are suspected as a cause of arm pain, the therapist should modify her handling. She should carefully limit her use of simultaneous tactile, proprioceptive, and kinesthetic input and move more slowly to give the nervous system time to receive and process the input from these systems. At the same time, she should rule out other causes for the pain, by carefully realigning the shoulder joint and decreasing the amount of stretch on tight tissues. If the patient continues to complain of discomfort, the therapist may have to end the treatment session and resume more carefully on her next visit. It is very important that the therapist treat the arm without causing pain, so the patient does not associate therapy with pain and thus resist arm treatment.

Shoulder-Hand Syndrome

Shoulder-hand syndrome in neurologic patients is similar to dystrophic syndromes that develop after orthopedic injuries. It begins with diffuse aching in the shoulder, arm, and hand and may progress to changes in skin and bone and muscle atrophy. The development of shoulder-hand syndrome is clinically associated with edema in the hand and with dense flaccid hemiplegia. Shoulder-hand syndrome, a chronic pain syndrome, may have its origins in painful episodes during treatment or begin with severe arm pain experienced during transfers or in bed. From these acute episodes, pain builds up in the arm until the arm hurts all the time and in places that were not initially painful. At its most severe, the affected arm cannot be touched or moved without pain, and the patient is reluctant to participate in therapy for fear of further pain. The treatment for shoulder-hand syndrome is described below.

Acute Versus Chronic Pain

Most instances of arm pain occur suddenly during treatment for the reasons discussed above or develop as a result of a fall or injury to the arm. If the therapist is able to diagnose the cause of the pain and is careful to change her handling to both avoid further pain and eliminate the problems that have contributed to the development of pain, acute shoulder pain should resolve quickly and not reappear. On the other hand, if the therapist continues with treatment activities that are painful to the patient, a chronic pain situation will develop. In chronic pain, all movements of the arm are painful, the arm and hand are often painful to the touch, and pain is present at night or at times during the day when there is nothing to provoke it. Arm treatment is more difficult with chronic pain, as the patient may come to associate therapy with pain and avoid treatment. However, it is important for therapists to treat the arm with chronic pain, with the goals of eliminating arm pain and preparing the patient to participate in active arm treatment without recurrence of pain.

The treatment of chronic arm pain has several important steps or stages.

1. *Eliminate pain from treatment and the patient's home routine.* Therapists often perform range of motion and other exercises that cause severe arm pain or prescribe painful exercises for the patient to do at home. Usually, the removal of painful exercises from the patient's treatment program results in an immediate and dramatic decrease in the intensity and frequency of pain. In our experience, self-range and range of motion exercises that are performed without appropriate shoulder mechanics are the most common cause of chronic shoulder pain. These exercises may be selected because of fears of losing range of motion or because of a misguided belief in the "no pain, no gain" philosophy. The pain associated with these exercises is often so severe that it leads to the very limitations in joint movement that it is designed to prevent. The elimination of painful movements is the important first step to eliminating pain. It demonstrates to the patient the therapist's commitment to resolving his problem.

2. *Desensitize the arm and hand to touch.* In chronic pain situations, even light touch to the affected arm or hand is perceived as painful. This tactile hypersensitivity must be decreased, so that the therapist can begin to touch the arm without causing discomfort. Most of the work of desensitization can be done outside of therapy by the patient or his family. The patient should be shown how to touch and lightly rub his arm and hand, gradually increasing the amount of pressure and the duration of touch until he is able to tolerate tactile input without discomfort. During treatment, the therapist follows a similar process until the patient does not find her touch aversive or painful.

3. *Eliminate hand edema.* Edema in the hand has been shown to be associated with shoulder pain and shoulder-hand syndrome. Edema also places the skin under stretch and blocks joint movement (Fig. 6-24H). Its removal increases blood circulation to the arm and increases available passive motion. Active treatment of edema begins as soon as the hand and arm have been desensitized to touch. Edema should be treated and eliminated so that the tissues of the lower arm and hand become soft, pliable, and easily moved. The patient and his family can be shown how to soften the edema using squeezing/compression and how to free the skin from connective tissue and bone. When the edema is soft and pitting and the skin soft and mobile, the therapist uses manual pressure to move the edema from the forearm and hand.

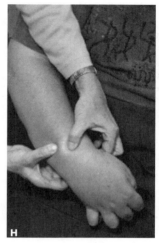

FIGURE 6-24H *(Continued)* (H) Edema in the hand and forearm.

4. *Introduce pain-free arm movements.* The above three steps prepare the arm and hand for a more active treatment program. Generally, the time spent in those stages will decrease the intensity of pain and establish a trusting relationship between patient and therapist. As the therapist begins to move the arm, it is important that she continue that trust by not causing pain. To do this, she begins treatment with activities that reestablish mobility in the scapula and avoids movements of the glenohumeral joint until the scapula has mobility in the planes of elevation/depression, abduction/adduction, and upward rotation. Sitting, supine, and sidelying scapula mobilization and forearm weightbearing are the best activities for this stage because they are different from the treatment activities that previously provoked pain. Once the scapula has regained mobility and the patient is able to tolerate scapula movements without pain, the therapist can introduce guided arm movements below 60 degrees of forward flexion.

5. *Gradually increase movement demands.* In the final stage of treatment, the therapist gradually increases the variety and complexity of arm movements that are used in treatment. To do this, she may increase the range of arm movement, ask the patient to be more active during weightbearing and movements in space, or teach the patient to incorporate his hemiplegic arm into activities of daily living and functional tasks. Secondary problems of joint hypomobility and muscle shortening are also addressed in this stage of treatment. The therapist should continue to be careful to avoid pain, as she gradually increases the tolerance of the patient for movement and sensory feedback. When this stage of treatment is complete, the arm is pain-free and the patient is able to fully participate in treatment without recurrence of pain.

Although the treatment program outlined above requires a major investment of treatment time, its long-term benefit to the patient makes the time expenditure worthwhile. In our practice, this program has been successful with almost 100% of patients with painful shoulders and shoulder-hand syndrome. The program also works with the less common but equally painful leg-foot pain.

Loss of Functional Performance

Neurologic patients with all levels of motor impairment experience loss of functional use of their involved arm. In the acute and flaccid patient, loss of functional use of the arm is directly related to the patient's inability to activate muscles with sufficient strength and/or coordination for task performance. However, motor recovery and muscle strength do not automatically translate into functional use of the arm. Many patients who have the ability to move their arm in functional patterns and to use their hand for grasp do not spontaneously incorporate these movements into life tasks. There are probably several explanations for this failure. Many patients are discouraged from using their hand by the slowness of their movements and the amount of effort necessary to move the hand. Other patients may have difficulty planning the correct sequences of movements involved in the task, even though the movements themselves are in their motor repertoire. The fact that learned disuse is so prevalent in the hemiplegic arm emphasizes the importance of combining movement reeducation with functional objects and tasks as quickly as possible, so that the patient learns to perform functional movements with his newly acquired motor control. The use of common household objects rather than therapy objects makes this training even more concrete.

ASSESSMENT GUIDELINES

The assessment of shoulder and arm movements and problems should focus on three general areas: (1) upper extremity alignment and mobility, (2) available movement patterns in the shoulder, arm, and hand, and (3) functional use in the arm and hand.

I. Assess alignment and mobility in the shoulder, arm, and hand.

Describe the resting alignment of trunk, scapula, and arm.

Correct trunk alignment and identify scapula and shoulder joint position.

Describe the resting alignment in the arm, forearm, and hand.

II. Assess control of movement

Describe available extended arm reach patterns and the range in which the patient has control.

Describe control of elbow flexion patterns.

Describe available movements in forearm, wrist, and hand.

Identify ability to combine distal movements, with shoulder and elbow patterns.

What additional movements or muscles are evident when you assist proximal and distal movements of the arm? What significant movement patterns cannot be performed?

III. Assess the impairments that affect the arm

Correct trunk position and subluxation if necessary. Identify the passive mobility of shoulder girdle with the arm by the side of the body.

Which movements are restricted? What is the available range?

What primary and secondary impairments are contributing to the changes in mobility?

Assess the alignment of the elbow, forearm, wrist, and hand. What problems are evident? Try to line up the axis of the shoulder with the forearm, wrist, and hand. Identify any impairments that interfere with this process.

Assess functional abilities

What functional uses of the hand or arm does the patient indicate that he can perform?

What problems limit this use? What functional movements of the arm and hand should the patient be prepared for?

THERAPY GOALS

Functional Goals

The treatment of arm problems and retraining of arm movements is necessary to help the patient achieve the following functional goals:

1. Establish postural control of the involved arm, so that the hemiplegic arm rests naturally by the side of the body and moves appropriately with the trunk during functional movements and task performance.

2. Establish control of movements necessary for use of the arm in bilateral and unilateral arm tasks.

3. Increase the performance of the hemiplegic arm in life tasks.

Treatment Goals and Techniques

Treatment Goal: Restore alignment to the subluxed shoulder and arm in preparation for movement reeducation.

Treatment Technique: Reduction of inferior subluxation. The therapist must correct the position of the scapula and glenohumeral joint and reseat the humerus in the fossa whenever the hemiplegic shoulder has an inferior subluxation. Before correcting scapula and humerus, the therapist must carefully assess the position of the patient's trunk and scapula. This assessment allows her to understand the relationship between trunk position and scapula alignment and to systematically correct both problems (Fig. 6-25A–G). Techniques for changing the position of the scapula/glenohumeral joint with anterior and superior subluxations are described in Figure 6-26.

Treatment Technique: Support of the subluxed shoulder and distal arm for movement reeducation. The therapist must be able to keep her correction of scapula-shoulder joint position and add control of the lower arm and hand to move the arm in space. To do this easily, she has to switch the position of her hands. With this technique, the therapist will use her back hand to control the scapula and shoulder joint, and her front hand to control the distal arm and hand (Fig. 6-25H–K).

FIGURE 6-25 (A) Right hemiplegia. The right humerus is subluxed inferiorly. (B) The starting alignment of the trunk and scapula. The right scapula appears lower than the left. The right scapula does not appear downwardly rotated, although downward rotation is the cause of inferior subluxation. The right side of the rib cage appears longer, and the ribs look flared and prominent on the right. Note how the lumbar spine appears to angle toward the right. (C) The therapist corrects the position of the trunk, by moving the right side of the rib cage down and in. This correction shows the true position of the right scapula. The right scapula now appears lower and downwardly rotated compared with the left scapula. (D) Having identified the true position of the scapula, the therapist will now correct the position of the right scapula and glenohumeral joint to remove the inferior subluxation. The therapist faces the hemiplegic arm. She will use her hand that is closest to the patient's back to control his scapula, and her front hand to support the glenohumeral joint. She slips her right hand between the patient's ribs and arm. Her left hand places the humerus in slight abduction to make a space for the right hand. (E) The therapist raises her right hand until it rests in the axilla between the ribs and the arm. She uses both hands to lift the shoulder girdle up slightly. This maneuver partially reduces the separation between the scapula and humerus. (F) The therapist moves her left hand to the scapula, so that her left fingers lie along the vertebral border and inferior angle of the scapula. She moves the inferior angle of the scapula laterally to rotate the scapula upward. As the scapula upwardly rotates, the therapist will feel the humerus slip back into the glenoid fossa. At this time, she should externally rotate the humerus to neutral. The subluxation has now been reduced. (G) The therapist's right hand is holding the scapula and shoulder joint in its corrected position, while her left hand tucks the right side of the rib cage. The position of the scapula has been re-marked to show the symmetry in the shoulders, spine, and rib cage. (H & I) To switch hand position without letting go of the shoulder joint, the therapist slips her left hand in the axilla so that the fingers overlap those of the right hand. This two-handed axillary grip can also be used to mobilize the scapula. (J & K) The therapist removes her right hand from the axilla and moves it to the patient's hand. The therapist's left hand holds the shoulder joint in a stable position, so that the joint does not move when the right hand is removed. She grasps the patient's hemiplegic hand with her right hand as if shaking hands with him. With this grip, the therapist is able to maintain good alignment of the shoulder, compatible positions between proximal and distal arm, and extension of the wrist. The grip allows her to lift and move the arm with elbow extension and to position the forearm in pronation, midposition, or supination during arm movements.

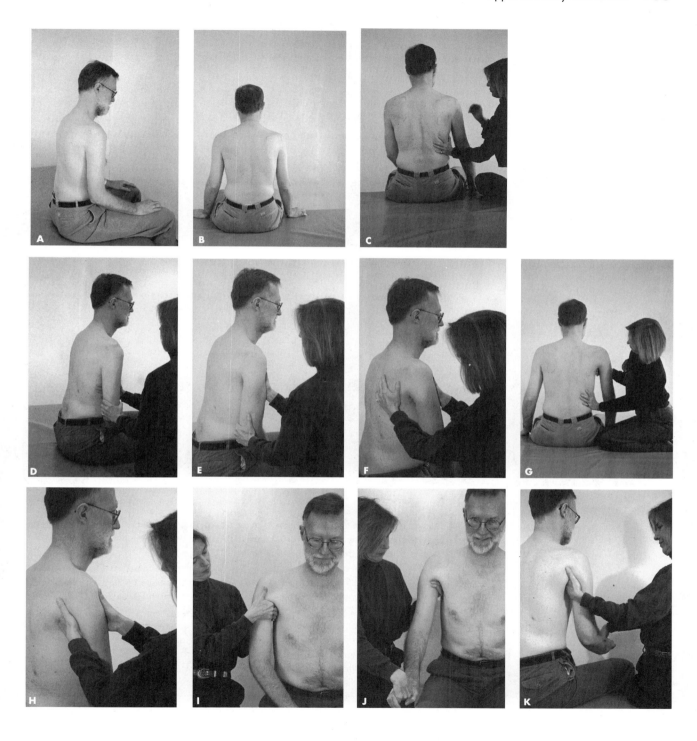

Treatment Goal: Increase scapula mobility and decrease hypertonicity to ensure normal scapulohumeral rhythm.

Treatment Technique: Shoulder girdle mobilization in sitting (Bobath treatment technique). Mobility of the scapula on the rib cage is a prerequisite for shoulder and arm movements and pain-free range of motion. The therapist should use the technique of scapula mobilization in sitting to check mobility in the scapula and ensure that it moves freely before beginning movement reeducation. Shoulder girdle mobilization in sitting is also one of the best techniques for quickly reducing flexor hypertonicity in the arm. This technique is also used for anterior and superior subluxations to restore the normal resting position of the scapula and humerus and decrease unbalanced muscle tension, so that these subluxations can be manually corrected (Fig. 6-26A–H).

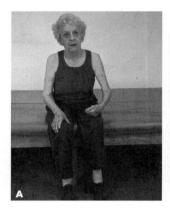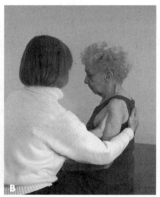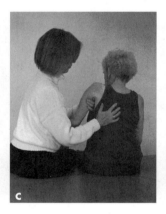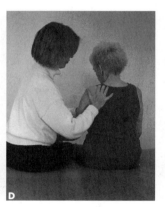

FIGURE 6-26 *(A)* The patient before treatment, left hemiplegia, anterior subluxation. *(B)* The therapist puts her left hand in the patient's axilla as described above in Figure 6-25E. Her right hand is placed on the scapula. The therapist will use her hands to increase mobility in the scapula in the planes of elevation/depression and abduction/adduction. These movements will also lengthen hypertonic or shortened muscles and bring the scapula in a more normal resting position on the rib cage. When the trunk position is extremely asymmetric, the therapist should correct trunk alignment before treating the hemiplegic shoulder. Trunk treatment is described in detail in Chapter 5. *(C)* The therapist moves the scapula into elevation. Her two hands move the scapula and shoulder joint up at the same rate and the same distance. The therapist stops the upward movement when the normal range of scapula glide is complete or when muscle tightness stops the motion. The therapist should always start scapula mobilization with elevation, even if the shoulder girdle is already elevated. The shoulder has a large range of glide into elevation. By bringing the shoulder girdle up, the therapist increases the range in which she can bring it down. *(D)* The therapist moves her left hand to the top of the scapula, so that her fingertips rest along the spine of the scapula. Her two hands move together to bring the scapula out of elevation to a normal resting position and, if possible, into slight depression. The movement into scapula depression lengthens tight scapula elevators, while the movement up lengthens the latissimus. The therapist should repeat these movements until muscle resistance is gone and the scapula moves freely in both directions. Often this movement will result in gradual decrease in hypertonicity in the elbow and lower arm. *(Figure continues.)*

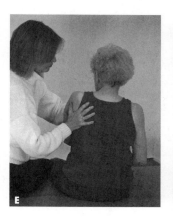
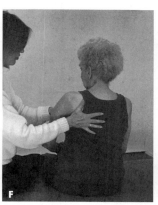
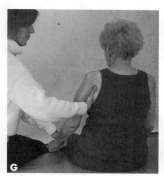
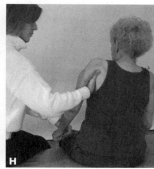

FIGURE 6-26 *(Continued)* *(E)* The therapist moves the scapula in the plane of abduction/adduction. Here her hands move the scapula and humerus forward into scapula abduction. As the shoulder girdle moves forward, the therapist allows the humerus to roll into internal rotation. This movement lengthens the muscles that connect the scapula to the spine. *(F)* The therapist moves the scapula back into adduction. During this movement, it is important that the therapist's left hand moves the front of the shoulder back and rolls the humerus into external rotation while the right hand moves the scapula toward the spine. This lengthens the pectoral and tight internal rotators of the shoulder. The therapist also repeats this movement until muscle hypertonicity or stiffness resolves. *(G & H)* Alternative hand placement. The therapist has moved her hands to the shaking hand grip described in Figure 6-25. This grip allows the therapist to hold the hemiplegic elbow in extension while moving the scapula. It makes it more difficult to control the movements of the scapula, as she has no direct control on the scapula. *(H)* Here her hands are elevating the scapula. Both hands maintain steady contact with the shoulder and hand and move up the same amount. To depress the scapula, the hand in the axilla relaxes its upward pressure and lets the shoulder down, while maintaining support of the axilla. The therapist must not use her control on the hemiplegic hand to pull the shoulder down, as this might distract the shoulder joint. *(Figure continues.)*

Treatment Technique: Lengthening hypertonic elbow flexors to gain elbow extension. Scapula mobilization usually results in decreased hypertonicity in the shoulder girdle. Often the elbow joint will release as well, since the movements of the scapula allow the therapist to reposition the glenohumeral joint. Scapula mobilization can be followed by specific techniques to decrease muscle tone in the elbow, forearm, wrist, and hand (Fig. 6-26I–O).

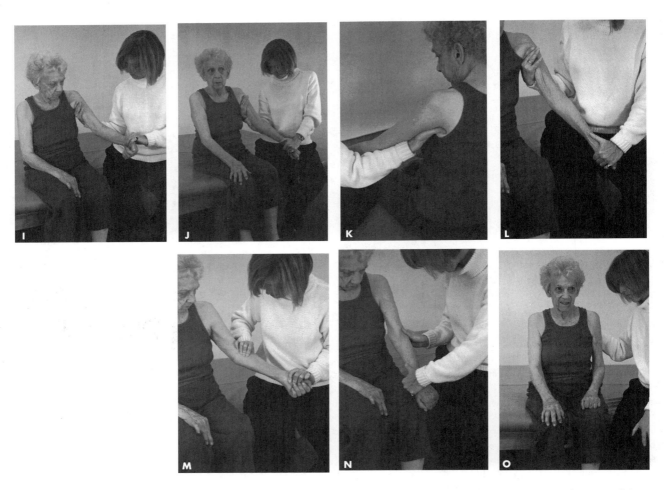

FIGURE 6-26 (*Continued*) *(I)* The therapist uses the shaking hand grip to maintain alignment of the shoulder and extend the elbow to its maximum available length. *(J & K)* She supports the back of the humerus against her right forearm and uses her left hand to pronate the patient's forearm and extend the elbow. This places the elbow flexors on stretch. *(L)* As the elbow flexors relax, the therapist gradually brings the elbow into full extension. Note the bands of muscle tightness in the biceps and in the forearm that are placed on stretch with this grip. *(M)* Once hypertonicity in the biceps has decreased, the therapist can supinate the forearm with the elbow in extension. Here she is doing soft tissue release on the tight tissues of the forearm. *(N)* The therapist holds the elbow in extension and returns the forearm to pronation. She is massaging the muscles of the elbow and top of the forearm. Note how the tissues have let go in the arm and forearm. *(O)* The position of the hemiplegic arm following scapula mobilization and elbow lengthening; compare to the starting position of the arm in Fig.A. The finger flexor muscles are still tight. (*Figure continues.*)

Treatment Technique: Opening a fisted hand. Decreasing wrist and finger hypertonicity should not be attempted until muscle tension in the shoulder, elbow, and forearm has responded to treatment. At this time, the therapist may lengthen hypertonic wrist and finger flexors and open the fisted hand (Fig. 6-26P–T).

Additional suggestions: shoulder mobilization in supine/side lying; forearm weightbearing.

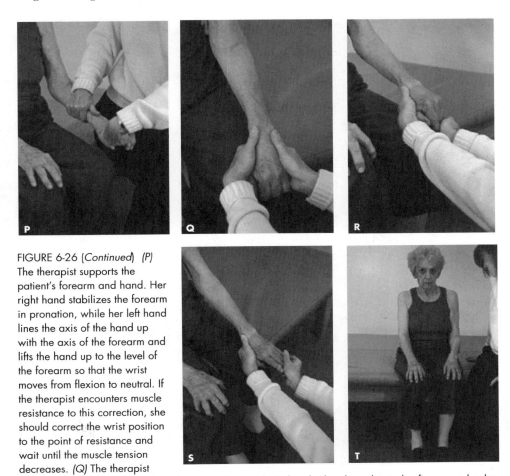

FIGURE 6-26 *(Continued)* *(P)* The therapist supports the patient's forearm and hand. Her right hand stabilizes the forearm in pronation, while her left hand lines the axis of the hand up with the axis of the forearm and lifts the hand up to the level of the forearm so that the wrist moves from flexion to neutral. If the therapist encounters muscle resistance to this correction, she should correct the wrist position to the point of resistance and wait until the muscle tension decreases. *(Q)* The therapist moves her hands to either side of the patient's hemiplegic hand. She places her index fingers under the carpal bones, her other fingers in the palm, and her thumbs over the top of the carpal bones so that the tips of the thumbs rest on the distal radius and ulna. The therapist uses her fingers to lift the carpal and metacarpal bones up until they are level with the distal forearm. When wrist and finger flexor tendons are shortened across the wrist, the therapist will meet resistance to this movement. She continues to hold this position against resistance until muscle pull across the wrist has decreased and the carpal bones are level with the radius. *(R)* The therapist stabilizes the position of the hand and wrist with her left hand. She uses the fingertips of her right hand to extend the interphalangeal joints of the fingers, keeping the metacarpophalangeal joints in flexion. When finger flexors are shortened in the palm, she will also feel resistance to this motion. The therapist should hold the fingers in a partially extended position until the resistance to extension disappears. *(S)* When finger resistance decreases, the interphalangeal and metacarpophalangeal joints are brought into full extension. *(T)* Following this technique the hand is open and relaxed. The therapist is now ready to begin movement reeducation. Again compare the position of the hemiplegic arm and hand to Fig. A.

Treatment Goal: Reeducate functional movements of the hemiplegic arm.

Treatment Technique: Reeducation of extended arm reach patterns (Fig. 6-27A–M).

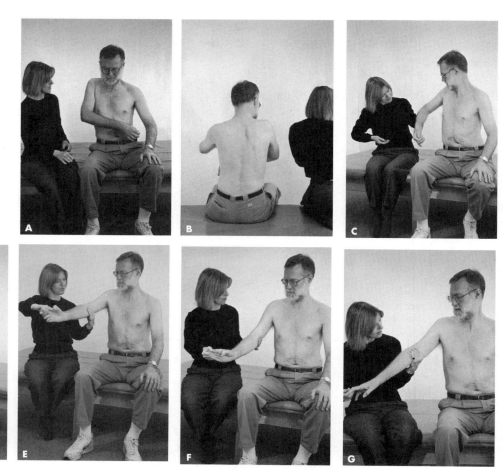

FIGURE 6-27 *(A & B)* Right hemiplegia. The patient is attempting to reach forward. He is able to activate scapula and shoulder muscles but lacks control of elbow extension. He initiates the movement with shoulder elevation and elbow flexion. *(C)* Abducted reach. He uses a combination of deltoid and trunk rotation to bring the arm to the side. Elbow extension is not available. *(D)* The therapist begins reeducation of extended arm reach patterns from this starting position. She is using the shaking hand grip described previously to hold the arm in extension before lifting it off the knee. *(E)* She moves the arm into forward flexion. As she moves the hand from the knee, she rotates the forearm from pronation into neutral rotation so that the hand is in a functional position for grasp. During these movements, the therapist asks the patient to first feel the movement, then to try to assist. When she feels the patient actively assisting her, she may also stop the arm movement and ask the patient to try to hold his arm briefly where she has placed it. *(F & G)* The therapist may also practice rotational movements of the shoulder joint. Here she is moving the arm from neutral rotation at the shoulder and forearm to internal rotation/pronation. Practice of these movements prepares the patient to approach objects efficiently and position his hand for different patterns of grasp. *(Figure continues.)*

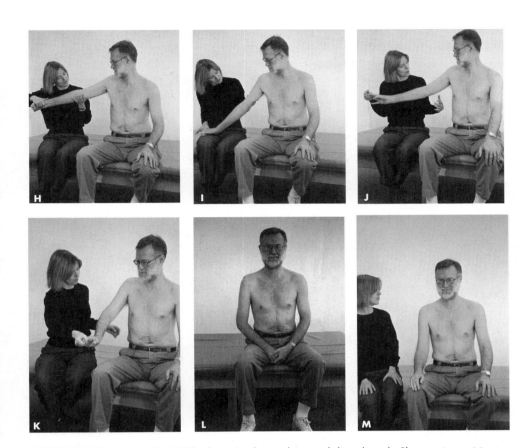

FIGURE 6-27 (*Continued*) (*H & I*) The therapist also reeducates abducted reach. She practices raising the arm from an abducted position by the side of the body and also moving from forward flexion into horizontal abduction. At the end of all extended arm patterns, the therapist should return the hand to rest on the knee or on the treatment mat, so that the patient learns to stop the muscle contraction when movement has been completed. (*J*) When the therapist feels that the patient is assisting her guided movements, she gradually lightens or removes part of her control. Here the therapist has removed her control of the shoulder girdle. Her right hand is supporting part of the weight of the lower arm, while the patient controls his shoulder and elbow position. Since the therapist has only light control of the hemiplegic hand, the patient is doing most of the work to hold this position of his arm. The therapist will move the arm to another position and ask the patient to hold the new position. (*K*) The therapist is now asking the patient to lower his arm to his knee. This activity is harder than the one in the previous figure because the patient has to use eccentric muscle activity to control the weight of his arm, rather than isometric control to stabilize a position. During this harder task, the hemiplegic shoulder has begun to elevate and internally rotate slightly. The quality of the patient's movements often decline slightly as the therapist removes some of her control, but this is a necessary part of motor learning. When the patient has an easier time performing this movement, the therapist will try to help him maintain external rotation while moving the arm. (*L & M*) The patient's shoulder position before and after treatment. Before treatment, the subluxation is evident, and after treatment the subluxation has almost disappeared. This improvement in shoulder alignment is not uncommon when treatment has successfully realigned the scapula and activated shoulder girdle muscles. The therapist has used movements of the arm above 60 degrees of flexion in this treatment series to increase appropriate use of scapula muscles and scapula rotation. In the short term, the subluxation is likely to reappear relatively quickly as the effects of treatment fade. However, as the shoulder muscles get stronger and the patient learns to move his hemiplegic arm with more normal scapulohumeral rhythm, the size of the separation is likely to diminish.

Treatment Technique: Reeducation of elbow and forearm movements. Arm movements that combine elbow flexion with shoulder movement and/or forearm rotation are extremely important for arm function close to the body. These movement patterns should be part of arm treatment from the earliest days of rehabilitation. Since the hemiplegic arm is often flexed at the elbow and elbow extension in difficult or impossible, therapists tend to focus early reeducation efforts on extended arm reach and neglect movements of elbow flexion. This is unfortunate, because practice of these movements in treatment helps the patient learn to recruit elbow flexor muscles appropriately and to quiet the elbow flexors once movement has been completed (Fig. 6-28).

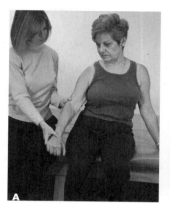
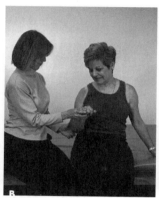
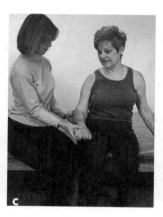
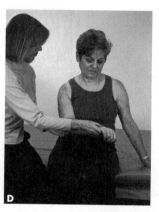
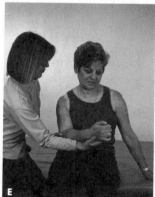

FIGURE 6-28 *(A)* Right hemiplegia. The therapist will reeducate elbow flexion, with the humerus stabilized by the side of the body and elbow flexion combined with shoulder movements. This treatment series also demonstrates practice of forearm rotation. The therapist begins with the elbow in extension. Her left hand holds the humerus stable with the shoulder in neutral extension or slight flexion. Her right hand holds the wrist in slight extension with the axis of the hand in line with the axis of the pronated forearm. The therapist will control the movements of the elbow with her right hand. Her left hand prevents inappropriate use of shoulder muscles during movements of the elbow. The therapist has chosen to start to reeducate elbow flexion with the forearm in pronation to avoid excessive use of the biceps muscle. Later, she can practice elbow flexion with the forearm in neutral rotation and in supination. *(B & C)* The therapist moves the elbow into flexion and back into extension. Initially, the patient is told to use her elbow muscles to bend the elbow and to relax these muscles gradually to extend the elbow. This part of training emphasizes concentric and eccentric muscle activation. Later, the therapist should help the patient actively fire her triceps to straighten the elbow by bringing the elbow into flexion and asking the patient to straighten it. Once this control is established, the patient may practice using elbow flexors to bend the elbow and then switching to elbow extensors to straighten it. *(D & E)* Reeducation of forearm pronation/supination should be introduced at the same time as elbow flexion. In this figure, the therapist has flexed the elbow to 90 degrees and is practicing forearm rotation from pronation to supination and back. Forearm rotation with the elbow in flexion is very important to position the thumb and fingers for grasp and manipulation. *(Figure continues.)*

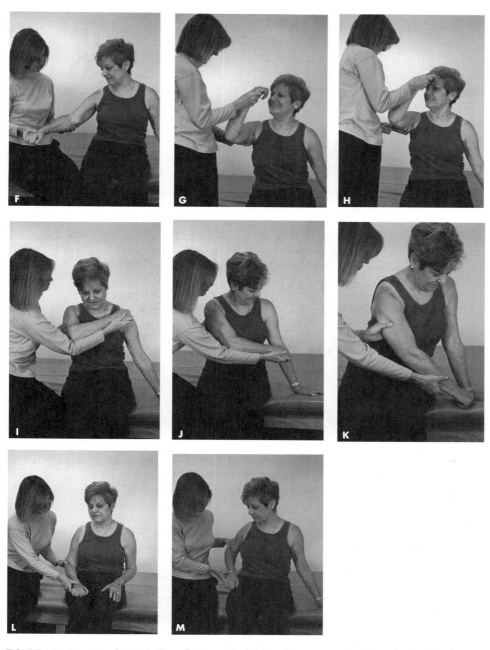

FIGURE 6-28 (*Continued*) *(F–H)* Elbow flexion with shoulder flexion is used to bring the hand to the mouth or hair. In this pattern, the forearm rotates from pronation toward supination as the shoulder and elbow flex. The therapist can have the patient focus on assisting one part of this complex movement at a time before putting all the pieces together. *(I–K)* Bringing the hand to the opposite arm combines humeral horizontal adduction with elbow flexion and pronation. In this series, the therapist practices extending the elbow with the arm across the body. As the hemiplegic hand touches the mat, the therapist lightly pushes the hand into the support and tells the patient to stop working with her arm muscles. Teaching the arm muscles to quiet after movement is as important to reeducation as teaching the correct sequence of movement reeducation. The therapist could also practice control of the shoulder by having the patient move the hand from the head to the opposite shoulder or from the head to the ipsilateral shoulder. *(L & M)* Practice moving the hand from the knee toward the hip or trunk is also an important functional pattern. The therapist's left hand moves the humerus into shoulder hyperextension while her right hand moves the hand backward, increasing elbow flexion. (*Figure continues.*)

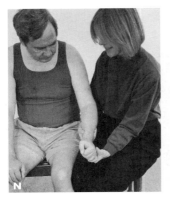
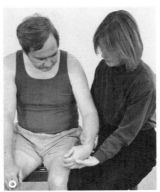

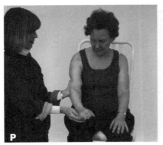
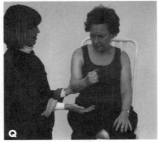
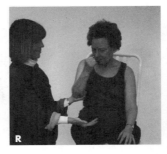
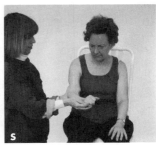

FIGURE 6-28 (*Continued*) *(N & O)* The therapist also reeducates movements of wrist flexion and extension. In these figures, she is assisting wrist movements with the forearm in midposition and the arm by the side of the body. Since wrist extension is one of the most difficult movements for hemiplegic patients, the therapist should reeducate wrist extension before wrist flexion. Movements of the wrist from extension into flexion are usually easier for the patient to perform and may be added once wrist extensors are able to stabilize the wrist in extension. Wrist flexion/extension should also be practiced with the forearm in pronation and the elbow in flexion. *(P–S)* Active-assistive movement reeducation is followed by independent practice of functional movements. In this sequence, the patient practices bringing her hemiplegic hand to her mouth. This movement sequence combines elbow flexion with forearm rotation and sustained wrist extension. She begins the movement with the forearm in pronation and the wrist in slight extension. As the elbow moves into flexion, she rotates the forearm from pronation to neutral rotation, maintaining the wrist in constant extension. To bring the hand to her mouth, she rotates the forearm into supination. As she returns her hand to rest on the therapist's hand, her elbow extends, her forearm rotates back into pronation, and her wrist stays in slight extension. The coordination of elbow flexion with forearm rotation can be varied by asking the patient to reach her hand to different parts of her body or for objects on a table.

Treatment Goal: Increase strength and control of arm movements in space. Once the hemiplegic arm is able to assist actively the therapist's guided movements, the therapist should gradually withdraw her assistance. The following treatment activities demonstrate three treatment variations in which the patient is more active during arm movements.

Treatment Technique: Bilateral arm movements with distal control. (Fig. 6-29).

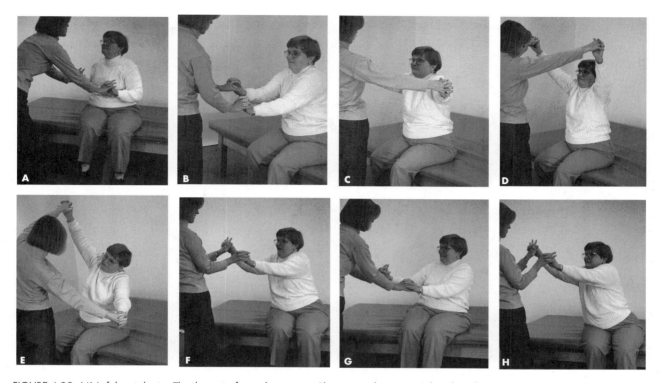

FIGURE 6-29 (A) Left hemiplegia. The therapist faces the patient. She grasps the patient's hands with her hands, palm to palm, fingers interlaced, and wrists extended. The therapist asks for patterns of forward reach that combine shoulder flexion with elbow extension and for extended arm reach patterns with trunk weight shifts. (B) The therapist begins by asking the patient to reach her arms forward and straighten both elbows. The therapist bends her elbows and moves her hands back as the patient reaches forward, so that their palms remain close together. The therapist can offer slight resistance to the patient's elbow extension during this movement. This resistance provides increased sensory information that helps the patient recruit elbow extensors and shoulder flexors. It will also increase muscle strength in the shoulder and elbow. (C & D) The therapist can also use this grip to train and strengthen extended arm reach patterns. In these figures, the therapist moves the patient's hands from the front of the body into horizontal abduction, then into elevation. During these movements, the patient's arm is maintained above 90 degrees of elevation with elbow extension. This requires that the scapula and triceps muscles work constantly against the pull of gravity. The patient is obviously active because the therapist maintains only light contact with the patient's hands.(E) The therapist is making the activity harder for the patient by adding an upper-body-initiated initiated lateral trunk movement to the demands on the arm. During this movement, the arms actually remain in a constant position while the trunk moves. (F–H) The therapist varies the activity by asking for movement sequences that combine arm reach with trunk weight shifts. (F) The therapist asks the patient to reach forward with her arms and weight shift onto her right hip in an extension rotation pattern. (G) The patient maintains her arms up and shifts her weight on a backward diagonal to her left hip. This produces flexion rotation in the trunk. (H) The patient shifts on a forward diagonal to the right. This treatment activity asks both the trunk and arms to work hard and prepares for bilateral reach patterns with trunk rotation. The combination of arm and trunk movements could also be repeated with the body in midline, so that the patient combines arm reach with lower-trunk-initiated anterior/posterior movements and with trunk rotation to the left.

Treatment Technique: Practice of arm movement on a wall. The therapist can use a wall to help the patient practice arm movements in difficult ranges and to increase the strength and endurance of the shoulder girdle and elbow (Fig. 6-30).

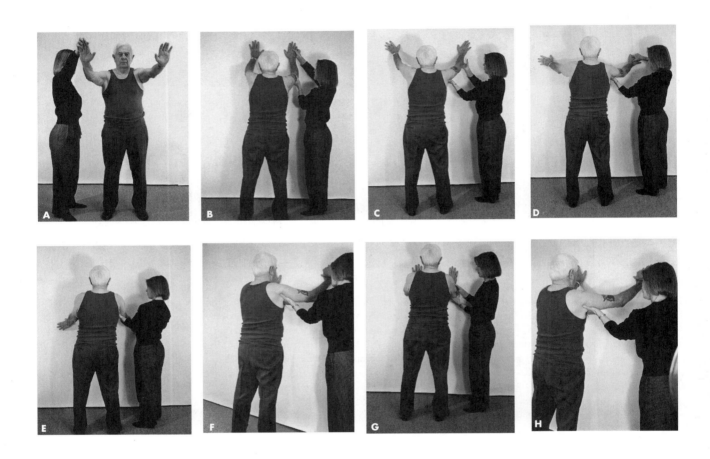

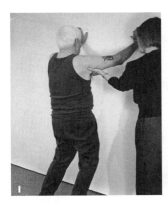
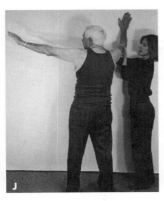
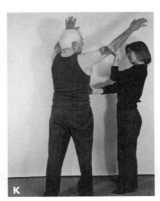
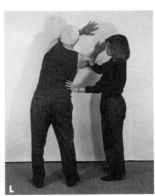

FIGURE 6-30 (*A*) Right hemiplegia. The patient has good motor recovery throughout the arm but has difficulty holding the arm above 90 degrees of elevation. The therapist will use the wall to build strength in the arm in this difficult range. (*B*) The patient faces the wall with his feet a comfortable arm's length away. The patient places his uninvolved arm on the wall, and the therapist assists the placement of the hemiplegic arm. In this treatment series, the therapist starts with the arm's at 120 degrees of shoulder flexion. This is higher than the patient can lift his arm independently. The amount of shoulder flexion could be decreased if muscle tightness restricted scapula rotation. (*C & D*) The patient moves his hands on the wall into horizontal abduction. The therapist is lightly supporting the humerus and forearm of the hemiplegic arm. Her support may be needed to prevent the arm from falling off the wall. It may also be needed to assist elbow extension and ensure the proper mechanical relationships among trunk/scapula, humerus, and distal arm. As the arm moves into horizontal abduction, the shoulder joint must externally rotate. Note the hemiplegic elbow is too flexed during this movement. This inappropriate elbow flexion occurs when the shoulder joint has not externally rotated sufficiently. (*E*) The therapist continues the movement below shoulder height. In this position, the shoulder must be fully externally rotated and the forearm supinated. Practice of moving in this arc of movement is one of the best ways to increase active control of shoulder external rotation. (*F*) The patient can also use the wall to practice and strengthen elbow extension. The therapist starts with the arm on the wall at approximately 90 degrees of shoulder flexion. (*G*) The patient bends his elbows and brings his upper trunk closer to the wall. (*H*) He straightens his elbows and pushes back from the wall. The therapist's hand in the axilla prevents excessive shoulder elevation and internal rotation during this movement. The following movements can be used to build endurance in the hemiplegic arm. (*I*) The patient performs knee bends while keeping both arms extended against the wall. (*J*) The patient holds his hemiplegic arm stable on the wall. He rotates his upper trunk to the left and reaches his left hand away from the wall to the side. As his trunk rotates away from the hemiplegic arm, the hemiplegic shoulder is placed in more abduction and external rotation. (*K*) The therapist lightly assists the right rotation of the arm and upper trunk. (*L*) The patient moves both arms to the right while the upper trunk initiates a lateral weight shift to the right. This movement should be repeated to the left. (*Figure continues.*)

FIGURE 6-30 (*Continued*)
(*M–O*) The therapist removes
her assistance, and the patient
moves his hands on the wall
independently. Note the slight
loss of external rotation in the
right shoulder during abduction.
(*P–R*) After treatment, the patient
is able to easily move his hemiplegic arm in space above 90
degrees of flexion. The wall
exercises would be a good
addition to his home program.

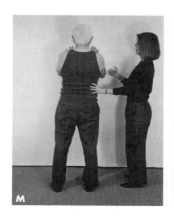

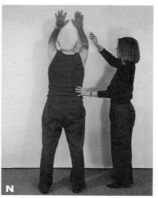

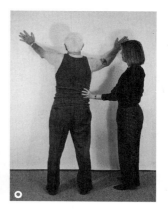

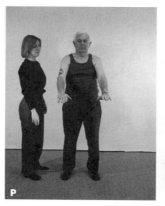

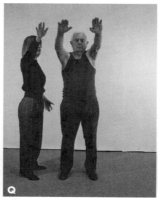

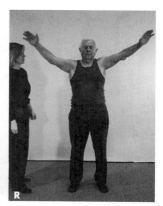

Treatment Technique: Independent practice—bilateral grasp. Cane exercises or similar movements using other objects such as balls or bolsters can also be used for independent practice and strengthening. In these exercises, the two arms move in symmetric patterns. The therapist may vary the position of the arms and the movement patterns that are performed through careful selection of objects. For example, cane exercises require arm movements with the forearm in pronation and the hand closed, while a large therapy ball places the forearm in neutral and the hand flat (Fig. 6-31).

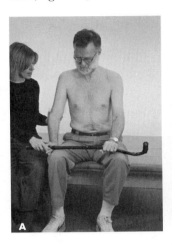
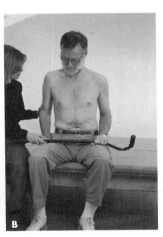
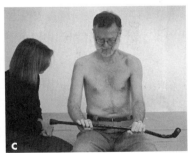
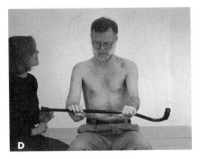

FIGURE 6-31 Right hemiplegia. (*A & B*) The therapist begins by helping the patient establish a proper grasp on the object. The therapist positions the cane in the palm of the hemiplegic hand and helps the patient close his fingers completely around the cane. Before lifting the cane, she brings the hemiplegic wrist into extension, so that the hand is aligned with the forearm and the movements of the cane will be initiated with the hands. If another object is chosen, the therapist should go through a similar process to establish grasp and appropriate wrist stability. (*B*) The therapist assists the first movements with the cane. This is done to teach the patient how much effort is necessary to move the cane and to maintain control of the timing and rhythm of the movement while the patient gains a sensory memory for the desired movements. The therapist practices the movements that are easiest for the patient first, before attempting more difficult movement patterns. The patient learns to move the cane from his knees toward his hips and back again. (Shoulder extension with elbow flexion.) The therapist keeps the cane close to the thighs so that the arms do not yet have to lift the complete weight of the cane. She may also practice lifting the cane with elbow flexion and lifting the cane with elbow extension and shoulder flexion. (*C & D*) The therapist removes her support so that the patient moves the cane independently and practices lifting the cane from the knees into the air. (Shoulder flexion with partial extension of the elbow.) Although the grasp pattern of the right hand is not ideal, the movements have a nice normal quality, and the two arms look symmetric. The patient is lifting the cane with distal initiation and moves into shoulder flexion without scapula elevation or internal rotation on the hemiplegic side. Compare the quality of the movement of the hemiplegic arm in this series to the movement in 6-27A for a demonstration of the value of bilateral exercise as a tool for training normal movements.

Treatment Goal: Prepare for functional use of the hemiplegic arm.

Treatment Techniques: Use of everyday objects to practice functional arm movements. In this treatment series, the therapist uses functional objects to provide movement reeducation for the distal arm and hand (Fig. 6-32).

Additional suggestions: trunk movements in sitting; trunk movements in standing; walking.

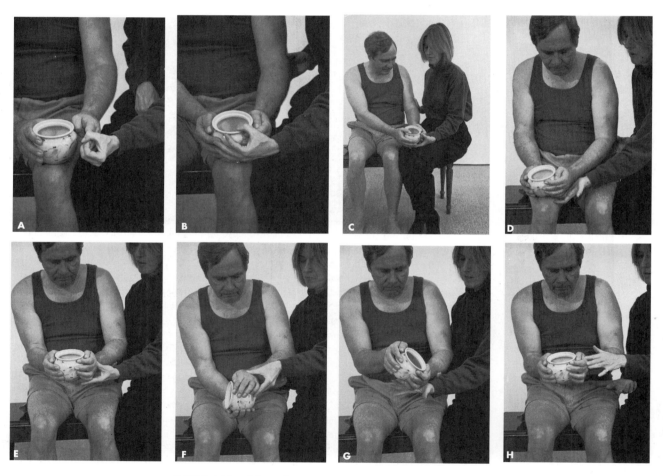

FIGURE 6-32 Left hemiplegia. (*A & B*) The therapist helps the patient establish grasp. The patient has no ability to extend his fingers to position the hemiplegic hand independently. During treatment, the therapist helps the left hand maintain grasp until the patient is able to maintain the hand in position without assistance. (*C–N*) The patient practices maintaining grasp and moving the bowl, using shoulder, elbow, forearm, and wrist movements. The therapist gradually withdraws her physical support and assistance. This treatment sequence demonstrates how an ordinary object can be used to help the patient develop functional movement strategies in the hemiplegic arm. Unilateral and bilateral patterns of static grasp are usually the first functional patterns that the patient acquires in his hemiplegic hand. *(Figure continues)*

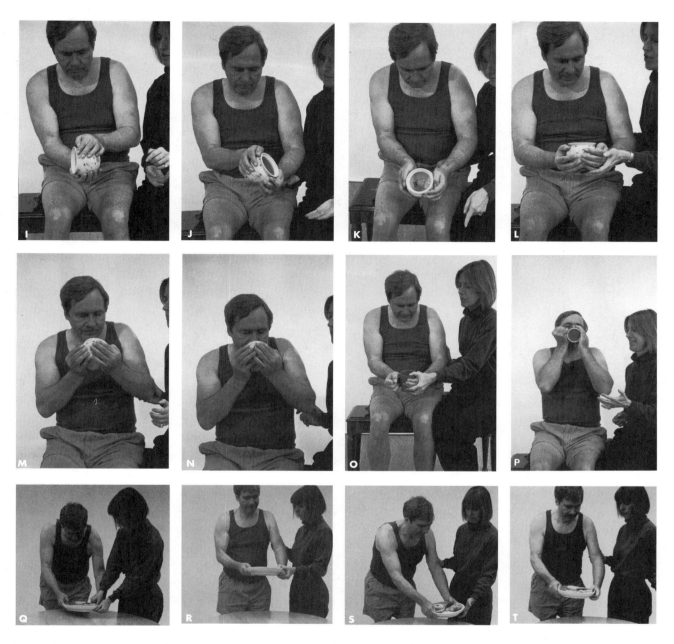

FIGURE 6-32 *(Continued)* Bilateral grasp and arm movement is easiest for the patient to learn because the hemiplegic side may learn from the performance of the uninvolved arm. Lateral similar movements can be practiced with unilateral grasp of the hemiplegic hand. Patients with more control of finger and thumb movements may also practice approach, grasp and release, and in-hand manipulation patterns with a variety of objects. *(O & P)* The therapist substitutes a mug for the bowl, so that the patient can practice using his hemiplegic hand to assist drinking. *(Q–T)* A similar treatment series in standing. The patient practices lifting the plate and performing upper-trunk-initiated weight shifts in standing to position the plate. The patient could also practice lifting the plate and carrying it to a new position. This exercise would provide practice combining arm movements with turning and walking.

REFERENCES

1. Codman EA: The Shoulder. Thomas Todd Co., Boston, 1934

2. Kapandji IA: The Physiology of the Joints. Vol. 1: Upper Limb. Fifth Edition. Churchill Livingstone, New York, 1982

3. Davies PM: Steps to Follow. Springer-Verlag, New York, 1985

4. Basmajian JV: Muscles Alive: Their Function Revealed by Electromyography. Balliere Tindall & Cox, London, 1962, pp 103–105

5. Sarhman SA, Norton BT: The relationship of volitional movement to spasticity in upper motor neuron symdrome. Ann Neurol 2:460–465, 1977

6. Caillet R: The Shoulder in Hemiplegia. FA Davis, Philadelphia, 1980

7. Inman VT, Saunders M, Abbott LC: Observations on the function of the shoulder joint. J Bone Joint Surg 26:1–30, 1944

7

Upper Extremity Weight Bearing Movements

Although support of body weight is a function most commonly associated with the lower extremities, weight bearing is also an important function of the upper extremity. In this book, upper extremity weight bearing is a very active and dynamic functional movement. Weight bearing on the upper extremities is used to support the weight of the trunk and upper body, to lift or move the body mass during transitional movements, such as sit to stand or sidelying to sitting, and to stabilize objects against a work surface for task performance. All these functions require movement in the trunk over the stable arm and activity in the muscles of the arm to maintain the arm on the supporting surface and simultaneously support the weight of the body. Our discussion of the upper extremity is focused on this active pattern of weight support. We do not discuss passive weight bearing in which the body leans on the arm without activity in the arm muscles or an active weight shift in the trunk.

This chapter presents an analysis of upper extremity weight bearing in sitting. In sitting, we have two common patterns of weight support on the arms. When seated at a table, we use the forearm and the hand for weight bearing on the table. We call this pattern *forearm weight bearing*. We also support body weight on our hands in sitting, when our arms are extended by the side of our body. We call this pattern of weight bearing *extended arm weight bearing*. The movement components, significant impairments, compensations, and treatment techniques differ for forearm and extended arm weight bearing. Consequently, we have divided this chapter into two parts and will discuss each type of weight bearing separately.

Forearm Weight Bearing In Sitting

CONCEPTS AND PRINCIPLES

Weight bearing on forearms is an important type of arm function in sitting that is used for activities at a table. We position our forearms on the table to support some of the weight of our upper body and to position the hand for function over and on the surface of the table. By using one or both arms for weight bearing, we make it easier to keep our upper body close to the table and our hands on the table surface, while resting the muscles of the trunk.

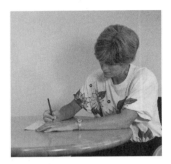

FIGURE 7-1 Forearm weight bearing while writing.

Weight bearing occurs when muscles in the trunk and shoulder girdle actively push or "depress" the forearms into the table. This muscle activity plants the forearms firmly on the table so that the arms are stable as the trunk moves around the arms. The active depression of the arms into the table that occurs with weight bearing is also used functionally in other ways. We use active depression of the forearm and hand to stabilize paper, books, or other objects positioned on the table. Table top activities such as eating, reading, and writing often combine weight support on one arm with hand and arm movements of the other arm (Fig. 7-1). An even more difficult form of shoulder girdle depression is required when we push into the table with our arms to lift our body up to standing or move our chair back from the table.

Forearm weight bearing is used in treatment in several different ways. With the acute patient who has poor muscular control of the trunk and a flaccid upper extremity, placing the upper extremities on a table in forearm weight bearing is one of the easiest ways to retrain trunk movements. In this treatment situation, the table is used to support the hemiplegic arm and maintain symmetry in the upper trunk while the therapist manually assists trunk movements and weight shift onto the hemiplegic side. As trunk control in sitting increases, the task of forearm weight bearing is used to activate muscles of the involved arm and train the arm to function in the task of weight bearing. The ability to weight bear on the forearm is one of the simplest functions of the arm and the easiest pattern of use to achieve in the hemiplegic arm because it does not depend on hand movements or control at the elbow, forearm, or wrist joints. Early functional use in weight bearing involves support of body weight on the arm and use of the forearm to stabilize objects. As control of the upper extremity increases, the patient may be taught to use active depression of the arm in more complex tasks and to use the arm in sit to stand.

Forearm weight bearing is also a very useful activity for treating problems that relate to primary and secondary impairments. The task of forearm weight bearing combines movements of the trunk, scapula, and arm. It can therefore be used to increase mobility in the scapula and lengthen tight muscles between the trunk and arm. Movements of the body over the arm are also a very effective treatment tool to decrease flexor hypertonicity of the arm and open a tightly fisted hand. As soon as weight bearing produces the desired changes in range, mobility, or tone, the focus of weight bearing treatment shifts to movement reeducation and functional training.

Uses of Forearm Weight Bearing

Retain trunk movements

Activate muscles of arm

Address secondary impairments

MOVEMENT COMPONENTS OF FOREARM WEIGHT BEARING

In forearm weight bearing, the body's base of support is increased to include the forearms and the area between the two arms, as well as the area defined by the lower extremities. Weight is supported on the elbow, forearm, and hand. As we work at a table, we automatically move our trunk around the weight bearing arms. When the trunk moves over the stable arms, the movement of the trunk changes the amount of weight placed on the forearms and the way that this weight is distributed. Trunk movements also change the position of the upper extremity relative to the trunk and are accompanied by changes in muscle length and different patterns of muscle activation in the arm. While the height of the table and distance of the body from the table do influence the patterns in the arm, the movement components that occur in the scapula and arm are the same components regardless of differences in body size and the varying heights of work surfaces.

The position of the hand on the table during forearm weight bearing is very important. When the hand rests on the table or participates in weight bearing, the palm is not flat in contact with the table. The longitudinal and distal arches of the palm are preserved during most weight bearing activities. The presence of these arches lifts the middle of the hand away from the top of the table. Weight is taken on the thenar and hypothenar eminences, the outside of the thumb, the outside of the fifth finger, and the fingertips. If the palmar arches are unnaturally flattened and the palm brought down to the table, the wrist flexes and the carpal bones come away from the table. This "flat hand" pattern, which encourages wrist flexion and collapse of the intrinsic arches of the hand, is a common treatment error.

Lower Trunk-Initiated Patterns

In the task of forearm weight bearing, most movements associated with function are initiated from the lower trunk. We describe these important functional movements in the section below.

Anterior Weight Shift

When an anterior weight shift is initiated in the lower trunk, the body moves closer to the table, increasing the amount of weight taken on the forearms. This movement results in a pattern of spinal extension. In the arms, the movement produces adduction and depression of the scapula, movement in the direction of extension, adduction and external rotation in the glenohumeral joint, and increased flexion at the elbow joint. The elbow and ulnar surfaces of the forearm and hand are in contact with the table and form the weight bearing surface of the arm (Fig. 7-2).

Functional Example

This movement is used to bring the center of gravity of the body closer to the table for functions such as writing or eating.

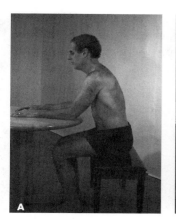 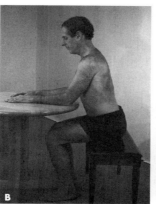 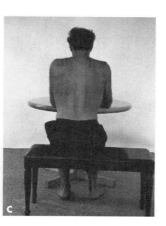

FIGURE 7-2 (A–C) Anterior weight shift.

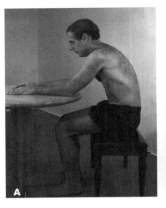
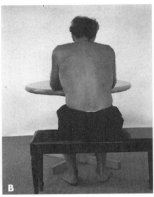
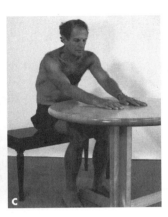

FIGURE 7-3 (A–C) Posterior weight shift.

Posterior Weight Shift

When a posterior weight shift is initiated in the lower trunk, the movement of the spine away from the table produces a posterior pelvic tilt and trunk flexion. Since the arms must remain on the table, the movement stops at the point where the arms would begin to move on the table. In the upper extremities, the posterior movement results in abduction and elevation of the scapulas, flexion, abduction, and internal rotation in the glenohumeral joints, and increased elbow extension. As the body moves farther back, the elbows partially extend and the weight bearing surface shifts from the forearms to the hands (Fig. 7-3).

Functional Example

This movement is used to move your spine back to rest it on the chair.

Lateral Weight Shift

A lateral weight shift initiated from the lower trunk to the right results in lateral flexion in the spine with the convexity of the curve on the right. The right arm and leg support increased body weight. In the right arm, the lateral weight shift results in scapula elevation and upward rotation, glenohumeral joint adduction and external rotation, and elbow flexion/supination with weight transfer to the ulnar side of the forearm and hand. On the left side, the movement of the spine away from the stable arm produces a pattern of downward rotation and depression in the scapula, abduction and internal rotation in the glenohumeral joint, partial elbow extension with pronation in the forearm, and weight transfer to the thenar side of the hand (Fig. 7-4; Table 7-1).

Functional Example

This movement is used to increase the weight on one side for support or to stabilize an object with one hand.

Upper-Trunk-Initiated Patterns

When the forearms are weight bearing, upper-trunk-initiated weight shifts bring the head and shoulder girdles closer to the table. While less commonly associated

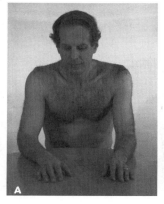 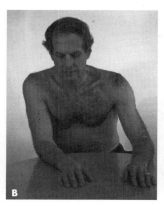 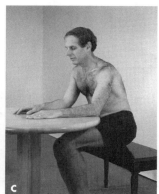 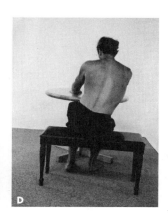

FIGURE 7-4 *(A–D)* Lateral weight shift.

with task performance than lower-trunk-initiated patterns, weight shifts initiated from the upper body are used functionally to rest the trunk during task performance at a table. Patients often substitute these weight shifts when lower-trunk-initiated patterns cannot be produced. For this reason, therapists need to be aware of how these patterns differ from the more functional lower trunk patterns (Table 7-2). Upper-body-initiated movements are also useful as treatment activities to increase flexibility in the spine and lengthen tight muscles between the trunk, scapula, and humerus.

Anterior Weight Shift

An anterior weight shift initiated from the upper body will bring the head forward and down toward the table. The movement forward produces flexion in the cervical and thoracic vertebrae. Spinal flexion is accompanied by elevation and abduction of the scapulas and abduction and internal rotation of the glenohumeral joints (Fig. 7-5).

TABLE 7-1 Movements Initiated from the Lower Trunk

	SPINE	SCAPULA	GLENOHUMERAL JOINT	ELBOW
Anterior	Extension	Adduction/ depression	Less flexion	More flexion
Posterior	Flexion	Abduction/ elevation	Flexion	Extension
Lateral				
Weight bearing	Convex	Elevation/ up rotation	Adduction/ external rotation	Flexion
Non-weight bearing	Concave	Depression/ down rotation	Abduction/ internal rotation	Extension

TABLE 7-2 Movements Initiated from the Upper Trunk

	SPINE	SCAPULA	GLENOHUMERAL JOINT	ELBOW
Anterior	Flexion	Elevation/ abduction	Less flexion	Flexion
Posterior	Extension	Depression/ adduction	Flexion	Extension
Lateral				
Weight bearing	Concave	Down rotation/ depression	Adduction	Flexion
Non-weight bearing	Convex	Elevation/ up rotation	Abduction	Extension

Functional Example

This movement is used to bring your head closer to your hands or the table.

Posterior Weight Shift

Upper-body-initiated posterior weight shifts are used in two different situations.

A posterior weight shift with the head and shoulders initiating the movement is used to return to upright sitting from the position described above. In this situation, extension in the spine occurs as the shoulders move back and up over the elbows. The movement produces depression and adduction in the scapulas, forward flexion with external rotation of the shoulders, and a decrease in the amount of weight placed on the elbows.

The posterior movement of the head and shoulders can also be performed from the starting position of forearm weight bearing. In this movement, the head and upper trunk move up and back away from the table, producing increased extension

FIGURE 7-5 *(A & B)* Anterior weight shift.

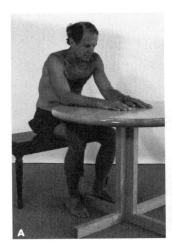
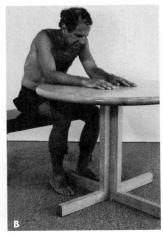

FIGURE 7-6 *(A & B) Posterior weight shift.*

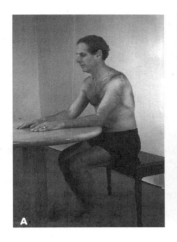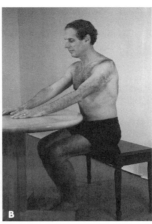

in the thoracic spine. For the arms to remain on the table during this movement, the shoulders flex and the elbows extend. Only the hands remain on the table when the movement is stopped by the length of the arms (Fig. 7-6).

Functional Example

This movement is used functionally to shift weight onto the hands prior to standing up.

Lateral Weight Shift

An upper-body-initiated lateral movement to the right produces lateral flexion in the spine with the concavity to the right. If the right forearm remains stable on the table, the right shoulder will move laterally past the elbow and then inferiorly. Side-bending to the right results in scapular depression and downward rotation, humeral adduction, and external rotation in the right arm. As the upper body moves closer to the table, the right elbow moves into extension, and the lateral aspect of the forearm becomes the weight bearing surface of the arm. On the left side, the trunk movements result in scapula upward rotation and elevation and humeral abduction with internal rotation. As the upper body moves farther to the right, the left elbow extends and leaves the table so that only the left hand remains on the table (Fig. 7-7).

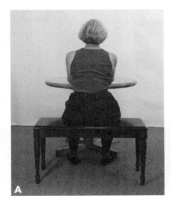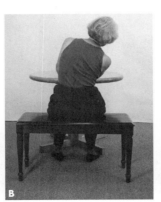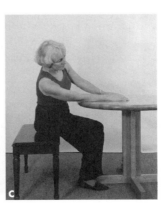

FIGURE 7-7 *(A–C) Lateral weight shift.*

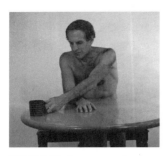

FIGURE 7-8 Rotation with arm movement across midline.

Functional Example

This movement pattern is frequently used in treatment to lengthen tight muscles in the trunk.

Rotational Patterns

When both forearms are weight bearing on the table and both femurs and feet are in contact with the chair and floor, slight rotational play is available in the middle of the spine, which allows us to twist one side of our rib cage slightly forward or back. This twisting results in rotation of the vertebrae on each other. For larger rotational movements to occur, it is necessary to move one arm out of weight bearing. Movement of one arm in horizontal abduction or adduction produces rotation in the spine and in the weight bearing arm at the shoulder joint. In this section, we will examine the rotational patterns that occur when one arm is weight bearing on the table and the other arm is moving.

Rotation with Arm Movement
Across Midline

If the left arm reaches to the right across the midline of the body towards the right forearm, the movement of the left arm is accompanied by spinal rotation to the right in a pattern of flexion rotation. The movement of the body produces scapula abduction with humeral adduction in the right (weight bearing) arm (Fig. 7-8). When the reaching hand stays close to the table, there is no change in the spine in the axis of flexion/extension. As the height of the reaching hand is raised from the table surface towards shoulder height, the increased elevation of the hand increases the extension in the thoracic spine.

Functional Example

These movements are used functionally to reach across the middle of the body. This is used in many feeding, cooking, and writing tasks.

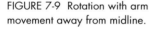

FIGURE 7-9 Rotation with arm movement away from midline.

Rotation with Arm Movement
Away from Midline

When the right arm reaches back and to the right away from the center of the body, the trunk movement is one of extension rotation. As the head and spine rotate to the right, the left shoulder joint moves forward, placing the scapula in adduction, the glenohumeral joint in abduction and internal rotation, and the forearm in pronation. The right scapula also adducts as the humerus moves into horizontal abduction (Fig. 7-9).

Functional Examples

This movement could be used to move an arm from the table to the arm of the chair or to reach behind for a coat.

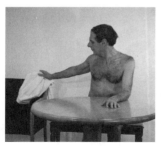

FUNCTIONAL APPLICATIONS OF FOREARM WEIGHT BEARING

Sit to Stand

Arms that are weight bearing on a table are often used to assist in the movement of sit to stand. To use the arms during sit to stand, the chair must be a sufficient distance from the table to allow the hips to come forward over the feet. To begin the movement, the lower trunk initiates an anterior weight shift movement that increases the amount of hip flexion and shifts more body weight onto the forearms and hands. As the shoulders come forward over the elbows, the elbows leave the table and partially extend, shifting the weight bearing surface of the arms to the base of the hand. As the hips leave the chair the shoulders continue to move up and forward and the elbows continue to extend. This shifts the weight off the distal forearm to the hand, resulting in increasing amounts of wrist extension. The hands can lift off the table as the legs move from partial flexion to extension, if a full stand is the goal. Or the hands may remain on the table as the legs extend. This pattern results in extended-arm weight bearing in standing with the hips in partial flexion (Fig. 7-10).

Stabilization of Objects

During task performance at the table, we often combine weight bearing to support partial body weight with weight bearing to stabilize objects. The weight bearing arm may stabilize objects with a flat open hand or with a partially closed grasp. A flat hand pattern of stabilization is used to hold paper down during writing or to keep a book open. Grasp is combined with weight bearing during such tasks as slicing and opening jars or bottles. To stabilize an object, weight must be shifted onto the stabilizing extremity. A downward force is delivered from the hand into the object to maintain it in a stable position.

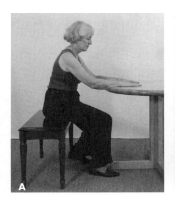 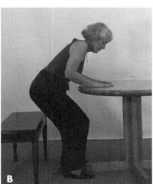 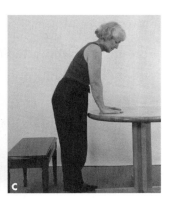

FIGURE 7-10 (A–C) Sit to stand.

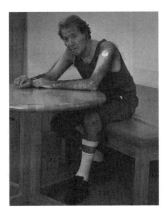

FIGURE 7-11 Excessive flexion in the upper trunk during forearm weight bearing.

SIGNIFICANT IMPAIRMENTS THAT INTERFERE WITH PERFORMANCE

Loss of Control of Critical Trunk Movements

Upper extremity weight bearing depends on the ability of the trunk to move around the table and the stable forearm. Two movements in the trunk are the most critical for forearm weight bearing: the ability to maintain thoracic spine extension and the ability to perform lower-trunk-initiated anterior and lateral weight shifts. Anterior trunk movements with spinal extension are necessary to bring the center of gravity closer to the table and establish weight on the forearms. From this anterior position with the thoracic spine extended, lateral trunk movements are used to shift weight to one arm and to assist the reaching movements of the non-weight bearing arm. Upper trunk extension control is also necessary to change the weight bearing surface from forearms to hands and to accompany the push with the arms that moves the body from sitting to standing.

Many neurologic patients have poor control of upper trunk extension in sitting and difficulty initiating trunk movements from the lower trunk. These problems are commonly associated with muscle weakness in the trunk, arm, and leg. They may also be present when hypomobility in the spine and hip joints along with associated soft tissue limitations interfere with normal trunk movement patterns. When the critical trunk movement patterns cannot be performed, the patient will be unable to support body weight on his forearms by using the normal components of weight bearing.

Patients without good trunk control in sitting may attempt to perform forearm weight bearing while maintaining flexion in the upper trunk (Fig. 7-11). This trunk posture results in atypical upper extremity movements of excessive elevation and internal rotation of the shoulder girdle rather than the normal appropriate patterns of shoulder girdle movement. Similarly, the patient with limited control of trunk movements or a stiff trunk may substitute upper-body-initiated lateral weight shifts for the more functional lower-trunk-initiated movements (Fig. 7-12). This movement substitution does not produce a normal weight bearing pattern in the hemiplegic arm.

Whenever inappropriate trunk postures and weight shift patterns are present during upper extremity weight bearing activities, the therapist must address the trunk problems before attempting to reeducate the muscles of the arm. Trunk problems are addressed first because the normal patterns of movement in the scapula and arm cannot occur without the appropriate trunk posture and move-

FIGURE 7-12 Inappropriate use of upper-trunk-initiated lateral weight shifts. *(A)* The patient is attempting to shift weight toward his hemiplegic forearm, using an upper trunk pattern. *(B)* The right forearm is not able to accept weight because of the excessive lateral movement of the upper trunk.

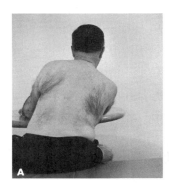
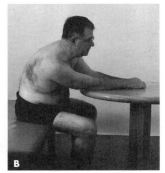

ment. With the forearms in weight bearing, the therapist uses handling to correct the position of the trunk and introduce the correct movement patterns in the trunk. During this time the arms are resting on the table, but the muscles of the involved arm may not be actively participating in weight bearing (Fig. 7-13). Once the trunk weight shift patterns have been established, the therapist changes her handling to use the task of forearm weight bearing to increase muscle activity in the arm and prepare for arm function in weight bearing.

Upper Extremity Weakness/Paralysis

Muscle activity is necessary in the shoulder girdle and arm to maintain the arm in a stable position on the table and support body weight. When the body moves around the weight bearing arm, the distribution of muscle activity in the arm changes to adapt to the new demands that the trunk position places on the arm. As the arms are loaded with increasing amounts of body weight, or the arms are used to push the body through space, increased amounts of muscle strength are necessary in the weight bearing arm. Similarly, when the weight bearing is used to stabilize an object, graded control of the amount of pressure that is delivered through the forearm and hand is necessary to maintain the object in the correct position. While it is possible to lean on the arms without muscle activity in the arm or trunk, this is a position of rest, not of function.

When the muscles of the arm are severely weak or paralyzed, forearm weight bearing is either not possible or performed with atypical movement substitutions because the arm muscles cannot participate appropriately in the task. The flaccid arm does not have sufficient muscle activity to stabilize the arm on the table, causing the arm to slide when the trunk moves. In cases of incomplete recovery in which some but not all the muscles of the arm have recovered strength and control, the arm will participate normally in some parts of forearm weight bearing and use muscle substitutions to replace the action of the missing motor components. Any movement deficits that exist in forearm weight bearing should be reeducated in treatment so that the patient may regain the functional use of weight bearing.

Forearm weight bearing is one of the first activities that is used with the flaccid arm to reestablish appropriate scapula alignment and reeducate control in the muscles that connect the scapula to the trunk and the arm. However, weight bearing will not produce these benefits unless the therapist manually structures the activity so that the arm is stable on the table and the scapula moves appropriately as the patient moves his trunk (Fig. 7-14). This early assistance by the therapist is necessary to teach the scapula and arm muscles to contract during weight bearing.

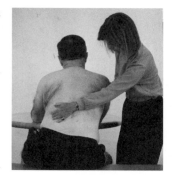

FIGURE 7-13 Retraining lower-trunk-initiated weight shift to the hemiplegic side. The therapist's hands stabilize the hemiplegic arm on the table, while assisting the correct trunk weight shift.

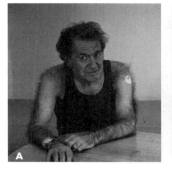 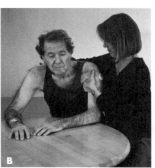

FIGURE 7-14 Assisting the hemiplegic arm during weight bearing. (A) Without assistance from the therapist, the hemiplegic arm slides onto the table as the trunk moves. (B) The therapist stabilizes the hemiplegic arm on the table and maintains good alignment in the shoulder while asking the trunk to move.

Once the patient can activate the correct arm muscles, the therapist can withdraw her input or decrease her level of assistance. As the patient learns to maintain his arm in a stable position on the table and shift his trunk over the arm, the task of weight bearing can be incorporated into functional activities and sit to stand.

Upper Extremity Hypertonicity

Hypertonic or spastic flexor muscles of the upper extremity maintain the arm in an unnatural posture that interferes with weight bearing. Upper extremity hypertonicity is commonly found in the scapula elevators, pectorals, elbow flexors, and wrist and finger flexors. Tension in the scapula elevators and pectorals maintains the forearm in an adducted position across the body and prevents the elbow and forearm from being placed in contact with the table. Similarly, when the wrist and fingers are held in a tightly flexed position, the wrist cannot be extended to neutral to allow the heel of the hand to rest on the table, and the fingers cannot be opened with the wrist in neutral to allow normal alignment of the hand on the table.

Hypertonicity restricts the ability of the arm to accept weight in two ways. First, hypertonus and associated muscle shortening prevent the arm from being positioned on the table with the hand and forearm in line with the shoulder and the correct areas of the forearm and hand in contact with the table (Fig. 7-15A). Second, hypertonicity in the muscles of the arm interferes with the free movement of the scapula on the rib cage and the humerus in the glenohumeral joint, both which must occur as the trunk moves around the weight bearing arm. When hypertonicity is present in the shoulder girdle, trunk movements result in atypical movements in the scapula and shoulder joint (Fig. 7-15B).

Forearm weight bearing is a useful and appropriate treatment activity for decreasing hypertonus and changing the resting posture of the arm. Since hypertonicity in the arm prevents normal placement of the arm on the table, the initial part of weight bearing treatment is structured to use the movements of the trunk to lengthen tight muscles and reduce muscle tone in hypertonic muscles. The hemiplegic arm is positioned on the table with the best alignment possible, and the therapist uses her hands to stabilize the arm while the patient moves his trunk in directions that will lengthen the spastic muscles. For example, when the pectoral muscles are shortened, the involved arm rests on the table in a position of internal rotation and adduction. Lat-

FIGURE 7-15 *(A)* Abnormal positioning of the hemiplegic right arm during forearm weight bearing. *(B)* Atypical movements of the hemiplegic right shoulder girdle during an anterior weight shift.

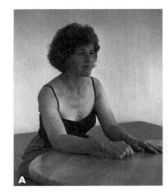
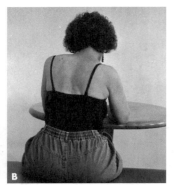

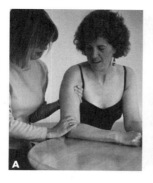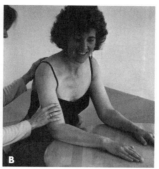

FIGURE 7-16 Using weight bearing to reduce hypertonicity. *(A)* The position of the arm at the start of treatment. *(B)* The position of the arm after treatment, showing reduction of muscle tension at the shoulder, wrist, and fingers.

eral trunk movements toward the involved arm will increase the amount of external rotation at the glenohumeral joint, and lateral movements away from the involved arm should help the therapist achieve length in the pectoral muscles. As the movements of the trunk elongate the tight tissues, the therapist should feel a release of tension in the arm. This release of tension allows her to gradually correct the position of the arm on the table and use her hands to guide the appropriate upper extremity patterns during movements of the trunk (Fig. 7-16). A similar treatment sequence may be used when the hemiplegic arm is in an unnatural position on the table because of soft tissue tightness in the muscles connecting the trunk, scapula, and humerus.

Once the position of the arm has been corrected on the table and the movements of the trunk result in appropriate changes in scapula and humerus position, the therapist should ask the patient to use his arm more actively in the task. For example, the patient could be asked to push with his hemiplegic arm while shifting weight towards his uninvolved side or to use the arm as an assist during sit to stand. At this point, the weight bearing is being used to reeducate muscle activity rather than change muscle tension. It is important to remember that reducing hypertonicity in the arm does not generally translate directly into improved arm function, nor does the reduction in tone last for long between treatment sessions when tone reduction is the only goal of treatment. Permanent reduction in upper extremity hypertonus is only achieved when there is a change in the patient's patterns of active movement. Active use of the hypertonic muscles of the arm in weight bearing may contribute to a permanent change in muscle tone by training appropriate patterns of muscle activation and relaxation.

Abnormal Upper Extremity Alignment

Abnormal alignment in the shoulder girdle is a common problem in the arm that causes abnormal joint mechanics and pain during forearm weight bearing. The alignment problems are generally present before the arm is placed on the table and are unchanged when the arm rests on the table. For example, inferior subluxation is a common example of an alignment problem of the glenohumeral joint. Since inferior subluxation is caused by loss of scapula alignment on the rib cage, the physical separation between the humerus and the shoulder joint may not disappear when the arms rest on the table, even though the table takes the weight of the humerus off the joint capsule (Fig. 7-17). The subluxation is only reduced when the therapist lifts the humerus up and upwardly rotates the scapula. This creates the correct starting position for weight bearing.

FIGURE 7-17 Inferior subluxation, right hemiplegia. *(A)* The subluxed shoulder before the arm is placed on the table. *(B)* In weight bearing, the right shoulder is lower and the scapula is downwardly rotated. *(C)* The therapist corrects the subluxation by upwardly rotating the scapula and lifting the humerus up into the glenoid fossa. Her correction of the hemiplegic shoulder restored symmetry to the two sides of the body.

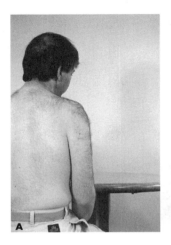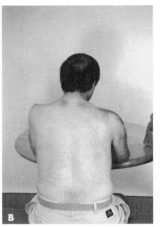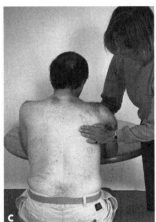

Alignment problems may also become evident for the first time when the arms are placed on the table. *Winging*, or displacement of a portion of the scapula from contact with the rib cage, often appears when the forearms are placed on the table (Fig. 7-18). Scapula winging develops when the position of the scapula and that of the trunk are incompatible, and thus may result from malalignment in both the trunk and shoulder girdle. Both subluxation and winging are most commonly associated with muscle weakness and hypotonicity. They may be present in arms with hypertonicity or soft tissue shortening as well.

Shoulder subluxation and scapula winging must be corrected before the hemiplegic arm is asked to accept weight. With subluxation, the position of the scapula and glenohumeral joint should be corrected before the arm is brought to the table and the integrity of the joint preserved as the forearm is placed in weight bearing. When winging is evident as the arm is placed in weight bearing, the therapist must correct alignment in the trunk and scapula before progressing further. It is important to establish the correct biomechanical relationships of the shoulder girdle before the arm accepts weight, so that movements of the trunk will produce normal movement components in the arm. If the scapula and shoulder joint are not correctly aligned, the movements of the trunk around the weight bearing arm will place tractioning and approximating forces on the abnormally aligned shoulder joint, leading to further joint instability and pain.

FIGURE 7-18 Winging scapula, left hemiplegia.

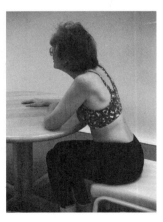

ASSESSMENT GUIDELINES

Assessment of forearm weight bearing should be directed toward three general areas. First, the therapist must identify problems with the position of the trunk and arm in the weight bearing position. When this is completed, the therapist should identify movement problems in the trunk and arm that become evident as the trunk moves around the weight bearing arms. The third area of assessment examines the causes for the alignment problems and movement problems by looking at the significant impairments that are influencing performance. General questions to assist problem solving in these areas are listed below.

Assessment of Forearm Weight Bearing

I. Place both arms on the table in forearm weight bearing. Describe the position of the trunk and involved arm. What problems did you encounter in bringing the involved arm to the table?

II. Ask the patient to initiate anterior, posterior, and lateral weight shifts from his lower trunk. What difficulties and atypical movements do you observe? What patterns can the patient perform relatively normally?

III. Place your hands on the patient's trunk and arm. Try to correct his posture and/or realign his shoulder and correct the position of the arm. What problems do you encounter? Where do you put your hands to make his body symmetric?

Then, try to maintain correct alignment in the trunk and arm and repeat the trunk movements. Which patterns improve? Which problems do not change easily?

IV. Identify the major impairments that are interfering with forearm weight bearing. How will you structure forearm weight bearing to work on those impairments? What other treatment techniques and positions will be useful to improve performance?

V. How will you use forearm weight bearing in treatment? What functional goals will this treatment activity help you to achieve? How will you help your patient incorporate forearm weight bearing into his daily life?

THERAPY GOALS

Functional Goals

Forearm weight bearing in sitting is used in treatment to help the patient achieve the following functional goals:

1. To be able to maintain the hemiplegic forearm on the table and support weight on it.

2. To be able to support the body weight on the arm during task performance and for rest.

3. To use the arm in weight bearing to stabilize objects.

4. To use the arm during sit to stand (see also Ch.13).

Treatment Goals and Techniques

Treatment Goal: Train the trunk components of forearm weight bearing.

Treatment Technique: (Fig. 7-19) Before beginning movement reeducation, the therapist uses her hands to provide appropriate trunk alignment and correct obvious asymmetries. She then maintains this alignment while assisting appropriate trunk weight shifts. The goal of this part of the treatment progression is to teach the patient to perform the trunk movement components of forearm weight bearing.

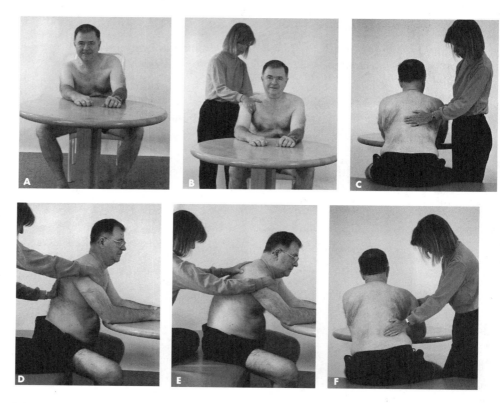

FIGURE 7-19 *(A)* Before treatment, the patient's hemiplegic right side appears shorter and the right shoulder appears lower. *(B)* The therapist uses an axillary/trunk grip to increase extension in the upper trunk, while supporting the right shoulder joint and maintaining the forearm in a stable position. This axillary grip or the alternate version shown in Figure 7-22 should always be used when the gleno-humeral joint is subluxed. *(C)* The position of the therapist's back hand. *(D)* The relative positions of the therapist's two hands. The hand on the front of the shoulder brings the upper trunk into extension. It also externally rotates the shoulder joint as the trunk is extended and delivers a slight downward pressure along the shaft of the humerus into the forearm to keep the arm on the table. At the same time, the hand on the spine delivers a compatible forward force to the trunk. The pressure from this hand tells the spine to extend as the patient moves his trunk forward toward the table. *(Figure continues.)*

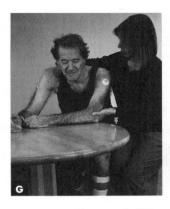
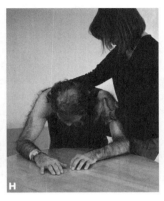
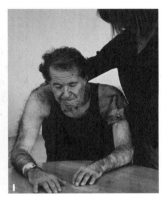

FIGURE 7-19 *(Continued)* *(E)* During a posterior weight shift, the therapist lightens her pressure on the spine to allow it to flex and shift weight backwards. Her hand that controls the hemiplegic shoulder joint delivers a backward message to the clavicle and front of the trunk to tell the trunk to move away from the table. As the trunk moves posteriorly, she allows the glenohumeral joint to rotate internally but continues to deliver a downward force into the elbow, so that the forearm stays on the table as the trunk moves away. *(F)* To train lower-trunk-initiated lateral weight shifts, the therapist maintains the same control at the patients hemiplegic shoulder but changes her hand control on the trunk. During a lateral weight shift away from the hemiplegic side, the therapist's hand moves to the hemiplegic side of the rib cage, where its pressure helps the ribs to tuck and move to the uninvolved side. As the patient moves farther to the left, her hand on the rib cage delivers a diagonal pressure down toward the patient's left hip. Similarly, to help the patient shift weight toward his hemiplegic hip, the therapist moves her hand to the uninvolved side of the trunk and assists the movements through that side of the rib cage.
(G) Patients with severe weakness in the trunk and arm may not be able to easily perform lower-body-initiated movements and maintain the arm on the table. With these patients, treatment often begins with upper-trunk-initiated movements. *(H)* The patient moves his upper trunk in an anterior direction, so that the upper trunk flexes. The therapist's hand in the axilla supports the shoulder joint and stabilizes the forearm on the table. The therapist's arm on the patient's upper trunk helps maintain his body in midline. *(I)* The patient extends his upper trunk. When these movements are possible with minimal assistance, the therapist begins to ask for lower-trunk-initiated weight shifts.

.Treatment Technique: A two-sided rib cage grip can also be used to train anterior/posterior and lateral weight shifts. There is no control of the hemiplegic shoulder joint with this hand placement (Fig. 7-20).

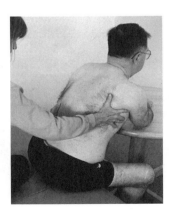

FIGURE 7-20 The therapist places her two hands on the lateral side of the back of the rib cage. The hands may be placed on the rib cage symmetrically or, as in this figure, in unequal heights so that they may be used to correct alignment in the spine/rib cage and to assist the desired movement. In this figure, the patient is asked to perform a lower-trunk-initiated lateral weight shift to the hemiplegic side. The therapist's right hand is lifting the hemiplegic side of the trunk, as her left hand tucks the patient's uninvolved rib cage and delivers a diagonal message into the hemiplegic hip to accept weight. The therapist may also hold this hand placement while asking for anterior/posterior movements.

Treatment Goal: Reeducate appropriate scapula/arm movements during trunk weight shifts. Reeducation of the upper extremity components of forearm weight bearing begins as soon as the patient is able to perform the necessary anterior/posterior and lateral weight shifts with his trunk with little or no assistance from the therapist. In this part of the treatment, the therapist uses hand placements that provide control of the scapula and arm. The goal of this part of the treatment progression is to activate appropriate muscles in the hemiplegic arm by assisting the movements of the scapula/glenohumeral joint.

Treatment Technique: Scapula mobility can be improved and correct scapula movements reeducated during the task of forearm weight bearing. Hand placements that control the scapula and axilla are the best way to begin this process (Fig. 7-21).

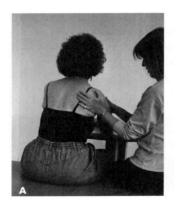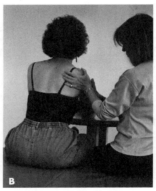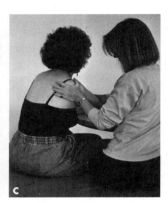

FIGURE 7-21 *(A)* The therapist's right hand is in the patient's axilla as described in the previous series. She places her left hand over the patient's hemiplegic scapula. *(B)* The patient performs an anterior weight shift. As the trunk moves forward, the therapist's hands give a message to the scapula to adduct and depress and to the glenohumeral joint to externally rotate. *(C)* The therapist changes her messages during a posterior weight shift to help the scapula abduct and elevate and the shoulder joint flex and internally rotate. This hand placement can also be used to facilitate appropriate scapula/arm movements during lower-trunk-initiated lateral movements.

Treatment Goal: Increase muscle activity in the arm.

Treatment Technique: Arm movements are most easily trained using an axillary/forearm or axillary hand grip (Fig. 7-22).

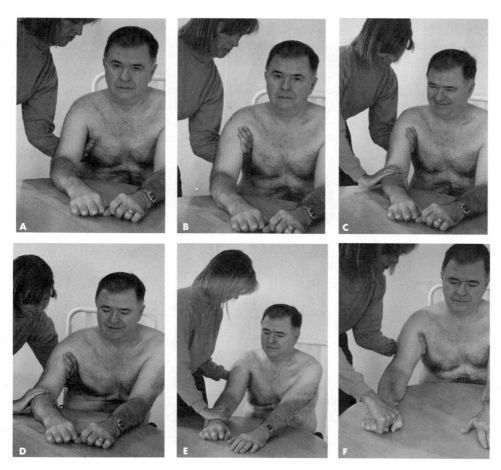

FIGURE 7-22 *(A)* The therapist faces the patient's hemiplegic side and places her back hand in the axilla. *(B)* This hand lifts the humerus into the fossa and externally rotates the joint to neutral, if possible. At the same time, the therapist delivers a slight downward message along the shaft of the humerus to the table. *(C)* The therapist places her front hand on the patient's forearm near the elbow joint. Her two hands together increase the message to the arm to depress into the table. If the patient has minimal weight on his hemiplegic side, she will have to bring the body towards her before proceeding further. *(D)* As the patient's weight shifts, the therapist's hands assist the appropriate patterns of movement in the shoulder, elbow, and forearm. Here the patient is shifting laterally away from his hemiplegic side. The therapist's left hand is assisting shoulder girdle depression, scapula downward rotation, and humeral abduction with internal rotation. Her right hand helps the elbow stay on the table and the forearm pronate. The same hand placement can be used for weight shifts toward the hemiplegic side and for anterior/posterior weight shifts. The therapist delivers compatible shoulder and arm messages during these movements, so that the patient learns to activate appropriate arm muscles. *(E)* The arm muscles become more active when the patient moves from forearm weight bearing to weight bearing on the wrist and hand. In this figure, the therapist is helping the patient extend his elbow and change weight bearing from the forearm to the wrist. The patient shifts his weight posteriorly. The therapist's left hand lifts the humerus up so that the elbow moves into extension. The therapist's right hand maintains the wrist on the table. *(F)* An alternate grip. The therapist's fingers are in the palm of the hemiplegic hand, where they help support the palmar arches. Her thumb lies along the top of the wrist joint.

Treatment Goal: Decrease secondary impairments in the trunk and shoulder girdle.

Treatment Technique: Hypomobility in the spine and rib cage interferes with normal trunk movements in weight bearing, especially lateral weight shifts. Upper-trunk-initiated lateral weight shifts may be used to increase mobility in the spine and rib cage and lengthen tight tissues between the trunk and pelvis (Fig. 7-23).

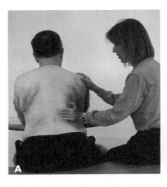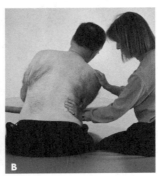

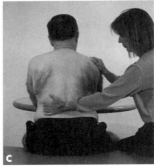

FIGURE 7-23   *(A)* To increase lateral flexion to the hemiplegic side, the therapist places one hand on top of the hemiplegic shoulder to stabilize the arm on the table. Her other hand is placed at the bottom of the hemiplegic rib cage. *(B)* As the patient moves his upper trunk laterally toward his hemiplegic side, the therapist tucks the hemiplegic rib cage so that the spine laterally flexes toward her. Her hand on top of the shoulder helps move the shoulder girdle laterally and down. *(C)* To assist the movement of lateral flexion toward the uninvolved side, the therapist moves her hand to the opposite side of the rib cage. While the patient moves his upper trunk toward his uninvolved side, her hands tuck the rib cage and guide the hemiplegic shoulder medially and superiorly.

Treatment Technique: Forearm weight bearing is a very effective way of lengthening tight muscles that connect the rib cage, scapula, and humerus (Fig. 7-24).

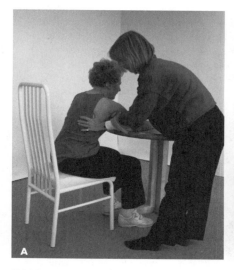 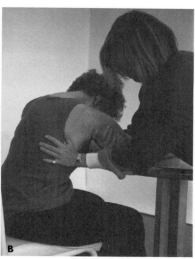

FIGURE 7-24 *(A)* To lengthen tight muscles in this area, the therapist uses one hand to stabilize the humerus on the table. With her other hand, she stabilizes the scapula in a position where the tight muscles are placed on slight tension. Here, the therapist's left hand is holding the inferior angle of the scapula against the rib cage. *(B)* The patient initiates a posterior weight shift. As her body moves back away from the humerus, the stretch between the therapist's two hands is increased.

Treatment Goal: Reduce flexor hypertonicity in the hemiplegic arm and hand.

Treatment Technique: Movements of the body over the weight bearing arm are a very effective way of gradually lengthening hypertonic muscles in the arm and realigning shoulder, elbow forearm, and wrist joints (Fig. 7-25).

FIGURE 7-25 *(A)* The position of the hemiplegic arm in weight bearing before treatment. *(B & C)* Weight bearing begins with the arm in an uncorrected position on the table. The therapist uses an axillary/trunk grip to increase mobility in the scapula and glenohumeral joint, as the patient performs lower-trunk-initiated weight shifts. *(D)* Increased mobility at the shoulder joint allows the humerus to be positioned in more external rotation and the forearm brought more into the line of the shoulder. The therapist shifts her hand placements to axilla/forearm control. *(E & F)* The patient performs anterior/posterior weight shifts. The therapist uses the anterior movements to increase mobility in external rotation. The posterior movements result in a release of elbow and wrist flexor tone. *(G)* During lateral weight shifts, the therapist's control on the hemiplegic forearm accentuates the rotation of the forearm. Following this segment of treatment, the humerus, elbow, forearm, and hand all lie in the same plane. *(H & I)* Upper-trunk-initiated lateral weight shifts are used to increase mobility at the distal forearm and wrist. The therapist moves her hand from the proximal forearm to rest over the distal forearm and wrist joint. As the patient moves toward her intact side, the pressure of the therapist's hand rolls the forearm into pronation. Her hand in the axilla lifts the shoulder up so that the hemiplegic elbow extends. This increases the amount of extension in the wrist. As the patient moves to her hemiplegic side, the therapist maintains the wrist in extension and the forearm in pronation. *(J)* Following this section of treatment, the entire forearm, wrist, and hand rest on the table. The fingers remain tightly flexed.

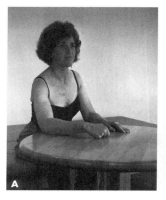

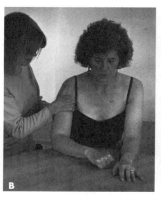

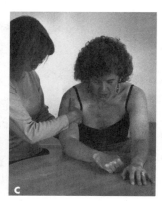

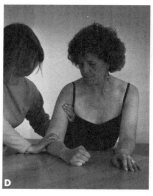

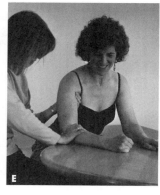

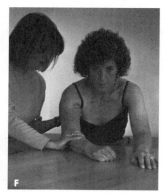

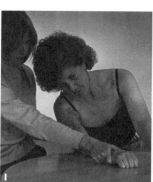

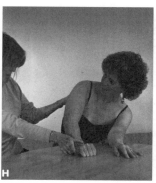

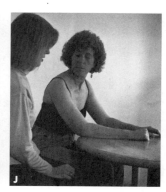

Treatment Technique: When the hand is fisted in weight bearing, but muscle tension is decreased at the wrist and more proximally, the therapist should attempt to open the hand (Fig. 7-26).

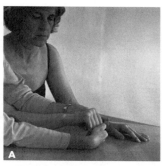

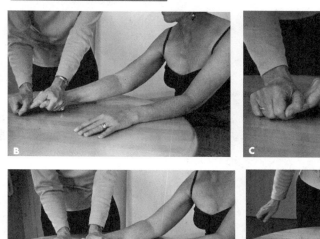

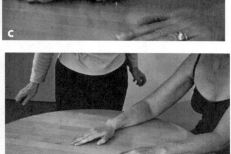

FIGURE 7-26 *(A)* The therapist stabilizes the hemiplegic wrist in neutral extension with her left hand. With her right hand, she brings the fingertips out of the palm, keeping the metacarpal joint in flexion. The therapist may encounter strong resistance to extension of the fingers. She maintains her grip on the fingers and waits for hypertonicity to release. She gradually brings the interphalangeal joints into extension as the flexor tension decreases. The hand is lifted slightly above the table during this part of the technique. *(B & C)* The therapist maintains her control on the wrist and fingers while slowly returning the hand to the table. The metacarpal joint is still flexed. *(D)* As tension decreases in the metacarpal joint, the therapist moves this joint into increased extension. *(E)* Tension in all the extrinsic wrist and finger muscles has decreased, allowing the relaxed hand to rest in an open, normally aligned position on the table. The palmar arches of the hand are preserved in weight bearing when the technique is performed correctly.

Treatment Goal: Increase functional use of forearm weight bearing in sit to stand.

Treatment Technique: The therapist uses the axillary/wrist grip to control the hemiplegic arm during the stand (Fig. 7-27).

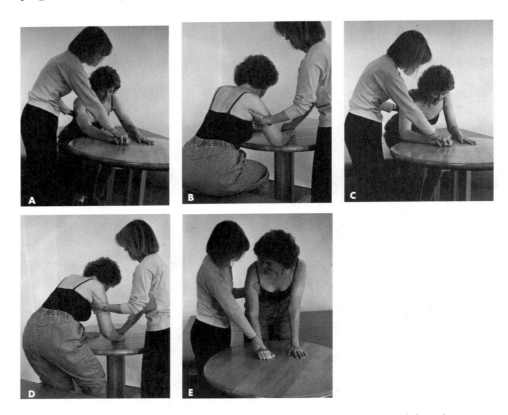

FIGURE 7-27 *(A)* The starting position. *(B)* The patient initiates an anterior weight shift, so that weight is shifted towards the feet. *(C)* The patient's shoulders continue to travel forward as the hips leave the bed. The therapist's hands move the hemiplegic shoulder at the same rate as the uninvolved side. Weight is still on both forearms. *(D)* As the legs begin to extend, the shoulders should continue to move forward and up. The therapist lifts the hemiplegic shoulder forward and up to allow the elbow to leave the table and partially extend. Weight is shifted onto the wrist and hand. The therapist maintains the hemiplegic hand on the table. At this stage of the movement, the therapist must also ensure that the patient keeps equal weight on both legs. If the patient shifts increased body weight to her uninvolved side during the stand, the hemiplegic arm will leave the table. *(E)* In full standing, the shoulders are positioned over the hands, and weight is supported on the extended wrist and palm. The therapist's hands maintain the elbow in extension and weight on the arm. The patient has weight on a fisted hand because of limited length in wrist and finger flexors. The activity can also be done with the fingers open in extension, if joint mobility and muscle length are adequate to permit full extension in the wrist and fingers.

Extended-Arm
Weight Bearing in Sitting

CONCEPTS AND PRINCIPLES

In this section, we continue our discussion of upper extremity weight bearing in sitting with an analysis of extended-arm weight bearing. In this functional movement, the weight bearing arms are extended by the sides of the body, and weight is supported on the hands. Extended-arm weight bearing is a more difficult movement pattern than forearm weight bearing. In forearm weight bearing, the table provides support and stability to the upper trunk. The muscles of the shoulder girdle must be active to stabilize the arm on the table and support partial body weight while the trunk moves, but these arm movements do not depend on activity in the elbow, wrist, or hand. During extended-arm weight bearing, the upper trunk is erect and unsupported, and the arm is extended. This requires increased control of trunk extension to maintain the upper trunk in alignment over the lower trunk and pelvis. It also requires strength and control in the shoulder girdle, elbow, and wrist to keep the arm extended on the supporting surface as body weight is shifted over it. For normal extended-arm weight bearing to occur, the muscles of the proximal and distal arm must be able to maintain the elbow in a rigid but not locked position while body weight is transferred to and supported by the arm and hand.

Extended-arm weight bearing also differs from forearm weight bearing in the ways that it is used for function. Forearm weight bearing is important for function at a table; extended-arm weight bearing as described in this chapter is used for functions in sitting that do not involve a table. We use weight bearing with our arms by the side of the body to increase the stability of our body when our balance is challenged. We shift body weight onto our arms and lean on them to rest the trunk muscles when sitting without back support (Fig. 7-28). And we use extended-arm weight bearing to help lift the body during the transition from sitting to standing and in part of the movement sequence of moving from sidelying to sitting.

Although many of the descriptions of normal movement components in this chapter involve bilateral weight bearing, we often place only one arm in the extended-arm weight bearing position. Unilateral upper extremity weight bearing leaves one arm free for movement so that the body weight can be supported on one arm while the other arm is engaged in functional performance. The use of one arm in weight bearing to stabilize an object is an essential pattern of bilateral coordination, used in such activities as slicing bread, chopping vegetables, or writing. In sitting, these activities usually occur with trunk rotation.

Because extended-arm weight bearing is such an important functional pattern, it should be included in every treatment program for the arm. The ability to accept weight on the extended arm allows the patient to use his involved arm for the functions described above and to adapt the movement patterns in the arm to perform related functions in other positions. For example, the motor components in the arm in sitting extended-arm weight bearing are similar to those used in standing extended-arm weight bearing, in quadruped, and in functions such as pushing a grocery cart and holding a railing while climbing stairs.

FIGURE 7-28 Extended-arm weight bearing.

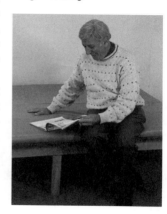

Extended-arm weight bearing is also an important treatment activity because it helps reeducate critical movement patterns in the trunk and arm. Extended-arm weight bearing in sitting is one of the best places to increase extension in the thoracic spine and gain strength in the adductors and upward rotators of the scapula. When these movement components have been reestablished in the patient's movement repertoire, they lead to improved upright control of the trunk in unsupported sitting, standing, and walking and to improved alignment of the scapula and glenohumeral joint. Similarly, extended-arm weight bearing is one of the first positions in which the patient is able to activate elbow extensors and wrist extensors in a pattern similar to that used during forward reach and to combine active arm patterns with appropriate trunk and lower extremity movements. Extended-arm weight bearing may also be used in treatment to lengthen tight or hypertonic muscles in the shoulder, elbow, wrist, and fingers and to increase mobility in the scapula and shoulder joint through active movement rather than passive stretching.

MOVEMENT COMPONENTS

When one or both arms are extended by the side of the body and resting on the support, the weight bearing hands expand the body's base of support in a lateral direction. The arms can be placed in weight bearing in different positions relative to the trunk. These variations are associated with different movement requirements in the trunk and arm and with different functions in daily life. While hand placement is largely selected in daily life according to the intended functional task, the length of the arms relative to the trunk varies widely among individuals and will affect how the arms can be positioned for weight bearing. In treatment, the position of the arms is selected according to the goal of the activity, the body proportions of the patient, and the status of impairments that influence trunk and arm posture.

During extended-arm weight bearing, the hands can be positioned at the edge of the mat with the fingers over the edge, laterally alongside the thighs or hips, or laterally behind the hips. At the edge of the mat, the weight bearing arms are optimally positioned to provide additional stability to the trunk and to assist in the transition of sit to stand. In this position the shoulders are aligned in front of the hips, placing the thoracic spine in slight flexion, the scapulas in abduction and elevation, and the glenohumeral joint in internal rotation (Fig. 7-29A & B). This position is used in treatment if muscle tightness limits the range in the arm in abduction and external rotation and when it is appropriate for the function being trained.

Moving the hands backwards toward the hip joints takes the spine out of flexion and changes the position of the scapulas and arms. When the hands are moved backwards from the edge of the seat toward the hip joints, the spine extends, the scapulas adduct and the shoulder joint moves into horizontal abduction with external rotation. This position is used functionally to support the trunk. It is also the arm position most often used in treatment to train lower-trunk-initiated weight shift patterns. As the hands move back further to a position behind the hips, spinal extension and scapula adduction increase even more. This position can only be used in treatment when the spine, scapulas, and shoulder joints are extremely mobile (Fig. 7-29C & D).

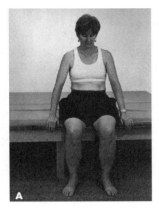

FIGURE 7-29 *(A & B)* Extended-arm weight bearing with the hands at the edge of the mat with the fingers over the edge. The shoulders are aligned in front of the hips, placing the thoracic spine in slight flexion, the scapulas in rotation and elevation, and the glenohumeral joint in internal rotation. *(C & D)* Trunk extension and scapula adduction increase as the weight bearing position of the hands changes from the edge of the mat to more abducted and posterior positions.

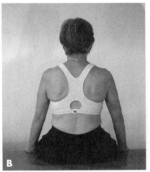
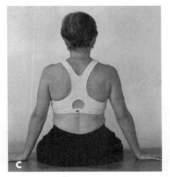
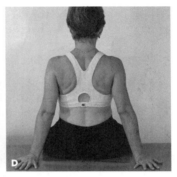

Upper-Trunk-Initiated Movements

Upper-trunk-initiated weight shifts are not particularly important for function in forearm weight bearing. However, in extended-arm weight bearing, upper-trunk-initiated patterns have important functional uses (Table 7-3). For the movement

TABLE 7-3 Upper-Trunk-Initiated Movements

	TRUNK	SCAPULA	HUMERUS	ELBOW	WRIST
Anterior	Flexion	Abduction/ elevation	Less flexion/ internal rotation	Slight flexion	Extension
Lateral					
Weight bearing	Lateral flexion Concave	Down rotation/ depression	Abduction	Flexion	Extension
Non-weight bearing	Convex	Elevation/ up rotation	Adduction	Extension	Leaves bed

FIGURE 7-30 *(A–C)* Anterior weight shift.

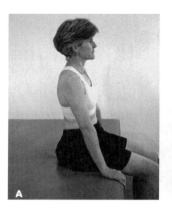 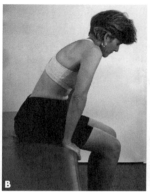 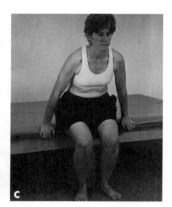

components described below, the weight bearing arms are positioned close to the edge of the mat, with the fingertips hanging over the edge.

Anterior Weight Shift

In an anterior weight shift initiated from the upper trunk, the head and shoulders move forward and down. This places the spine in flexion and the shoulders in front of the hands. As the shoulders move forward, increased body weight is shifted onto the hands. The muscles of the shoulder and elbow must be active to stabilize the elbow in extension so that the wrist, not the elbow, is the fulcrum of the movement. The movement of the body over the fixed arm causes the scapula to elevate and abduct, the humerus to internally rotate, and the wrist to extend (Fig. 7-30).

Functional Example

This movement is used for sit to stand with the arms assisting in the movement.

Lateral Weight Shift

When the upper trunk moves laterally to the right so that the right side of the trunk shortens, the weight of the upper trunk is shifted over the right arm, and the left arm leaves the support. As the spine laterally flexes toward the right, the right elbow flexes, and the shoulder and elbow move down. In the right arm, the movement results in downward rotation of the scapula and abduction of the humerus. To bring the elbow to the support, the trunk must slightly rotate backwards. The left hand may come across the body to rest on the bed near the right knee as the trunk rotates, to help support the trunk as it moves down (Fig. 7-31).

Functional Example

This movement is one of the common ways to lie down.

Lower-Trunk-Initiated Movements

For the movement components described below (Table 7-4), the hands are positioned close to the thighs about level with the hip joints. The fingers of the hands point laterally away from the body. This position places the spine in extension, the

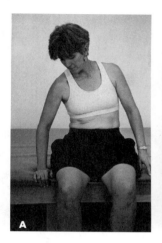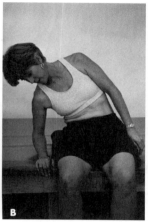

FIGURE 7-31 *(A & B)* Lateral weight shift.

scapulas in adduction, and the extended arms in abduction and external rotation. We have chosen this position for the arms because it is the easiest position for the lower-trunk-initiated movements to occur. It is also the position most often used in treatment to increase control of trunk and arm extension.

Anterior Weight Shift

During an anterior weight shift initiated in the lower body, the pelvis and lumbar spine move forward. This forward movement increases the amount of flexion at the hips and produces extension in the thoracic and lumbar spine. As the body moves forward and more body weight is transferred to the hands, the scapulas adduct and depress and the shoulder joints externally rotate. The elbows remain in extension. This results in full extension at the wrist and a slight flattening of the palmar arches in the hand (Fig. 7-32).

TABLE 7-4 Lower-Trunk-Initiated Movements

	TRUNK	SCAPULA	HUMERUS	ELBOW	WRIST
Anterior	Extension	Adduction/ depression	Less flexion/ external rotation	Extension	Extension
Posterior	Flexion	Abduction/ elevation	Flexion/ internal rotation	Extension	Less flexion
Lateral					
Weight bearing	Lateral flexion Convex	Elevation/ up rotation	Adduction/ external rotation	Slight flexion	Extension
Non-weight bearing	Concave	Depression/ down rotation	Abduction/ internal rotation	Extension	Less extension

FIGURE 7-32 *(A & B)* Anterior weight shift.

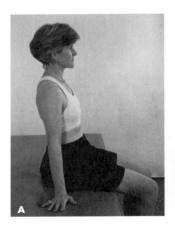 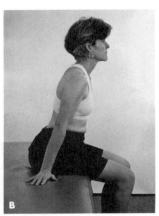

Functional Example

This movement could be used as part of scooting forward or back on the support.

Posterior Weight Shift

When the lower trunk initiates a posterior weight shift, the lower spine flexes and the pelvis moves backwards so that the hips are in less flexion. As the spine moves away from the stable arms, the scapulas abduct and elevate, while the shoulder joint moves into slight flexion with internal rotation. The elbow remains in extension, and the amount of wrist joint extension is decreased as the forearm moves backwards. Weight shifts to the ulnar side of the hand (Fig. 7-33).

Functional Example

This movement is used to scoot the hips back on the bed.

Lateral Weight Shift

When the lower trunk initiates a lateral weight shift to the right, the right arm accepts more body weight, but the left arm stays in contact with the bed. The movement begins with a lateral movement in the pelvis. The left side of the pelvis elevates and moves to the right, while the right side of the pelvis moves to the right and down. This places the spine in lateral flexion with the concavity on the left. As the right side of the rib cage lengthens and moves to the right, the right shoulder moves sideways and up until it is over the right hand. This movement produces scapula elevation and upward rotation, glenohumeral joint external rotation, humeral adduction, wrist extension with weight on the heel of the hand. On the left side, the rib cage shortens, and the left shoulder moves to the right. This results in downward rotation and depression of the scapula, shoulder internal rotation and abduction, elbow extension, and movement of the wrist out of extension. As the body moves away from the left arm, the heel of the hand leaves the support, but the fingers remain in contact when the length of the arm is proportional to the length of the trunk (Fig. 7-34).

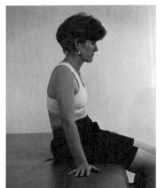

FIGURE 7-33 Posterior weight shift.

Functional Example

This pattern could be used to cross one leg over the other or to shift weight to one arm to rest the trunk or free the other arm for function.

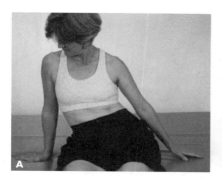
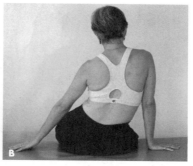

FIGURE 7-34 *(A & B)* Lateral weight shift.

Rotational Movements

When both hands are in weight bearing by the hips, the trunk cannot rotate very much before one hand loses contact with the mat. Only small rotations of the head and shoulders are possible in this position. For more functional rotational movements to occur, one hand is taken out of weight bearing to move with the trunk as it rotates, while the other arm remains in contact with the supporting surface. Three patterns of movement that combine trunk rotation with extended arm weight bearing are described below.

Upper Trunk Rotation on a Stable Lower Trunk

Very little change in spinal position occurs when one hand is moved across midline and placed in weight bearing on the same side of the body as the other arm. In this rotational pattern, the hand stays close to the level of the mat as it crosses midline. As the left hand crosses midline, the trunk rotates to the right with slight flexion in the upper trunk. As the left hand approaches the right leg, increased body weight shifts to the right hip. The rotation causes the right side of the rib cage to rotate backwards. This places the right scapula in greater abduction. (Fig. 7-35).

Functional Example

This movement is used to bring both hands to the same side of the body for a functional task involving weight bearing. It is also a common treatment activity.

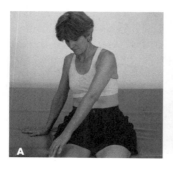
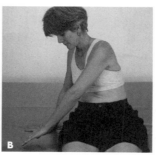

FIGURE 7-35 *(A & B)* Upper trunk rotation to place both arms in extended arm weight bearing on the right side.

FIGURE 7-36 *(A & B)* Rotation with trunk flexion.

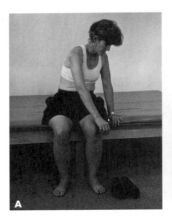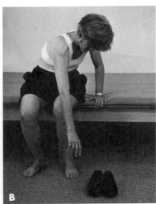

Rotation With Trunk Flexion

Rotation with trunk flexion occurs when the non-weight bearing arm moves across midline and reaches for an object lower than the supporting surface. In this pattern, trunk rotation is combined with an upper-trunk-initiated anterior weight shift, resulting in flexion rotation. When the right arm moves across midline and the left arm remains in weight bearing, the spine rotates to the left, and weight is transferred onto the left hip. In the weight bearing arm, the initial movement components are the same as described above. As the right arm reaches down and the upper trunk flexes further, the left elbow flexes and the humerus hyperextends and internally rotates to allow the trunk to move forward and down (Fig. 7-36).

Functional Example

This movement is used to pick something off the floor. The weight bearing arm provides additional postural stability.

Rotation With Trunk Extension

An extension rotation pattern is used when the arm rotates across midline to reach for something that is positioned high above the level of the supporting surface. To initiate this pattern of rotation to the left, the right hand reaches up and forward as the trunk begins to rotate. The raising of the hand is accompanied by increased extension in the upper trunk. As the right hand approaches midline, the right side of the rib cage rotates forward and the left side rotates back. Increased body weight is transferred to the left hip and the left arm. As the right arm continues to reach up and to the left, the right side of the trunk is lengthened. For the left arm to stay on the mat, the left side of the trunk is shortened. In the left arm, the scapula is downwardly rotated and depressed, the shoulder joint is flexed and slightly internally rotated, and the elbow is partially flexed. The left wrist is fully extended with the weight shift (Fig. 7-37).

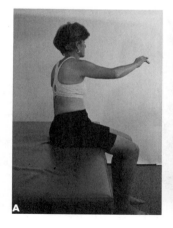 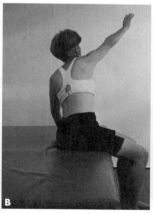 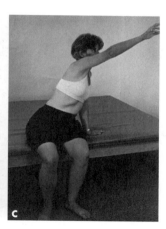

FIGURE 7-37 (A–C) Rotation across midline with trunk extension.

Functional Example

This movement is used for reaching across midline for high objects. The weight bearing arm adds stability to the trunk.

SIGNIFICANT IMPAIRMENTS THAT INTERFERE WITH PERFORMANCE

Extended-arm weight bearing is a difficult functional pattern for neurologic patients. The task is difficult because it requires muscle strength and control in muscles of the trunk and arm that are frequently weak or paralyzed. It is also difficult because it requires soft tissue length in muscle groups of the arm that shorten quickly in the months after stroke. The most common impairments that interfere specifically with extended-arm weight bearing are discussed below. Additional impairments that are included in the chapters on forearm weight bearing and arm movements may also be relevant.

Upper Extremity Hypertonicity

Extended-arm weight bearing by definition requires extension in the arm. This pattern of extension includes relative extension in the thoracic spine, adduction of the scapulas, abduction and external rotation at the shoulder, and extension in the elbow, wrist, and fingers. For the extended arm to accept body weight as the body moves over it, full extension range is necessary in the elbow, wrist, and fingers. Hypertonicity in the arm usually affects the flexor muscles of the elbow, wrist, and fingers, as well as powerful muscles connecting the arm to the trunk. These muscles maintain the arm in a flexed position close to the body and resist lengthening, making it difficult for the arm to be passively extended or placed in the abducted weight bearing position (Fig. 7-38). When hypertonicity has been present for several weeks or months, these muscles may develop soft tissue shortening and, eventually, contractures.

The arm with flexor hypertonicity cannot be placed into the position for extended-arm weight bearing until the abnormal muscle tension is decreased. As the tension in the hypertonic flexor muscles is reduced, the arm may be passively

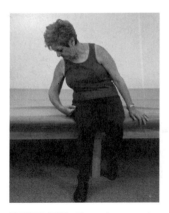

FIGURE 7-38 Flexor hypertonicity in the hemiplegic arm prevents the arm from being placed in the position for extended-arm weight bearing.

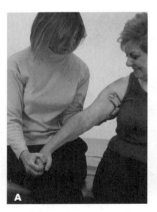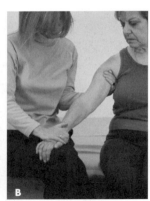

FIGURE 7-39 *(A)* Weight bearing on the therapist's leg can be used when tension in the wrist and fingers prevents the hand from being placed on the mat. The therapist begins weight bearing on a fisted hand. *(B)* Further reduction of hypertonicity in the wrist and fingers after weight bearing on a fisted hand.

extended at the elbow and wrist and the arm gradually moved into position for weight bearing. Upper extremity spasticity is decreased using techniques such as scapula mobilization in sitting or supine and forearm weight bearing. These techniques produce the release of muscle tension necessary to extend the arm passively and prepare for extended-arm weight bearing. Once the arm is passively extended, weight bearing on the hand can be used to reduce muscle tension further, open a fisted hand, and activate muscles in normal patterns.

When the muscles of the wrist and fingers are hypertonic, full extension of the elbow, wrist, and fingers may not be immediately available when abnormal muscle tone has been reduced at the shoulder and elbow. In this case, the therapist must alter the position of the arm in weight bearing. For example, she may place the hand in weight bearing over the edge of the mat or on her leg, decreasing the need for full muscle length at the shoulder, wrist, and fingers, or use her hand under the patient's palm to decrease the range of wrist extension (Fig. 7-39A). Movements of the trunk over the weight bearing hand can be used to lengthen wrist and finger muscles, allowing gradual improved range and position during weight bearing treatment (Fig. 7-39B). Whenever hypertonicity is present, the patient should be active during weight bearing so that the task recruits appropriate muscle contractions in hypertonic muscles and their antagonists. The prolonged stretch on muscles that occurs with passive propping on an extended arm frequently leads to shoulder and wrist pain and tendonitis.

Upper Extremity Weakness

In extended-arm weight bearing, the position of the arm is maintained by muscle activity in the shoulder girdle, elbow, and wrist. The elbow extensors must contract to stabilize the elbow joint in extension, connecting the humerus with the forearm into one functional unit. This muscle activity around the elbow joint allows body weight to be transferred down the arm to the hand and makes the wrist joint the fulcrum for movements of the trunk over the weight bearing arm. In addition, the shoulder depressors deliver a downward force along the shaft of the arm to keep the hand on the support.

When the involved arm is weak, the patient is unable to produce some or all of these essential movement components. Most patients with weakness have difficulty contracting the triceps muscle with adequate force to extend the elbow or to keep it extended as body weight is shifted on the arm. When the elbow is not held in extension as the patient attempts to perform lower-trunk-initiated movements, the elbow flexes as the shoulder comes toward the hand (Fig. 7-40). Other patients may be able to hold the elbow in extension but have difficulty using the shoulder girdle muscles to push the arm onto the support. This causes the arm to slide or lift off the support as the trunk moves, so that no weight is transferred to the hand.

Many patients with muscle weakness in the arm learn to perform extended-arm weight bearing using atypical movements to stabilize the arm on the support and mechanically lock the elbow. Neurologic patients learn to use one of two patterns to lock their elbow mechanically. The elbow may be mechanically locked when the shoulder is rotated forward with internal rotation at the glenohumeral joint. In this position, the elbow is stable, but the trunk is sheared to the uninvolved side and the thoracic spine is in flexion (Fig. 7-41A). The strong forward rotation of the humerus and forearm over the hand places a rotatory force on the center of the hand that collapses the palmer arches (Fig. 7-41B). The second atypical compensation places the elbow joint in hyperextension. Although weight is shifted onto the arm with this pattern, the muscles of the arm and trunk are not active, and weight is supported on the arm by "hanging on ligaments" rather than active muscle contraction.

To reeducate extended-arm weight bearing for the patient with weakness in the arm, the therapist selects hand placements that allow her to establish normal alignment in the trunk and arm and assist the action of the weak muscles (Fig. 7-42). The assistance of the therapist allows that patient to learn the appropriate sequences of muscle activity and to participate actively in the task to the extent possible. Assisted practice often results in increased muscle strength and independent

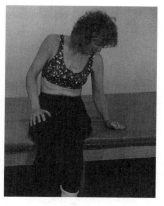

FIGURE 7-40 Inability to maintain extension at the elbow. The patient is attempting to shift weight toward her hemiplegic arm.

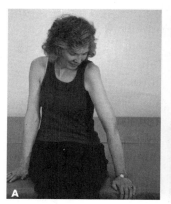
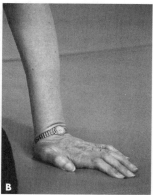

FIGURE 7-41 (A) Mechanically locking the elbow in extension by rotating the shoulder joint forward. (B) Collapse of the palmar arches, caused by atypical patterns in the proximal arm.

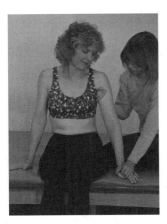

FIGURE 7-42 Reeducating extended-arm weight bearing. The therapist's hand placements allow her to control the position of the trunk, shoulder, elbow, and hand as the patient actively moves her trunk.

performance. If the therapist does not assist the weak muscles, the patient will learn to perform the movements using an atypical pattern to stiffen the involved arm. These undesirable movements block the use of normal trunk and arm patterns.

Soft Tissue Restrictions

While often associated with spasticity, soft tissue shortening and associated joint hypomobility are frequent secondary complications in patients with hypotonia/flaccid paralysis and with good recovery of muscle strength and control. These problems may be present in the trunk, in the shoulder girdle, and in the lower arm and hand. The most common problems that interfere with performance are loss of mobility and tissue length between the trunk and scapula, between the scapula and humerus, and loss of muscle length at the wrist and fingers.

When soft tissue and joint mobility restrictions are present, the therapist modifies the position of weight bearing so that tight tissues are lengthened without placing destructive forces on joints. For example, loss of muscle length in the long finger flexors may prevent the hand being placed flat on the mat for weight bearing. The therapist may have this patient weight bear on a fisted hand to avoid flattening the palmar arches and creating alignment problems in the hand (Fig. 7-43). If the arm cannot be comfortable positioned for extended-arm weight bearing, the task should not be used until tissue length and joint mobility has increased through the use of other treatment activities. Forearm weight bearing and supine treatment are good places to lengthen tight muscles between the arm and trunk and between proximal and distal arm segments. Suggestions for using extended-arm weight bearing to increase muscle length and range are discussed below.

ASSESSMENT GUIDELINES

Assessment in extended-arm weight bearing should focus on the position of the arm and trunk during the activity and the ability to perform the movements with the correct movement components. Placing the arm into the extended-arm weight bearing position will be difficult for many patients. When the arm cannot be posi-

FIGURE 7-43 (A) Tightness in the finger flexors results in atypical hand position during weight bearing. (B) Allowing the fingers to be fisted results in a more acceptable hand position.

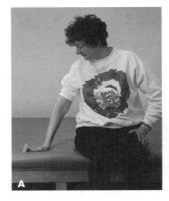
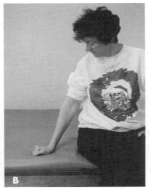

tioned correctly for the task, the therapist should try to determine the impairments that are interfering with the task. These impairments should be addressed in treatment so that extended-arm weight bearing can be used for treatment and function.

ASSESSMENT GUIDELINES

Assessing Extended-Arm Weight Bearing

I. Position the involved arm in extension and place the hand on the mat. Describe any problems that interfere with placing the hand in weight bearing. Identify the position of the involved trunk, scapula, glenohumeral joint, elbow, wrist, and fingers when the arm rests on the mat.

II. Assess the control of the arm as the patient initiates upper and lower body movements. Identify movements that are performed with atypical or compensatory patterns and any movement patterns that cannot be performed.

What problems do you observe in the arm and the trunk during those difficult movements?

III. Use your hands on the patient's trunk and arm to correct position and assist these movements. Which movements or problems improve with your handling? Where did you put your hands to make these changes?

What problems or movements did not change with handling?

IV. List the major primary and secondary impairments that are interfering with extended-arm weight bearing. What treatment techniques will you use to address these problems and improve extended-arm weight bearing?

V. For what function are you preparing with this activity?

THERAPY GOALS

Functional Goals

The task of extended-arm weight bearing will be useful to the patient in meeting the following functional goals:

1. To be able to support body weight on an extended arm to rest or support the trunk.

2. To be able to use weight bearing in task performance either to stabilize objects or to assist in postural control.

3. To be able to use weight bearing in sit to stand.

Treatment Goals and Techniques

Treatment Goal: Reeducate components of extended-arm weight bearing.

Treatment Technique: Reestablish normal alignment in the hemiplegic arm. Before the hemiplegic arm can be placed in extended-arm weight bearing, the therapist must realign the shoulder joint and move the elbow and wrist into extension with the axis of the humerus in line with the forearm and hand (Fig. 7-44).

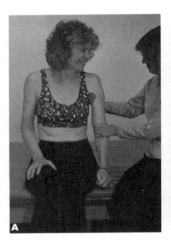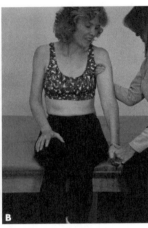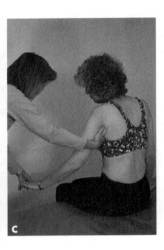

FIGURE 7-44 The therapist uses an axillary/hand shake grip to align the hemiplegic arm. *(A)* The shoulder joint is positioned first. The therapist's hand in the axilla lifts the shoulder joint up and back, increasing thoracic extension. At the same time, she externally rotates the humerus. *(B)* She takes the hemiplegic hand in her other hand, as if shaking the hand. With this hand, she brings the elbow into extension and lines the forearm up with the humerus. *(C)* Maintaining this grip, the therapist moves the hemiplegic arm into horizontal abduction to prepare for extended arm weight bearing.

Treatment Technique: Teach active shoulder depression. Since extended-arm weight bearing combines trunk movements with those of the upper extremity, it is a difficult activity for most hemiplegic patients. It is often easier for the patient to learn and practice the important movement components of the hemiplegic arm before attempting to combine these movements with trunk weight shifts. In this portion of treatment, the therapist teaches the hemiplegic arm to be active in weight bearing (Fig. 7-45).

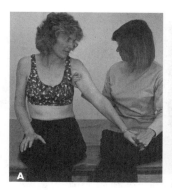 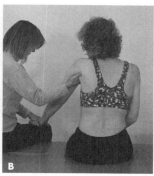 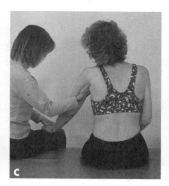 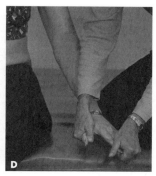

FIGURE 7-45 *(A)* To train the upper extremity components of shoulder depression with elbow extension, the therapist uses the axillary/hand shake grip and places the hemiplegic hand in weight bearing on her thigh. This weight bearing position for the hemiplegic hand is critical for two reasons: (1) The therapist uses her leg to push back into the hand, providing it with increased sensory input, and (2) by using her leg, the therapist is also better able to feel whether the patient is pushing with her hemiplegic arm in the desired pattern. *(B)* To prepare for active depression of the arm, the therapist uses her hand in the axilla to elevate the hemiplegic shoulder. As she lifts the shoulder, she also lifts her leg slightly, so that the hemiplegic hand remains against her leg and the elbow remains extended. *(C)* The therapist then asks the patient to push her hand into her leg, while at the same time her hand in the axilla helps the shoulder girdle to depress. She uses her leg to give a slight resistance to the movement but moves her leg down as the shoulder moves down, so that the elbow remains extended. After the patient has felt the movement several times, she should be encouraged to be more active. The therapist may tell her to push her leg away. *(D)* When the patient is able to depress the shoulder girdle actively and maintain elbow extension, the hemiplegic hand may be moved to a weight bearing position on the mat for the next stage of weight bearing treatment. The therapist grasps the fingers and the thumb of the hemiplegic hand. She maintains the wrist in extension while moving the hand.

Treatment Technique: Reeducate elbow extension in weight bearing. Activity in the elbow extensors is necessary during weight bearing on the hemiplegic arm. The movement of elbow extension can be practiced in isolation before asking for elbow extension with trunk movements (Fig. 7-46).

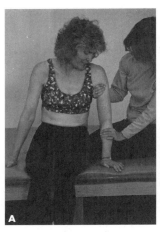 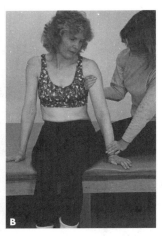

FIGURE 7-46 *(A)* The patient with assistance of the therapist practices elbow flexion, without moving her trunk laterally. The therapist's hand moves the humerus slightly back to initiate flexion. Her hand on the forearm maintains a steady downward pressure into the hand to keep it stable. *(B)* The patient actively extends the elbow. The therapist may assist the extension if necessary, by using her hand in the axilla to lift the shoulder girdle up and back. Later, this elbow movement may be combined with upper-trunk-initiated lateral weight shifts, to prepare the arm to be active in the transition of sidelying to/from sitting.

Treatment Technique: Activate trunk movements with the hemiplegic arm in extended-arm weight bearing (Fig. 7-47).

FIGURE 7-47 In this segment of treatment, the therapist asks the patient to move his trunk actively, while she assists the hemiplegic arm in the appropriate movement components. The goal is to help the patient learn to combine trunk and arm movements. *(A)* The therapist controls the hemiplegic arm using an axillary/palmar grip. *(B)* She can also use an axillary/forearm grip. Her two hands stabilize the position of the shoulder and elbow joints and provide a downward pressure along the humerus and forearm into the hemiplegic hand. *(C–E)* The therapist asks the patient to perform lower-trunk-initiated lateral weight shifts. As the patient moves toward her left side, the therapist's hand in the axilla lifts the scapula and guides the shoulder joint over the hand, keeping the humerus externally rotated. Her opposite hand stabilizes the hand on the mat. When the patient shifts toward her uninvolved side, the therapist depresses the hemiplegic shoulder and pushes from the humerus down into the hand. The patient is encouraged to push actively with the arm as weight is shifted to the other side. Similar hand placements are also used to combine lower-body-initiated anterior/posterior movements with the arm in extended-arm weight bearing. *(F)* The therapist may move her hand from control of the patient's distal arm to the trunk. Here the therapist's hand on the trunk is bringing the bottom of the rib cage forward to increase trunk extension. *(G)* The therapist uses her hand on the patient's rib cage to increase lateral flexion of the spine as the patient shifts weight to her uninvolved side.

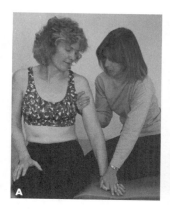
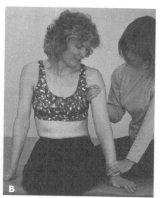

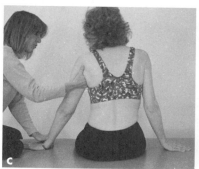
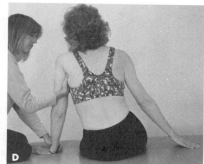
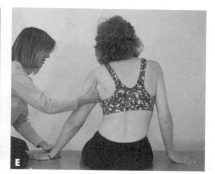

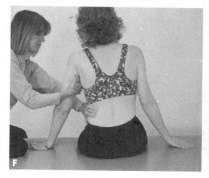
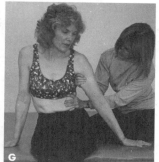

Treatment Goal: Reduce flexor hypertonicity and/or lengthen shortened tissues in the hemiplegic arm.

Treatment Technique: Extended-arm weight bearing can be used to reduce muscle tension systematically and lengthen tight muscles. The stages of treatment are similar to those described above and in the section on forearm weight bearing (Fig. 7-48).

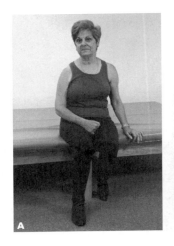
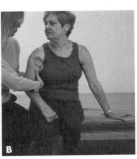
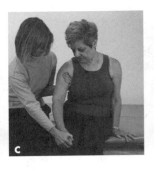
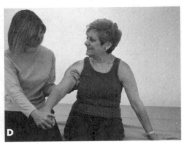
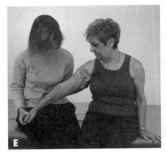
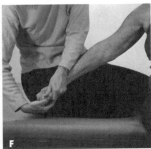
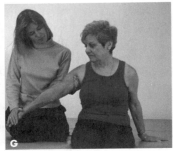
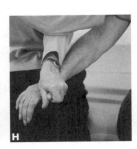

FIGURE 7-48 *(A)* Right hemiplegia before treatment. *(B)* The therapist uses an axillary grip to mobilize the scapula in the planes of elevation/depression and abduction/adduction. *(C)* As the movements of the scapula result in decreased tension at the elbow, her other hand guides the elbow into more extension. *(D)* The arm is moved into abduction and placed on the therapist's knee. Since the flexor tone in the wrist and fingers is too high to allow extension, the hand is placed in weight bearing with slight flexion at the wrist and fisted fingers. The patient is asked to perform lower-trunk-initiated weight shifts while the arm is in weight bearing. *(E)* As muscle tension decreases, the arm is moved into a greater range of horizontal abduction with external rotation. Note position of wrist and fingers. *(F)* As muscle tension in the distal arm decreases, the therapist opens the hand. *(G)* Weight bearing on an open hand. *(H)* The fingers drape naturally over the therapist's leg when muscle tension at the wrist and hand is reduced. At this point, the hand may be placed in weight bearing on the mat. *(Figure continues.)*

FIGURE 7-48 *(Continued)* *(I)* To move the hand from her knee to the mat, the therapist lets go of control of the glenohumeral joint and uses both hands to lift the open hand. *(J)* The hand is lowered to the mat. *(K)* Once the hand has been placed on the mat, the patient is asked to perform trunk movements.

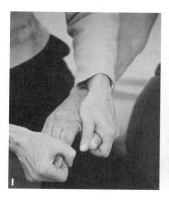
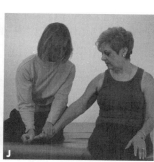
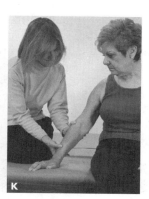

Treatment Technique: A fisted hand may also be placed directly on the mat for weight bearing. This may be necessary if the muscles at the wrist and fingers lack enough length for the fingers to be fully extended with wrist extension (Fig. 7-49).

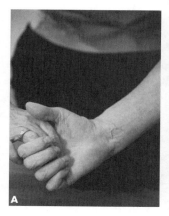
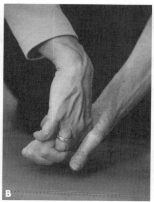
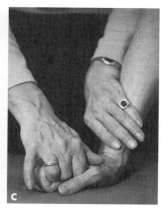

FIGURE 7-49 *(A)* The therapist places her fingers into the palm of the hemiplegic hand and her thumb on the back of the hand. *(B)* Pressure between her thumb and fingers allows her to bring the wrist into extension. *(C)* The therapist retains this grip on the hand while it is in weight bearing. Her control on the palm prevents collapse of the hand with weight bearing. It also allows her to feel for release of tension in the fingers, which would allow her to open the hand on the mat.

Treatment Goal: Incorporate extended-arm weight bearing in functional patterns.

Treatment Technique: The practice of rotational trunk movements toward the hemiplegic side prepares the patient to support weight on his hemiplegic arm while using his uninvolved arm for task performance. This activity requires that the patient be able to assist in the easier task of lower-body-initiated lateral weight shifts to the hemiplegic side (Fig. 7-50).

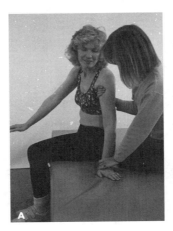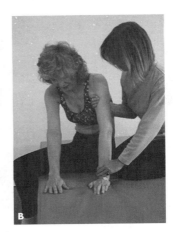

FIGURE 7-50 *(A)* The therapist supports the hemiplegic arm with the axillary/forearm grip. The patient rotates her head and shoulder girdle toward the hemiplegic side. As the hemiplegic shoulder rotates back, the patient lifts her uninvolved arm off the mat. *(B)* The uninvolved arm is placed in weight bearing position, with the trunk in flexion rotation. In this position, the patient's hemiplegic shoulder girdle tends to collapse forward, flexing the elbow. The therapist's hand in the axilla lifts the shoulder girdle up and back to maintain the arm in extension with the correct pattern of trunk rotation. The patient may practice shifting weight forward over the hands and back in this position.

Treatment Technique: Extended-arm weight bearing can also be trained in the function of sit to stand. For this activity, the arm is placed in weight bearing on the edge of the treatment mat. The patient practices upper-body-initiated anterior weight shifts with active depression of the hemiplegic arm. When the patient can perform this pattern with minimal assistance, he is asked to lift the hips slightly off the mat while pushing with the arm (Fig. 7-51 A–C).

FIGURE 7-51 *(A–C)* Use of the arms in weight bearing during sit to stand.

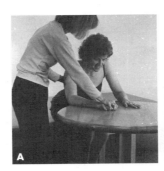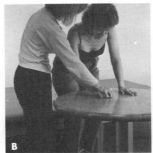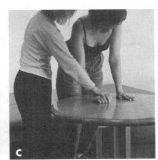

8
Lower Extremity
Movements in Sitting

In sitting, the legs are used as an active base to support movements of the trunk and limbs, to move the body around, and to interact with the environment. As with upper extremity weight bearing in sitting (Ch. 7), weight bearing movements in the legs are a dynamic process that is a response to active trunk movements. The concept of weight bearing that we feel is critical to effective treatment of stroke patients is one in which these trunk movements allow a weight shift of the center of gravity, which results in active contraction of supporting muscles in the leg. These trunk movements may be used for an arm task (reaching for an object beyond arms length), an arm and leg task (reaching for a shoe and putting it on), or a mobility task (moving from sitting to standing). In treatment, reeducation of trunk movements in sitting results in increased hip and knee strength and control, if appropriate trunk and leg alignment is maintained while hip and knee muscles are activated. Prerequisites for muscle activation include sufficient muscle length across the lower trunk and hip joints to allow the femur to be seated in an appropriate position in the acetabulum, active firing of muscles during the weight shifts, and enough trunk control to allow the upper trunk to respond to and follow movements initiated by the lower trunk.

Patients with neurologic impairments have difficulty with lower extremity movements and function in sitting. These problems are related to primary and secondary impairments of the leg, but they are also related to trunk impairments. In the early stages of recovery, trunk weakness and lack of postural control result in problems of abnormal spinal and rib cage alignment and, since the pelvis is linked to the lower trunk in sitting, problems of pelvic obliquity. These alignment and movement problems in the trunk and pelvis influence the alignment and pattern of muscle return in the hip, knee, ankle, and foot. Muscle weakness in the leg interferes with both weight bearing and non-weight bearing movement patterns of the leg in sitting. The secondary impairments of muscle shortening, muscle shifting, and hypertonicity contribute to the loss of lower extremity control and to loss of function.

This chapter analyzes normal and abnormal *weight bearing movements* of the lower extremity, *non-weight bearing movements* of the lower extremity, and a functional example of the combination of the two patterns: *scooting.* Although the description that follows is limited to the trunk and lower extremity, the active use of the upper extremities can be added to the analysis of this movement. The upper extremities are frequently used to assist in balance and stability so that we can shift weight over our legs with greater ease.

Lower Extremity Weight Bearing in Sitting

CONCEPTS AND PRINCIPLES

In sitting, the weight bearing area of the legs include the ischial tuberosities, the portion of the thighs that are in contact with the supporting surface, and the feet. Active trunk weight shifts result in relative movement of both hip joints. The feet accept additional weight when they are more directly underneath the pelvis or knees and less weight when they are more in front. The thighs accept additional weight as the trunk moves anteriorly and less weight as the trunk moves posteriorly; the left thigh accepts more weight and the right thigh bears less weight as the trunk shifts to the left and vice versa.

It is important to remember that active movements of the upper and lower trunk in sitting are the basis for this description of relative lower extremity movements (see Ch. 5 for a review). As the trunk moves while the legs are supported by a chair, bed, or bench, the movement of the trunk changes the amount and distribution of weight placed on the legs. This changes the demand on the leg muscles and alters the state of muscle activation. As a result, the use of these weight bearing movement patterns is a part of the muscle reeducation and strengthening techniques of therapy.

LOWER EXTREMITY WEIGHT BEARING MOVEMENT COMPONENTS

Lower-Trunk-Initiated Leg Weight Bearing Patterns

Anterior Weight Shift—Hip Flexion Increases

When an anterior weight shift is initiated in the lower trunk, the spine extends and the center of gravity moves forward, increasing the amount of weight taken by the femurs and the feet. As the anterior superior iliac spine (ASIS) of the pelvis moves anteriorly, the movement of the body on the fixed femur produces an increase in hip flexion (Fig. 8-1A).

Functional Example

This movement is used to extend the reach of the arms forward and up; to initiate a sit to stand.

FIGURE 8-1 *(A)* Lower-trunk-initiated anterior weight shift results in increasing hip flexion. *(B)* Lower-trunk-initiated posterior weight shift results in decreasing hip flexion.

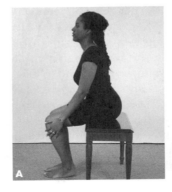 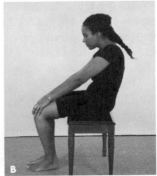

FIGURE 8-2 *(A & B)* Lower-trunk-initiated lateral weight shift to the right results in increasing right hip adduction and left hip abduction.

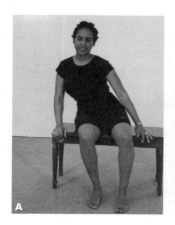
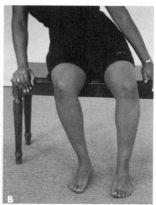

Posterior Weight Shift—Hip Flexion Decreases

When a posterior weight shift is initiated in the lower trunk, the lower spine moves into more flexion, the pelvis moves posteriorly, and there is less weight on the thighs and feet. This posterior movement of the body on the fixed femur produces a decrease of hip flexion in relation to the starting position (Fig. 8-1B). Active trunk weight shifting through the extremes of these two movements—anterior and posterior—is used to improve and strengthen movement control of the hip.

Functional Example

This movement is used to move the body away from an object or a surface, such as a table, and to move the body back to rest against a chair.

Lateral Weight Shift—Hip Adduction and Abduction

A lateral weight shift initiated from the lower trunk to the right results in lateral trunk flexion with the spinal convexity on the right and the spinal concavity on the left. Increased weight is shifted to the right hip and thigh, with a decrease of weight on the left hip and thigh. The right pelvis lists downward/depresses and the center of the pelvis translates laterally to the right; as the left pelvis lists upward/elevates, it also translates medially to the right. This lateral movement of the trunk and pelvis on the femurs results in relative right hip adduction and left hip abduction (Fig. 8-2).

FIGURE 8-3 Feet unsupported, lower-trunk-initiated lateral weight shift to the right.

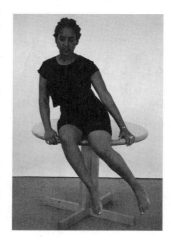

Functional Example

This movement is used to extend the reach of the arm to one side or to use the extended arm for support by the side of the body.

Weight Shifts With the Feet Unsupported

If the feet are not supported during these movements, the movements of the leg are more evident and the trunk must be more active because the base of support is smaller (see Chapter 5). During anterior/posterior lower-trunk-initiated weight shifts, there will be more knee movement, and during lateral movements, the hip rotational components are more obvious (Fig. 8-3; Table 8-1).

TABLE 8-1 Movement Summary: Movements Initiated from the Lower Trunk

	TRUNK	PELVIS	HIP
Anterior	Extension	Moves forward	Flexion
Posterior	Flexion	Moves backward	Less flexion
Lateral weight bearing	Convexity spine	Depression with lateral translation	Adduction
Lateral non-weight bearing	Concavity spine	Elevation with medial translation	Abduction

Upper-Trunk-Initiated Leg Weight Bearing Patterns

Upper-trunk-initiated movements influence the lower extremities in sitting to the degree the movement influences the lower trunk. Body structure, flexibility, and strength determine how, or if, the upper trunk movements influence the lower trunk. When the spine is flexible, an increase in upper trunk extension causes the lower trunk to extend, but if the spine is less flexible, this upper trunk movement may not result in a movement change in the lower trunk.

FIGURE 8-4 *(A)* Upper-trunk-initiated anterior weight shift results in increased hip flexion. *(B)* Upper-trunk-initiated lateral weight shift to the right results in increased weight on the right hip.

Anterior Weight Shift—Hip Flexion Increases

An upper-trunk-initiated anterior movement results in flexion of the upper trunk. The pelvis moves forward and hip flexion increases. If the upper trunk flexion translates down into the lower trunk, the lower trunk will flex as the pelvis moves forward. If the upper trunk flexion does not move down into the lower trunk, the spine will remain in neutral as the pelvis moves forward. Increased body weight is shifted forward onto the thighs and the feet (Fig. 8-4A).

Functional Example

Reaching to the floor.

Posterior Weight Shift—Minimal Change in Hip Position

Upper-trunk-initiated posterior weight shift in sitting moves the spine into extension. Since this extension rarely moves down into the lower trunk and pelvis, the influence on the lower extremities is minimal. While there may be no movement of the lower trunk over the leg, there may be increased activity in the hip muscles to provide additional balance control.

Functional Example

Looking at the ceiling.

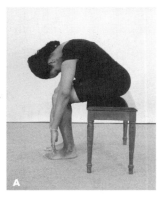
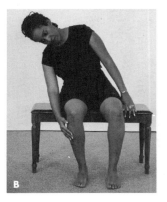

Lateral Weight Shift—Increased Weight on the Hip

Upper-trunk-initiated lateral weight shifts move the spine into lateral flexion with the concavity on the side the trunk moves toward. The upper body moves over the pelvis, but the pelvis stays on the bed through the movement range. This means that increased weight is transferred onto the weight bearing leg and may activate muscular control to assist with additional balance demands (Fig. 8-4B; Table 8-2).

TABLE 8-2 Movement Summary: Movements Initiated from the Upper Trunk

	TRUNK	PELVIS	HIP
Anterior	Flexion	Moves forward	Flexion
Posterior	Extension	Little change	Little movement
Lateral weight bearing	Concavity spine	Remains level	More weight
Lateral non-weight bearing	Convexity spine	Remains level	Less weight

Functional Example

Reaching down to one side; lying down.

SIGNIFICANT IMPAIRMENTS THAT INTERFERE WITH PERFORMANCE

Lack of Hip Control and Weakness

In hemiplegia, if there is weakness or lack of control at the hip joint, the hip will be unstable, and unsupported sitting will be difficult. The patient will avoid placing weight on that side during sitting or during sitting weight shifts. This results in asymmetric trunk and pelvic positions. If the trunk shifts or shears laterally, there is more of a spinal concavity on the hemiplegic side, and that side of the pelvis elevates. This contributes to uneven weight distribution on the thighs and an increase in hip abduction or external rotation (Fig. 8-5). If the trunk is excessively flexed and shifted laterally, and the hip is weak, the avoidance of weight on the affected hip often results in backward rotation of the pelvis. The femur moves into abduction. The abducted femoral position blocks lateral weight shift, thus decreasing the possibility of using trunk movements to strengthen the weak hip muscles.

With severe hip weakness and secondary tightness, lateral weight shifts to the unaffected side result in the hemiplegic side of the pelvis rotating forward and the femur passively moving with it into adduction.

When hip weakness is a problem, the therapist must correct asymmetries and assist the patient with compatible lower trunk and pelvic movements so that the hip

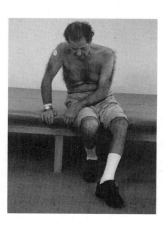

FIGURE 8-5 Patient with a longstanding left hemiplegia with severe hip weakness and loss of control. His weight is shifted to the right, his spine is laterally flexed with the concavity on the left, and the left side of the pelvis is elevated. The left hip joint is not on the surface of the mat. The left thigh is in excessive abduction and external rotation.

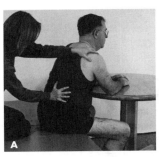

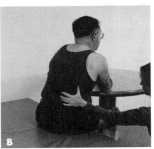

FIGURE 8-6 *(A)* Therapist uses forearm weight bearing to support the upper trunk as she helps the patient learn how to initiate a lower trunk lateral weight shift to begin to reeducate weight bearing movements of the hip. The therapist's right hand directs a downward and lateral message from the lower trunk on a diagonal into the right hip. Her left hand guides the upper body up and laterally and helps it follow the lower-body-initiated movement. *(B)* As the patient learns the trunk portion of the task, the therapist's hands move to correct hip joint alignment. Her right hand is assisting the position of the thigh while her left hand is reminding the lower trunk to initiate the movement. During treatment, the therapist grades the amount of lateral movement the weak hip can support.

muscles have a chance to be reeducated. The trunk-initiated movements must be trained with the appropriate hip alignment and movements (Fig. 8-6). During muscle reeducation, the therapist must grade the range of trunk movements to eliminate overshifting or leaning. Overshifting or leaning of the trunk results in "hanging" on hip ligaments or stretch weakness of the hip abductors. To strengthen weak hip muscles in sitting, the therapist must reeducate trunk and leg patterns with as much symmetry as possible.

When weak hip muscles result in an abnormal hip position during sitting, this proximal alignment problem will result in alignment disturbances in the lower leg and foot. If the hip falls into abduction and the foot remains on the ground, the lower leg will be in a varus position relative to the foot. This position of the lower leg increases the tension on the anterior compartment muscles of the foot and eventually results in the beginning of midfoot supination (Fig. 8-7).

Loss of Trunk Control and Alignment

Trunk weakness, lack of control, postural asymmetries, and the resultant atypical movement patterns are associated with an uneven distribution of weight on the pelvis (see Fig. 5-16A–F). Common patterns include lateral trunk shearing with elevation and rotation backward of the pelvis, resulting in excessive hip abduction; rib cage rotation backward and pelvic rotation forward, which leads to excessive hip adduction; excessive trunk flexion and pelvic rotation backward with hip abduction. Initially, these atypical hip positions exist because of compensatory weight shifts away from the hemiplegic side due to loss of trunk control. But, the hip muscles in these patients are also weak. If the trunk asymmetries are left untreated, they will compound the difficulty of reeducating trunk movements over the hip. During treatment, it is important that the therapist assess trunk/hip relationships before beginning treatment (Fig. 8-8).

FIGURE 8-7 *(A & B)* Right hip weakness with a position of hip abduction and external rotation. This asymmetry leads to an altered lower leg/foot relationship. Correction of pelvis and thigh results in a correction of ankle/foot position.

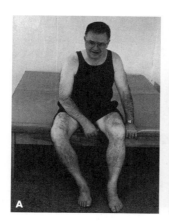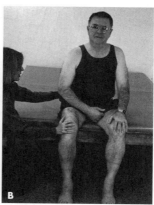

Trunk asymmetries and weakness patterns are often masked by pelvis and hip impairments. If the impairments are not identified in relationship to one another, the therapist may structure a treatment plan that does not result in functional improvement (Fig. 8-8).

Treatment of weight bearing leg movements in sitting must begin with a correction of trunk alignment and the reestablishment of trunk movement patterns. This is especially true during lateral movements. If lower trunk lateral movements are practiced without correcting the spinal alignment, the lateral hip muscles cannot be reeducated and strengthened. These lateral muscles do not get stronger because if the spine is too flexed as lateral movement is attempted, the center of gravity moves behind the hip joint, not over it. The compensatory movements of the upper trunk and pelvis prevents the activation of lateral hip muscles (Fig. 8-9).

FIGURE 8-8 *(A)* Patient with a right hemiplegia in sitting. The pelvis on the right appears elevated, and more weight is on the left hip. *(B)* The therapist corrects pelvic and hip position. With the pelvis in a neutral position, the trunk position becomes clearer. The upper trunk is laterally flexed, with the concavity on the right, and is rotated forward of the pelvis. *(C)* The therapist corrects both the pelvic and trunk positions before beginning the reeducation process. From this position of more appropriate alignment, she will ask the patient to practice trunk initiated movements to reeducate hip strength during weight bearing situations. Her left hand is directing a lateral and downward message into the patient's right hip. The therapist's right hand is on the upper axilla and on the anterior surface of the trunk. This hand is giving a message to the upper trunk to rotate back up to neutral and to come up out of lateral flexion. Counter pressure for this movement comes from her left hand.

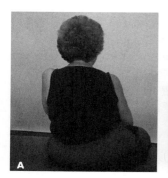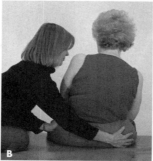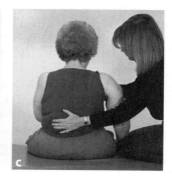

FIGURE 8-9 *(A)* Patient with a right hemiplegia trying to initiate lower trunk lateral movements with the spine in excessive flexion. Note the inappropriate upper body movement and the posterior position of the right side of the pelvis. *(B)* Therapist's right hand is on the patient's lower thoracic spine, encouraging spinal extension, while her left hand is assisting lateral hip stability as she begins to teach the patient lower-body-initiated movements.

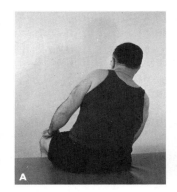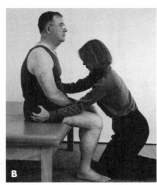

Hypertonicity

In sitting, during lower-trunk-initiated lateral weight movements, shifting past the available length in a tight tensor fascia lata muscle results in knee extension. This knee extension is often labeled as spasticity when, in fact, it is hypertonicity from poor alignment and excessive stretch. During attempts at lower-trunk-initiated posterior movements, the patient's knee may unexpectedly extend. This strong extensor knee movement, during a weight bearing movement, is due to tightness in the rectus femoris muscle. As the patient leans back with her knee bent and the foot on the floor, the available length of the rectus femoris is exceeded, and the knee strongly extends (Fig. 8-10).

Muscle Shortening and Abnormal Alignment of the Hip

FIGURE 8-10 Patient with a right hemiplegia trying to perform a lower trunk posterior movement. The knee moves into extension as a result of tightness in the rectus femoris muscle.

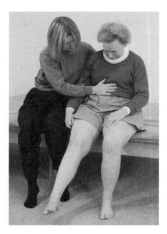

Abnormal alignment in the hip joint is an impairment that interferes with movement recovery and balance control. In sitting, alignment of the hip joint depends on trunk alignment and control. When trunk and hip alignment is not reestablished, muscle shortening of pelvic, hip, and knee muscles follows. Muscle shortening becomes a secondary impairment that then interferes with efficient muscle activation, strengthening, and functional retraining of both the trunk and hip. The alignment problems of the hip in a patient may be different in sitting than they are in standing in the same patient, because the length of the large two-joint muscles that cross the hip and knee joint are affected and altered by hip and knee joint position. This results in varying alignment disturbances related to whether the hip is flexed or extended. Shortened trunk/pelvic muscles also cause abnormal alignment of the hip in sitting. During lower-trunk-initiated anterior weight shifts, as the trunk moves forward, tight hamstring muscles are stretched across the pelvis, resulting in strong knee flexion on the hemiplegic side. In patients with tightness in the quadratus lumborum muscle, upper-body-initiated forward movements are performed with rib cage rotation backward or pelvic rotation backwards. In both cases, the pelvis is elevated and the hip and thigh are not secure on the surface.

Alignment problems in the pelvis and hip become more evident when the patient sits with little or no weight on the involved hip and thigh. These hip, pelvic, and trunk alignment problems must be corrected before muscle reeducation can increase strength (Fig. 8-11).

FIGURE 8-11 *(A)* Patient with a right hemiplegia. Right leg is abducted as a result of lateral thigh tightness. *(B)* As the therapist adducts the femur, the band of lateral muscle tightness becomes visible. The lateral tightness causes the pelvis to rotate forward as the femur is adducted.

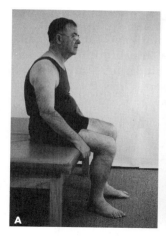 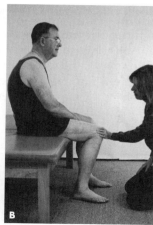

ASSESSMENT GUIDELINES

Assessment of leg movements during trunk initiated weight shifts should be preceded by an assessment of trunk movements in sitting (see below).

Assessing Leg Weight Bearing Movements

I. Describe the position of the trunk, pelvis, and hip during sitting.

II. When you correct the pelvic position, does the trunk position change? If so, describe the trunk position. Does the position of the femur/hip joint change? If so, how?

III. During trunk initiated movements, what accompanying leg movements occur? What hand placements result in improved leg/trunk relationships?

IV. Does the leg posture during the trunk initiated movements? Describe the

---

THERAPY GOALS

Functional Goals

The retraining of leg weight bearing movements in sitting is necessary to help the patient achieve the following functional goals:

1. Establish the ability to safely sit and respond to trunk and arm movements without losing balance.

2. Establish the ability to safely perform functional tasks in sitting.

Treatment Goals and Techniques

In acute treatment, the therapist needs to maintain alignment and mobility in the leg and trunk so that the patterns of trunk control are established, strength in the leg restored, and secondary impairments prevented. In intermediate and long term treatment settings, the therapist may have to set treatment goals to address the problems of muscle shortening, spasticity, and poor joint alignment as well as the movement deficits.

Treatment Goal: Correct trunk and hip alignment during trunk initiated movements to reeducate and strengthen hip and knee weight bearing movements.

Treatment Technique: Correction of upper body on lower body through support of the hemiplegic arm and correction of leg position to allow patient to strengthen hip in weight bearing movements (Fig. 8-12).

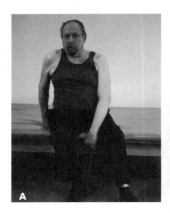 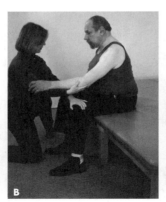 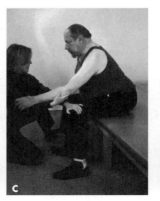 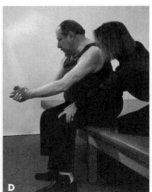

FIGURE 8-12 *(A)* Patient with left hemiplegia and severe weakness. Trunk and leg asymmetries result in less weight on left leg in sitting. *(B & C)* Therapist supports patient's forearm on her right arm and corrects the excessive internal rotation of the shoulder. Her right hand also directs an upward message through the humerus to the upper trunk to correct upper trunk forward flexion/lateral flexion. The therapist's left hand adducts the femur to a neutral position and directs a downward message through the tibia into the foot. She then asks the patient to initiate a lower trunk anterior movement, which results in increased hip flexion. If the patient shifts off his left side during the movement, she can use both hands to assist him to move both his trunk and leg back to midline. *(D)* As patient learns to control the trunk and leg position during the anterior/posterior weight shift, the therapist lets him provide the upper trunk correction through a symmetric arm position and moves behind him to assist leg position. From this position with the trunk and leg active, the patient is ready to practice scooting or sit to stand movements.

Treatment Goal: Lengthen shortened muscles to allow more range so weak muscles can be strengthened more easily.

Treatment Technique: Lengthen tight lateral leg muscles and activate and strengthen hip adductors and abductors by correcting trunk and pelvic position during upper-trunk-initiated movement (Fig. 8-13).

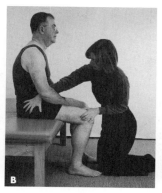
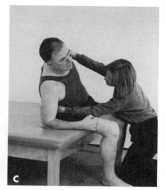
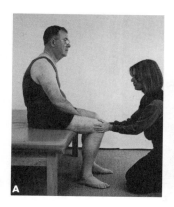
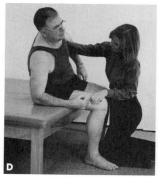
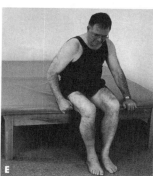

FIGURE 8-13 *(A)* Therapist adducts leg and assesses degree of tightness in lateral hip muscles. *(B)* Therapist's right hand directs downward messages to patient's right hip to provide stability so it will not spin forward as she adducts the distal end of the femur. Her two hands together gently apply a lengthening force to the tight lateral muscles. *(C)* The therapist teaches an upper-trunk-initiated lateral movement. *(D)* She then applies an adduction message to the right femur to lengthen the tight muscle as the patient performs the upper trunk movement that increases the amount of weight placed on his right hip. *(E)* After treatment to lengthen tight lateral muscles, the patient is able to practice hip adduction movements. The movement is still difficult, and he is concentrating and trying hard as evidenced by forward upper trunk movement, but this movement was impossible before treatment.

Treatment Technique: Forearm weight bearing to allow patient to practice lower-trunk-initiated patterns to activate and strengthen leg muscles. Therapist lengthens tight lateral leg muscles while the patient activates and controls the lower-trunk-initiated lateral movements. It is the movement of the trunk over the hip that changes the pelvic/hip position and allows a stretch of the tight leg muscles (Fig. 8-14).

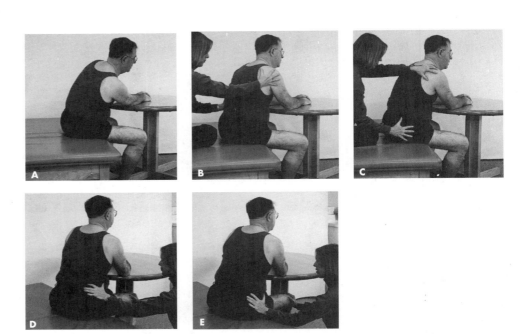

FIGURE 8-14 *(A)* Patient with right hemiplegia attempting to perform lower-trunk-initiated lateral movements to the right in forearm weight bearing. *(B)* Therapist corrects trunk alignment and teaches the patient the movement pattern. Her left hand is over the lateral aspect of the left lower rib cage. Her left hand gives a lateral and downward message into the patient's right hip. Her right hand is assisting the right upper body to prevent it from over-shifting to the right. The two hands together help the patient learn to activate the trunk pattern and to grade the movement over the right hip. *(C)* The therapist's right hand is helping the patient learn to control the movement of his pelvis over his right hip. Her left hand is correcting upper trunk position. *(D)* Now that the trunk movement has been practiced, the therapist moves to her goal of lengthening tight lateral hip and knee muscles. She uses her left hand to provide stability to the pelvis while her right hand begins to move the femur to stretch the muscle. *(E)* She holds the muscle in a slightly lengthened position and asks the patient to perform the lateral trunk weight shifts. As he initiates the movement, the right side of the pelvis translates laterally, which places an increased stretch on the lateral hip muscles. Note the change in the right spinal convexity as he moves to the right.

Treatment Goal: Reeducate trunk and leg movements in a functional task. Reeducate trunk and hip components during lower-trunk–initiated lateral movements and upper-body-initiated anterior movements. Lengthen tight hip and knee muscles to decrease knee extension hypertonicity.

Treatment Techniques: Train trunk and leg components during the functional task of putting on shoes (Fig. 8-15).

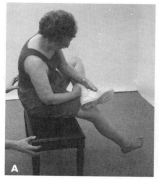
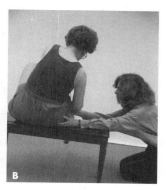
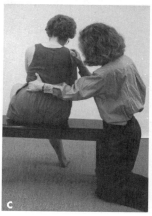
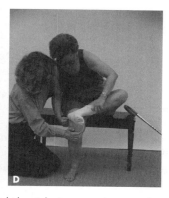

FIGURE 8-15 *(A)* Patient with a right hemiplegia attempting to perform a lower-trunk-initiated right lateral weight shift to put on her left shoe. Right knee is extending and right foot is off the floor because of extensor hypertonicity. (Her balance is precarious.) *(B)* Posterior view. Incompatible trunk components: a lower-body-initiated right lateral weight shift should result in a right spinal convexity. The patient is unweighting her left pelvis, the right spinal concavity is present, and her right leg is extending off the ground. *(C)* Therapist assists patient with the trunk weight shift as she crosses her left leg over her right leg. The therapist's left hand helps the patient learn how to initiate a lower trunk lateral weight shift. As the left side of the pelvis elevates, she directs a diagonal downward message into the right hip. As weight is appropriately taken on the right hip, the right leg does not extend but remains on the floor. The therapist's right hand is assisting the movement of the right upper body upward and over the right hip as the spine shifts laterally with a right convexity. *(D)* The therapist moves to the side of the patient. Her left hand continues to assist with the lower-trunk-initiated movement and her right hand keeps the lower leg on the floor as the patient leans forward to pull her sock on. The therapist can grade the amount and speed of the lateral movement so both hands together can provide a gradual stretch to both the medial hamstring muscles and the tensor fascia lata.

Lower Extremity Movements

CONCEPTS AND PRINCIPLES

In sitting, we move our legs for comfort or to change body position in daily activities. We move our legs to move an object away from us or toward us, for dressing as we put on socks, shoes, and pants, and to scoot on a bench.

As described in the last section, active weight shift of the trunk and contraction of the hip muscles on the weight bearing side is necessary to provide a stable base for the moving leg. One of the most important prerequisites for non-weight bearing movements of the leg in sitting is adequate trunk control. The trunk must be active and stable in sitting to provide stability for the leg as it lifts up. As one leg lifts off the supporting surface, the base of support for the trunk becomes smaller. The upper trunk must remain aligned over the lower trunk as the trunk moves and balances over one leg. Additional trunk control is also needed to adjust and adapt to demands of the moving leg.

In patients with hemiplegia, lifting the hemiplegic leg is difficult because of weakness and poor control of both the leg itself and the trunk muscles that provide balance and stability for that leg. It is also difficult for the patient to pick up his unaffected leg if there is not sufficient trunk or leg control to support body weight on the involved side.

The analysis below describes the movement components of the leg as it initiates movements in sitting and reviews the relationships between the trunk, pelvis, and leg during these non-weight bearing movements.

LOWER EXTREMITY MOVEMENT COMPONENTS

Hip Movement

Flexion

Hip flexion movements lift the thigh off the sitting surface. During the first few degrees of hip flexion from the sitting position, the pelvis remains stationary. As hip flexion continues, and the thigh lifts up, the trunk moves back as the pelvis moves toward a posterior tilt. As the leg lifts higher, body weight continues to shift back, the thoracic spine follows the movement of the pelvis and begins to flex (Fig. 8-16). We can flex the hip and lift the foot off the floor in a variety of patterns: We can flex the hip with knee flexion, thus keeping the foot under the knee, or we can flex the

FIGURE 8-16 *(A)* Initial hip flexion in sitting. *(B)* Increasing hip flexion occurs with posterior weight shifts of the trunk and pelvis. *(C)* Continued hip flexion is accompanied by flexion of the spine. Note active dorsiflexion of the foot.

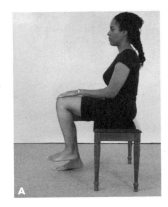 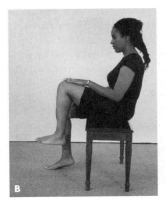 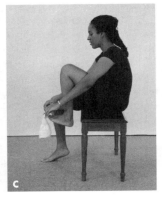

hip with a straight knee. This moves the foot forward and away from our body. While variability of knee and foot patterns during lower-extremity-initiated movements is critical for functional independence, it is usually the functional activity that determines the specific pattern we select. As the hip flexes and the leg lifts up, the ankle dorsiflexes to lift the foot up off the floor.

Functional Examples

Hip and knee flexion: to cross one leg over the other; to bring the foot up to tie a shoe. Hip flexion and knee extension: to lift the leg up onto a foot stool.

Abduction and Adduction

With the thigh supported on the sitting surface, the hips at 90 degrees flexion, adduction of the hip is possible to approximately 60 degrees and adduction to 30 degrees. As the hip moves in this plane, the thigh slides on the support and the pelvis remains still. As the femur moves laterally over the stationary foot, relative eversion accompanies hip abduction. When the femur moves medially, the foot is in relative inversion (Fig. 8-17).

When the thigh lifts up off the surface and the hip abducts, the hip abduction occurs with increasing degrees of external rotation and hip adduction. With the thigh off the surface, hip adduction occurs with increasing degrees of internal rotation. (Figure 8-18).

Functional Examples

To move the thigh in or out for comfort or to adjust foot position.

Knee and Ankle Flexion and Extension

Unlike the movements of the hip, which are associated with or influence pelvic and trunk movements, knee and ankle movements in sitting do not have as much influence on the trunk. Knee flexion and extension is possible in all hip patterns (Fig. 8-19).

Ankle dorsiflexion and plantar flexion movements also occur with the foot remaining in contact with the floor. When the foot is on the floor and the ankle dorsiflexes, additional weight is placed on the heel (Fig. 8-20A). When the foot is on the floor and the ankle plantar flexes, the heel lifts up and weight shifts to the

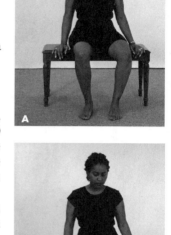

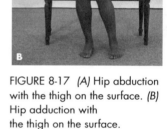

FIGURE 8-17 *(A)* Hip abduction with the thigh on the surface. *(B)* Hip adduction with the thigh on the surface.

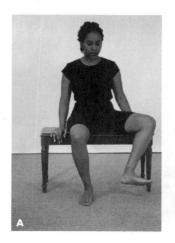

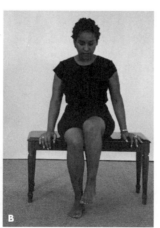

FIGURE 8-18 *(A)* Hip abduction with the thigh lifted off the surface. *(B)* Hip adduction with the thigh lifted off the surface.

FIGURE 8-19 *(A)* Knee extension and ankle dorsiflexion. *(B)* Hip and knee flexion with ankle dorsiflexion.

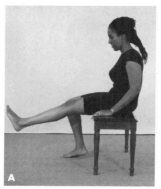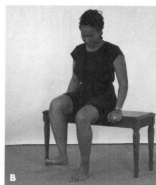

ball of the foot. This movement lifts the thigh off the bed a bit and flexes the hip (Fig. 8-20B).

Ankle dorsiflexion control is used when the leg lifts off the floor. This dorsiflexion movement assists with the control of weight and alignment of the foot as the leg changes position.

Functional Examples

To position the foot on the floor. To put the foot into shoes or slippers.

Combinations of Movements

Combination of patterns of movement occur when we cross one leg over the other. As we begin to cross the right leg over the left leg, the right hip flexes, externally rotates, and abducts. As the right hip adducts across the left leg, the right knee extends to clear the thigh and then flexes again. The right ankle dorsiflexes to lift the foot during the movement. If the leg initiates the movement, the pelvis remains level and the thighs accept an even amount of weight, but if the lower trunk initiates the lateral movement, the pelvis elevates as the leg crosses over (Fig. 8-21). If the pelvis elevates on the right side to help the leg cross over, the left hip and thigh will support more body weight. In this example, a non-weight bearing movement of the right leg is combined with a lower body lateral weight shift to the left and the corresponding weight bearing movements of the left hip.

FIGURE 8-20 *(A)* Ankle dorsiflexion with the heel on the floor. *(B)* Ankle plantarflexion with hip flexion.

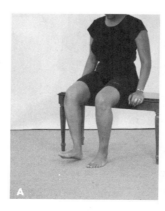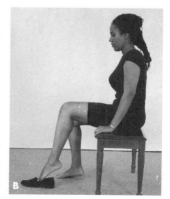

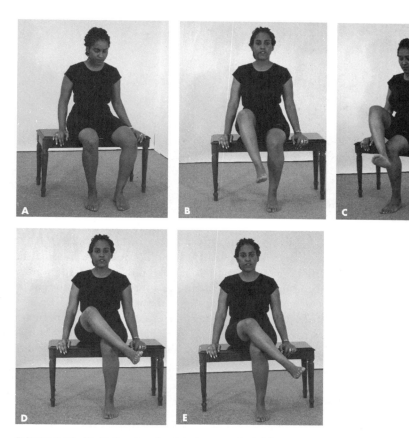

FIGURE 8-21 *(A–E)* Crossing the right leg over the left leg.

SIGNIFICANT IMPAIRMENTS THAT INTERFERE WITH PERFORMANCE

Weakness in the Leg

Muscle activity and strength in the leg is necessary to properly initiate and control non-weight bearing movements of the leg in sitting. Patients with a hemiplegia often are unable to recruit hip flexor muscles to lift the thigh up with hip and knee flexion. To compensate, they shift the trunk and pelvis back to assist in their attempts to move the leg. This excessive trunk movement often leads to the patient's learning to activate the rectus femoris, which results in knee extension with weak hip flexion (Fig. 8-22). Other patients compensate by leaning or pulling to the uninvolved side and using pelvic elevation or trunk rotation to move the leg. With these compensations, the hip flexes with abduction.

Weakness in the foot and ankle add to the heaviness of the lower leg and make it even harder to strengthen weak hip and knee movements. When the thigh lifts off the bed, the foot and ankle muscles are an active part of the movement initiation and position the foot for the desired function. In hemiplegia, the foot and ankle muscles are weak and do not move the foot at the start of an activity, or the move-

FIGURE 8-22 *(A & B)* Patient with right hemiplegia and leg weakness trying to move the leg up with hip and knee flexion. As she tries, she leans her trunk and pelvis back. The leg does not move with hip and knee flexion, but the knee begins to extend.

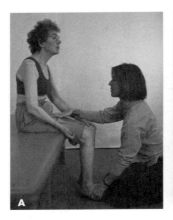
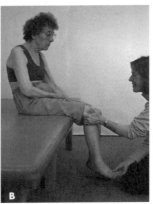

ment of the leg adversely affects the starting position of the foot (Fig. 8-23A). If the gastrocnemius muscle has shortened because of weak ankle dorsiflexors and the patient extends the knee, the movement of knee extension puts the gastrocnemius on stretch. This pull, at the distal end of the shortened muscle, moves the ankle into plantarflexion and the calcaneus into equinus and varus (Fig. 8-23B). The patient then has even more difficulty using or strengthening weak ankle dorsiflexor muscles to hold the foot up as the leg changes position. Specific muscle reeducation must focus on allowing the distal segment to be aligned and active as the hip and knee muscles move the leg (Fig. 8-24).

Loss of Trunk Control and Alignment

Movements of the leg in sitting depend on the ability of the trunk to remain upright, to provide stability for, and respond to, leg movements. Loss of trunk control results in loss of stability for leg movements. As the patient attempts to move the leg, the trunk moves, and the patient has more difficulty recruiting strength to perform the movement (Fig. 8-25).

Trunk asymmetries lead to atypical movements of the lower trunk and pelvis (see Ch. 5). These atypical movements result in uneven weight distribution and in loss

FIGURE 8-23 *(A)* Patient with weak ankle dorsiflexor muscles trying to lift her foot up. *(B)* As patient tries to move her right foot up, she extends her knee. As the knee extends, the calcaneus moves into equinus and varus. This places the foot in an inverted position.

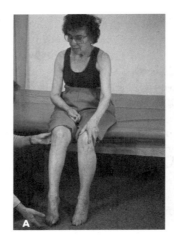
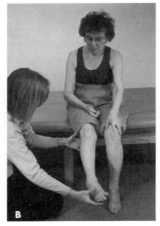

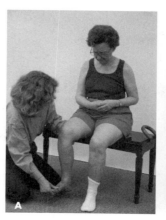 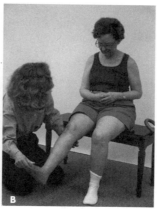

FIGURE 8-24 *(A & B)* Therapist holds foot and ankle to maintain alignment and to allow activation of ankle muscles as she helps the patient reeducate hip and knee movements.

of stability for leg movement. Weakness of the trunk and compensatory strategies that favor the use of the nonaffected side for function result in trunk asymmetries that over time result in severe muscle tightness or joint contracture. Trunk asymmetries cause rotational changes in the pelvis and change the relationship of the hip joint on the sitting surface. Treatment aimed at reeducation of leg movements becomes difficult unless the mechanical relationships between the trunk and leg can be restored.

Therefore, if a goal of treatment is to reeducate movements of the leg in sitting, the most important prerequisite is reestablishment of trunk control in sitting to provide stability for the moving leg. Trunk alignment and movement reeducation can be carried out in sitting or during upper extremity weight bearing (see Chs. 5 and 7).

Hypertonicity

Arm Hypertonicity

The most common cause of hypertonicity in the arm during movements of the leg in sitting is excessive recruitment of muscles because of leg weakness or insufficient muscle firing patterns. As the patient tries to lift his hemiplegic leg, he

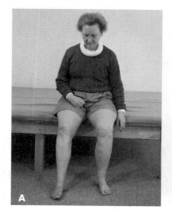 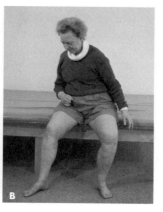

FIGURE 8-25 *(A & B)* Patient with a right hemiplegia with trunk asymmetries and weakness trying to abduct her right leg. As she moves it out into abduction, her trunk rotates to the right with the leg movement.

FIGURE 8-26 *(A)* Starting position; patient with a right hemiplegia. *(B)* Patient attempts to cross his right leg over his left leg. The leg does not have enough strength or control to perform the movement, and the right arm postures in flexion as he tries to compensate for the leg weakness.

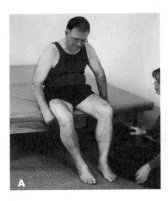
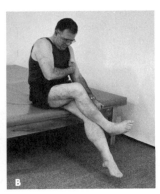

uses not only the return pattern and strength in the leg but also tries to help the leg by using available patterns in his trunk and arm. The arm postures in patterns that would be available if you asked him to initiate arm movements. When he stops trying to lift his leg, the arm will stop posturing and move back down to his side (Fig. 8-26).

Leg Hypertonicity

Hypertonicity in the leg can be a result of poor alignment from muscle tightness. This is evident in the foot. In sitting, tightness in the lateral hamstring and/or tensor fascia lata muscles can result in external rotation of the lower leg. This rotation of the lower leg increases tension on the anterior tibialis muscle and causes supination of the foot during leg movements (Fig. 8-27).

Leg hypertonicity in sitting can also be the result of either incomplete or unbalanced activation patterns or a combination of muscle shortening with resultant poor alignment and leg weakness. Atypical activation patterns in the hip and knee occur because of patterns of motor return or trunk asymmetries and loss of control and their resultant effect on the ability of the leg to regain strength and variety of muscle return. If the lower trunk and pelvis are rotated backward and the femur abducted as a result of muscle shortening, a flexion abduction external rotation pattern occurs when you ask the patient to lift his leg. This is not flexor spasticity, but an active recruitment, in a flexor pattern, of

FIGURE 8-27 *(A)* Patient with lateral thigh muscle tightness lifting his leg in a flexion/abduction/external rotation pattern. The right foot is supinating. *(B)* As the therapist lengthens the tight lateral hip and knee musculature, the foot supination decreases during attempts at lifting the leg.

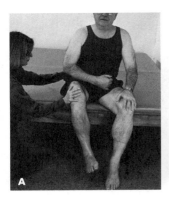
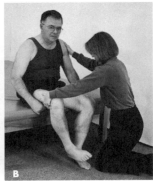

FIGURE 8-28 *(A)* Patient lifting his leg with activation of lateral hip flexors/abductors. *(B)* Patient lifting her leg with activation of knee extensors.

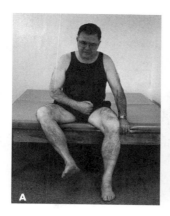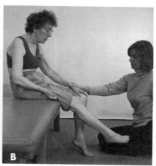

available unbalanced muscle firing. These patients can place their leg back on the floor and quiet the muscle firing (Fig. 8-28A). Patients with trunk and leg weakness who have the ability to fire the quadriceps muscle will lift their hemiplegic leg in an "extensor" pattern. They use whatever return they have (knee extension) to try to lift their leg up. When asked to stop lifting the leg, it moves back down to the floor. This active recruitment of muscle tension in available leg muscles is often labeled "spasticity" and thought to be undesirable. Perhaps we should think of it as beginning muscle return, insufficient for the desired movements, and note which additional muscles require reeducation to improve functional patterns in the leg (Fig. 8-28B).

ASSESSMENT GUIDELINES

Assessing Leg Movements

I. Describe the movements of the leg in sitting that can be performed independently. Which movements can be performed with assistance? Which movements cannot be performed?

II. If you provide stability to the lower trunk, are additional leg movements possible or does the range of movement increase?

III. What hand placements result in activation of new leg movements?

IV. Does the leg/foot posture when you ask the leg to move? What movements result in leg/foot posturing?

THERAPY GOALS

Functional Goals

The reeducation of non-weight bearing movements of the lower extremity in sitting are necessary to move and position the lower extremity for functional task performance and comfort.

Treatment Goals and Techniques

Treatment Goal: Reeducate proximal and distal leg movements in sitting. Strengthen weak or missing muscles.

Treatment Technique: Identify weak muscles and use handling to reeducate muscle firing patterns (Fig. 8-29).

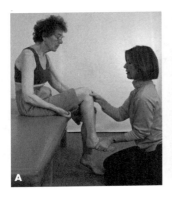
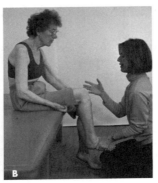

FIGURE 8-29 *(A)* Therapist provides a model of the desired hip and knee flexion movement. She uses her right hand to assist hip flexion while her left hand corrects the ankle position and prevents knee extension. She asks the patient not to straighten the knee but to keep the foot under the knee. (See Fig. 8-28B.) *(B)* As the patient recruits the muscles, the therapist feels the leg get lighter and removes her right hand to allow the patient to practice with less assistance.

Treatment Technique: Lengthen tight muscles, correct alignment, and reeducate weak ankle and foot muscles (Fig. 8-30).

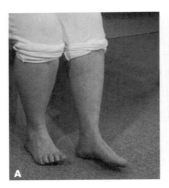
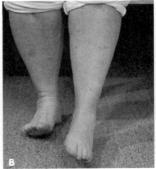
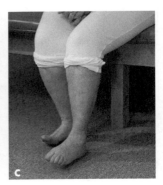

FIGURE 8-30 *(A–C)* Patient with a left hemiplegia trying to dorsiflex her left ankle in sitting. Left foot inverts; ankle remains plantarflexed, and toes do not dorsiflex, but anterior tibialis muscle fires. *(Figure continues)*.

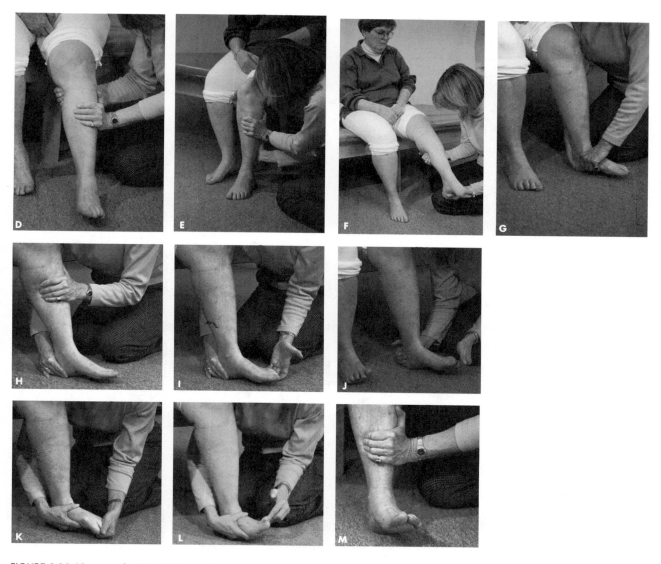

FIGURE 8-30 *(Continued)* *(D & E)* Therapist lengthens gastrocnemius muscle with knee flexion. Her left hand stabilizes the lower leg and directs a downward pressure into the foot to keep the heel in contact with the floor, while her right hand glides down the back of the calf, softening and lengthening the muscle tissue. *(F)* Therapist's right hand continues to lengthen the muscle tissue while her left hand holds the calcaneus and slowly extends the knee. She then lengthens the muscle with the knee extended. As the muscle lengthens, she corrects first the calcaneal equinus, then the calcaneal inversion. *(G)* With the heel firmly on the floor, the therapist's right hand holds the calcaneus in neutral, and the web space of her left hand, placed on the talus, directs pressure on a downward diagonal into the heel. This continues the lengthening of the gastrocnemius tendon and increases ankle joint dorsiflexion range. *(H)* With the heel stabilized, the therapist corrects the rotational component of the tibia on the foot. *(I & J)* Reeducation of active assistive ankle joint movements. Therapist holds the rearfoot position and asks the patient to lift the foot. *(K & L)* Therapist reeducates toe movements. *(M)* At the end of treatment, the therapist stabilizes the lower leg and asks the patient to lift her foot: the foot lifts up in a balanced position with both lateral and medial muscles firing (compare with Fig.B).

Treatment Goal: Increase trunk symmetry and lengthen tight leg muscles to allow reeducation of leg movements.

Treatment Technique: Correct lower trunk and pelvis to allow lengthening of tight hip abductors before reeducating hip and knee flexion movements with compatible trunk movements (Fig. 8-31).

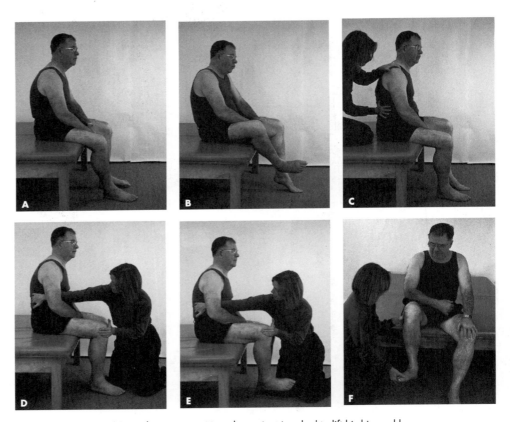

FIGURE 8-31   *(A & B)* From the sitting position, the patient is asked to lift his hip and knee up. The leg moves up, but with excessive abduction and external rotation. The trunk flexes as the pelvis posterior tilts and rotates back. *(C)* The therapist corrects the lower trunk position with her right hand while her left hand realigns the upper trunk. Both hands together encourage the patient to extend his spine to a neutral position. *(D)* While the therapist's left hand slowly lengthens the tight lateral muscles, her right hand helps the patient keep the pelvis and lower trunk from rotating back. Correction of the lower trunk and thigh provide a stretch at both ends of the tight muscle. *(E)* As she feels the muscle begin to lengthen, she asks the patient to initiate the hip and knee flexion. *(F)* The therapist's hands move more distally to correct the foot. Lengthening the tight thigh muscles allows the patient to practice strengthening additional hip muscles that will let him move the leg with less effort and more variety.

Treatment Goal: Select movement strategy that allows most efficient movement pattern to be practiced.

Treatment Technique: Teach patient to cross hemiplegic leg over the unaffected leg (Fig. 8-32).

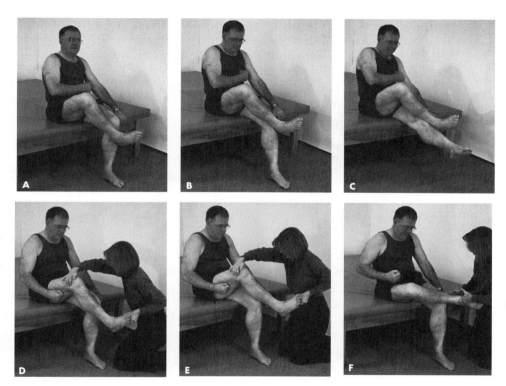

FIGURE 8-32 *(A–C)* Patient lifts hemiplegic right leg in a flexion/abduction pattern. As he attempts to cross it over his left leg, the loss of adduction range results in increased posterior trunk weight shift and eventually the left leg extends and comes off the floor to keep the right leg crossed. This results in poor balance, since both feet are in the air, and he grabs the mat with his left hand. *(D & E)* Therapist assists the adduction movement and gives verbal reminders to keep the left leg on the floor. *(F)* Since hip adduction is such a limiting factor, the therapist helps the patient practice crossing the leg with the hip in more abduction. This requires practicing knee flexion to keep the right leg on the left leg.

Scooting

CONCEPTS AND PRINCIPLES

Scooting is the term for moving the body in a sitting position on a supporting surface. In sitting, we scoot our hips forward and back to position the hips relative to the edge of the chair or bed. Scooting sideways is used to move the hips left or right on a seat or bench. There are two patterns of scooting: a lower-body-initiated pattern, with either lateral or rotational variations, and a partial stand pattern. Scooting forward or backward can be performed with any of the patterns, while scooting sideways is usually performed with the partial stand pattern.

Scooting movement components are used in treatment to help patients learn how to move in chairs or in bed without standing up. Like transfers, it is an activity that is taught to patients to allow independence at a wheelchair level and in the later stages of recovery is used to treat weakness in specific muscle groups or to treat secondary impairments of shortened muscle length or poor joint alignment.

MOVEMENT COMPONENTS

Lower-Body-Initiated Scooting Patterns

Lateral Weight Shift

To use this pattern, the upper trunk remains aligned over the lower trunk as the lower trunk initiates a lateral weight shift. To scoot forward with the left leg moving first, the lower trunk shifts laterally over the right thigh and hip. The pelvis depresses on the right, and the trunk flexes laterally so the convexity of the curve is on the right. Activity in the hip, knee, and foot lifts the left thigh off the chair or bed. The leg is held up as the left side of the trunk, pelvis, and thigh move forward. The right hip joint, the fulcrum of the movement, rotates as the left side of the body moves forward. This places the left shoulder, hip, and knee slightly anterior to the right shoulder, hip, and knee. The pelvis and femur move back down to the surface as the trunk becomes symmetric. To continue to scoot forward, the lower trunk initiates a lateral weight shift to the left, and the right side of the pelvis elevates. The non-weight bearing lower extremity pattern described above is repeated on the right. Scooting backward is the reverse of this pattern (Fig. 8-33).

Rotational Weight Shift

When we use a lower-trunk-initiated rotational pattern to scoot forward with the right leg, the upper trunk and shoulders face forward as weight shifts (lower-trunk-initiated) to the left hip and the lower trunk rotates to the left. The right leg moves forward along with the right side of the pelvis until the right hip is forward of the right shoulder. This movement places the right iliac crest anterior to the right shoulder and the left iliac crest posterior to the left shoulder: the lower trunk rotates on a stable upper trunk.

To move the left leg forward, we shift (lower-trunk-initiated) weight to the right hip and rotate the lower trunk to the right. The left side of the pelvis moves forward of the left shoulder. The thigh and pelvis move back to the supporting surface as the activity stops or continues to the opposite side.

During scooting, the foot can come off the floor with the thigh or the foot may stay in partial contact with the floor. When the toes and ball of the foot remain on the floor and the heel lifts up, the movement of the ankle helps lift the thigh off the surface.

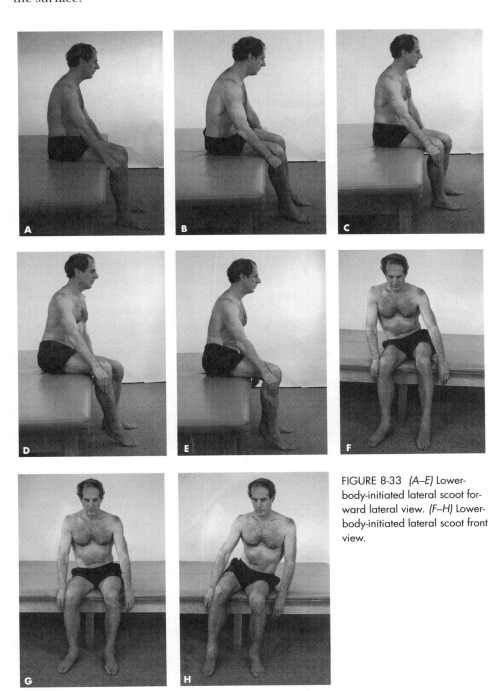

FIGURE 8-33 *(A–E)* Lower-body-initiated lateral scoot forward lateral view. *(F–H)* Lower-body-initiated lateral scoot front view.

FIGURE 8-34 *(A–C)* Partial stand scoot backward.

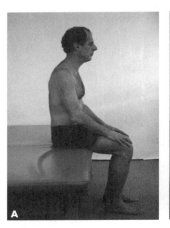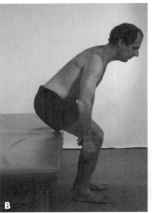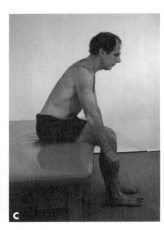

Partial Stand Scooting Pattern

The third type of scooting is done using a partial sit to stand movement. To scoot backward, the lower trunk initiates an anterior weight shift. As the trunk moves forward and up, the hips leave the supporting surface. The hips and knees are extending, and the ankles and toes dorsiflex to control the position of the lower leg. In this partial stand, the hips adjust to move back from the edge of the support. Control of knee flexion and ankle dorsiflexion is an important component of this hip adjustment. Eccentric control of the hips, knees, and ankle allows the hips and thighs to move back down to the surface. During the scoot, the feet do not move forward or back (Fig. 8-34).

To scoot forward, this pattern is reversed. Frequently, we use our arms to assist us in the scoot forward or back by pushing into armrests or the chair seat to reinforce the hip, knee, and lower leg control. This partial stand scooting pattern is also used to move sideways. During the partial stand, the hips and lower legs make a lateral adjustment over the feet to move the hips closer to the right or left. When scooting to the right, the right hip moves into relative adduction and the left hip moves into relative abduction. Eccentric control of the hips, knees, and ankles is again used to lower the trunk and pelvis back down to the surface.

SIGNIFICANT IMPAIRMENTS THAT INTERFERE WITH PERFORMANCE

Trunk and Leg Weakness

One common problem during scooting is difficulty moving the uninvolved leg forward or backward because of difficulty initiating a lower trunk weight shift. Without an appropriate weight shift, it is hard to unweight the moving leg. Patients have difficulty moving their uninvolved leg forward because they cannot initiate a lower trunk weight shift to the hemiplegic side. This inability to shift onto the hemiplegic side is due to either loss of trunk control and/or weakness and instability of the hemiplegic hip (Fig. 8-35A). A second problem is the inability to lift the hemiplegic leg enough to allow the thigh and pelvis to move forward or backward (Fig. 8-35B & C). Patients can often activate pelvic and hip muscles

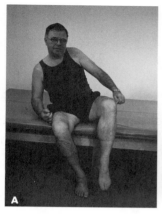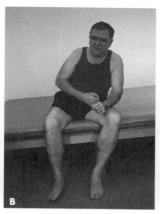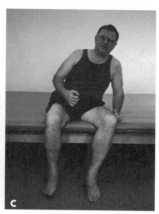

FIGURE 8-35 *(A)* Patient attempting to perform a lower-trunk-initiated lateral scoot. He is trying to weight shift to the right, but the trunk component is incorrect, and his right hip is not strong enough to support the weight shift. As a result, his body is falling to the right. *(B & C)* Patient performing a lower-body-initiated lateral scoot. He is shifting his weight to the left and attempting to lift his hemiplegic right leg. Even when he assists with his left arm, he cannot lift the right leg enough to move it on the mat.

to lift the proximal leg segment but have great difficulty using muscles of the lower leg to lift the lower leg and foot. The postural prerequisite for this task, control of the upper trunk over the lower trunk as the pelvis initiates the movement, is a third problem that frequently occurs. Practice of trunk initiation patterns and leg movements, both weight bearing and non-weight bearing, are necessary to strengthen the trunk and legs to train independent scooting.

Loss of Balance Control

During partial stand scooting movements, patients have difficulty controlling the descent because of weakness in the legs and incompatible trunk and leg movement patterns (Fig. 8-36).

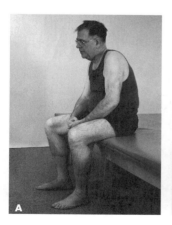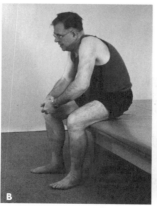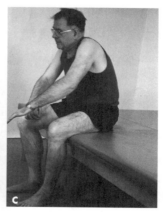

FIGURE 8-36 *(A & B)* Patient using a lower-trunk-initiated partial stand scoot backward. His trunk is excessively flexed for this initiation pattern, which makes it more difficult for him to use his legs effectively. *(C)* Patient losing his balance as he sits back from the scoot.

FIGURE 8-37 *(A–C)* Undesirable compensatory lateral scoot pattern.

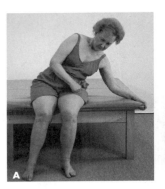 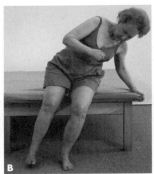 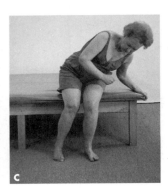

UNDESIRABLE COMPENSATORY PATTERNS

Scooting patterns that require lifting of the legs are extremely difficult for patients in the early stages of recovery because of the control demands of the trunk and the leg. Since it is difficult to control the weight shift onto the affected leg and to control the trunk as weight shifts onto the unaffected leg, the patient usually has a difficult time scooting either leg forward.

Figure 8-37 demonstrates a strong use of unaffected side to pull body laterally.

ASSESSMENT GUIDELINES

Assessing Scooting

I. Describe how the patient scoots forward/back, left/right. Which trunk initiation pattern does he use? How does he use his legs to assist?

II. Does the patient initiate the scoot with the appropriate trunk and leg components? If not, does the patient require more assistance with the trunk or leg components to learn to perform the activity?

III. Does the arm and/or leg posture during the activity? If so, during which part of the activity does the posturing begin. What hand placements result in a decrease in posturing?

THERAPY GOALS

Functional Goals

Functional goals for scooting for the acute stroke patient are designed to help them move in bed or to a wheelchair. Goals for higher-level patients are designed to help them complete their functional independence in all activities.

1. To scoot forward in a chair to prepare for sit to stand or transfers. To scoot backward in a wheelchair to position the body comfortably during wheelchair activities.

2. To scoot forward and backward in bed or on mat safely and independently.

3. To change body position for comfort in deep armchairs or sofas, to move along bench seats in restaurants, theaters, or in church, or to adjust in exercise equipment.

Treatment Goals and Techniques

Treatment Goals: To provide a model of the task.

Treatment Technique: Facilitate the movement sequence with upper body support and assistance to trunk and leg movements (Fig. 8-38).

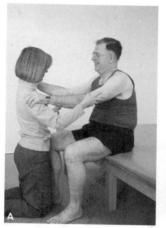
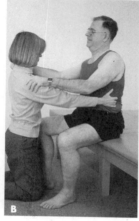
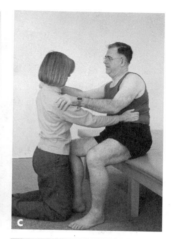
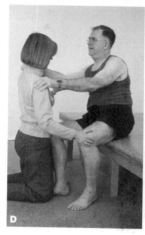
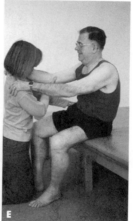

FIGURE 8-38 *(A)* Starting position for a patient with a right hemiplegia. Therapist uses her left hand to support the patient's arm, to correct alignment, and to keep it positioned on her left shoulder. He places his left hand on her right shoulder; his weight is shifted back behind his hips. *(B)* Therapist uses her right hand to encourage him to shift forward to a neutral starting position. *(C)* With his upper trunk supported through his arms, the patient initiates a lower trunk lateral weight shift. The therapist's right hand directs diagonal downward pressure from the lower left rib cage into the right hip. *(D)* As the patient completes the lateral weight shift and unweights the left thigh, the therapist assists the backward movement of the left leg as he scoots back. *(E)* The therapist changes her hand position to assist in the weight shift to the left. Her right hand moves to support his hemiplegic arm while her left hand moves to the lateral aspect of the right pelvis. Her left hand assists the movement of the pelvis up and medially as he initiates the trunk portion of the scoot.

Treatment Goals: Correct trunk asymmetries and reeducate trunk control during lower-trunk-initiated lateral scoot pattern.

Treatment Technique: Teach lower-trunk-initiated lateral pattern from behind the patient (Fig. 8-39).

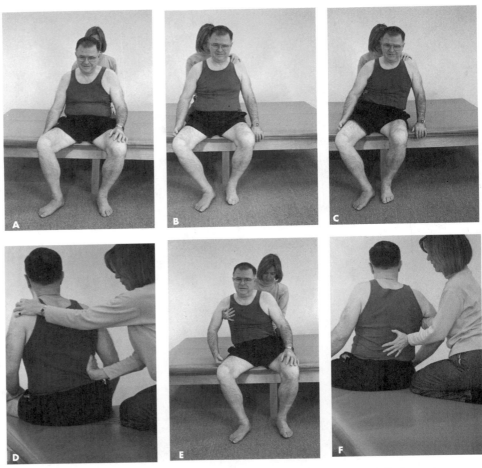

FIGURE 8-39 *(A)* Patient with right hemiplegia. Starting position with excessive trunk flexion and upper body rotated to right. *(B)* Therapist asks patient to sit straight; her left hand is on top of his left shoulder, directing a message to rotate back. Her right hand is on the bottom of his rib cage, directing a message forward. These two hand placements correct the upper body rotation and simultaneously encourage spinal extension to neutral. *(C & D)* Therapist assists the lower-trunk-initiated left lateral weight shift. Her right hand directs pressure on a downward diagonal into the left hip. Her left hand helps the upper body follow the movement of the lower body; as the weight shifts laterally, the convexity of the spinal curve is on the left and the left shoulder moves up and laterally but does not move past the left hip joint. *(E & F)* Therapist assists the lower-trunk-initiated right lateral weight shift. Her left hand is on the lower trunk, assisting the right lateral weight shift while her right forearm and hand is under his right axilla, encouraging the upper trunk to respond appropriately to the movement of the lower trunk. Her two hands together are moving the trunk over the hip so that the convexity of the spinal curve is on the right.

Treatment Goal: Allow patient to practice trunk component with verbal reminders and leg movements with assistance.

Treatment Technique: Active assistive non-weight bearing leg movements (Fig. 8-40).

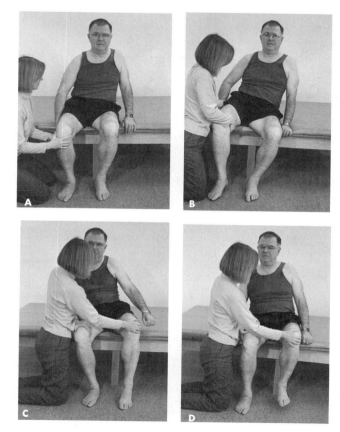

FIGURE 8-40 *(A)* Patient performs lower-trunk-initiated lateral movement. *(B)* Therapist places her left hand on the patient's hip, and her right hand is under the distal thigh to assist as he tries to lift it up. *(C)* The therapist holds the patient's right thigh on the bed as he initiates a lower trunk lateral movement to the right. *(D)* While patient can lift his left leg up, he cannot scoot his left side back, even when the therapist helps provide stability to his right leg. With the therapist assisting his leg movement, he does not have enough trunk or leg weight bearing control to perform the task. To learn to scoot, he needs the trunk and leg components to be reeducated together.

9

Lower Extremity Movements in Standing

CONCEPTS AND PRINCIPLES

Lower extremity function in standing is based on the ability to coordinate control between the legs and trunk. Lower extremity strength and coordination are necessary for both task performance and support of the body. Lower extremity control is the ability to support body weight on both legs, to transfer weight from one leg to the other, to stand on one leg and move the other, and to adapt to movements of the trunk and arms. Trunk control in standing gives us the ability to remain upright and aligned as body weight is shifted between the feet, to respond to movements of the leg so that the body remains balanced, and to initiate and respond to upper extremity functional movements. We use both lower extremity and trunk control for balance and safety in standing, during upper extremity tasks, and while walking.

Movement patterns in standing are initiated by either the legs or the upper trunk. Lower-extremity-initiated movement patterns result in a weight shift between the legs, a weight shift onto one leg, or movement of a leg in space. Upper-trunk-initiated movement patterns result in movement responses of the legs to adjust and maintain balance. The initiation pattern we select is determined by our functional needs. We select lower extremity patterns as we walk, when we change our position for comfort or balance, and when we need to move our legs for daily functional activities, such as putting on trousers. We select upper-trunk-initiated patterns when we use our arms for function or during upper body movements. For the arms to function in standing, the lower trunk and legs must be stable and support body weight, yet adapt to upper body movements.

Trunk control is a prerequisite for each of these initiation patterns. *Trunk control in standing* includes the ability to perform trunk movements, to control the upper trunk over the lower trunk, to produce small changes in trunk posture that are used as postural adjustments to leg movements, to coordinate trunk and leg movements in functional sequences, and for complex movement patterns, power production, speed, and balance. The precise interaction between trunk and leg components allows the mobility, balance, and postural control that we need to walk, jump, and run independently, and safely.

Independent, safe standing is an important functional goal for our patients. However, the ability to control the legs and trunk in standing is an extremely difficult task for patients with neurologic dysfunction. The task is difficult because it requires not only appropriate lower extremity strength, alignment, muscle firing, and sequencing patterns, but also the postural control in the trunk to initiate movements and to adapt and balance during both upper- and lower-extremity-initiated movements. Patients have difficulty in standing because of loss of trunk movements and because of the inability to use the involved leg to support weight and move in functional patterns. When these abilities are lost, balance is precarious, and the patient is unable to perform functional activities in standing. When balance is precarious, the patient is often unable to walk without assistive devices or the assistance of an individual.

Since control in standing is critical for both upper and lower extremity tasks and in preparation for walking, it is an important part of early treatment. When patients cannot stand and balance, the most important goal of treatment is to reeducate control in the trunk in conjunction with the related weight bearing movement components in the leg. Therapists must not ignore this basic element of standing treatment because it is a precursor for independent walking. While it may seem easier to immediately provide the patient with a hemiwalker or quad cane, it is more important for long-term independence and safety to help the patient regain these critical prerequisites of standing control. To prepare for walking or to improve gait patterns, standing treatment must retrain lower extremity weight bearing movements with appropriate weight shift patterns, must reeducate trunk control patterns to allow the trunk to remain stable and to respond appropriately to leg movements, and must retrain specific non-weight bearing leg movements. Canes may be necessary for safety, but balance will always be precarious and walking nonfunctional if the basic standing movement components are not a part of the patient's movement repertoire.

This chapter describes the movement components of the leg that are used to produce functional movements and to support body weight and that contribute to balance control. The chapter is divided into two sections. The first section analyzes the important movement components of the leg and trunk during lower-extremity-initiated non-weight bearing movements. The second section analyzes the movement components that occur in the legs during lower-extremity-initiated weight shifts and during upper-body-initiated movements. The description of lower extremity weight shifts analyzes leg stance patterns that are used during walking. This information about the legs and trunk in standing is essential for initial gait training and for improving balance and efficiency in patients with existing gait problems. It is also a critical part of the reeducation of arm movements and task performance in standing.

KINESIOLOGY

In standing, the trunk is defined as the spine and rib cage and their muscular attachments. The lower extremity includes the pelvis, femur, tibia, fibula, and foot. The lower extremity is attached to the trunk at the lumbosacral and the sacroiliac joints and through muscular attachments among the pelvis, spine, and rib cage. This definition of the trunk and lower extremity differs from that described in the sitting position. In sitting, the pelvis functions as part of the lower trunk, while in standing it functions as part of the leg.

To balance in the standing position, the trunk and legs must remain controlled during all planes of motion. As the body's line of gravity shifts through the hip, knee, ankle, and foot, the requirements for muscle force production and capsular and ligamentous tension change. The foot and ankle are critical joints in standing because they are the fulcrum of weight bearing movements and provide the base for changing positions of the knee, hip, and pelvis. In standing, the line of gravity falls anterior to the ankle joint. This means that activity in the posterior calf is necessary to prevent the body from falling forward. The line of gravity falls anterior to the knee joint, thus assisting with knee extension. At the hip, the line of gravity moves either through the joint or slightly anterior or posterior to the joint. The sacroiliac joints distribute the weight of the trunk between the two legs. In adults, the curves of the spine are well balanced over the pelvis.[1]

As lower extremity movement occurs, whether during weight shifts or non-weight bearing leg movements, there are coordinated sequences of movement, a rhythm, among the femur, pelvis, and spine. These sequences of leg movement patterns are similar to the relationships found in the shoulder girdle during arm movements. The terms we use for describing the movements of the pelvis and femur are found below.

Pelvic Movements

The pelvis has mobility in three planes of movement:

1. Elevation/depression (Fig. 9-1)
2. Anterior tilt/posterior tilt (Fig. 9-2)
3. Rotation forward/backward (right pelvis rotates left/right pelvis rotates right) (Figs. 9-3 and 9-4)

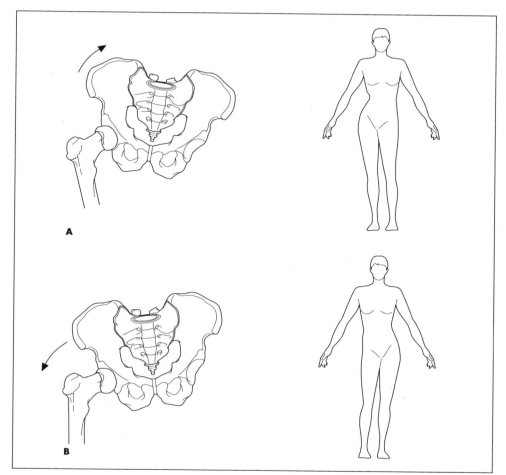

A

B

FIGURE 9-1 (*A*) Right hip elevation. (*B*) Right hip depression.

FIGURE 9-2 (*A*) Anterior tilt. (*B*) Posterior tilt.

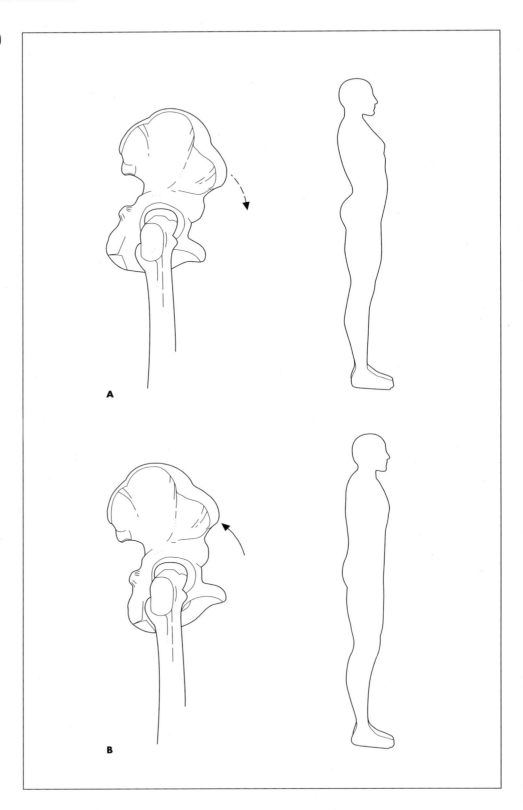

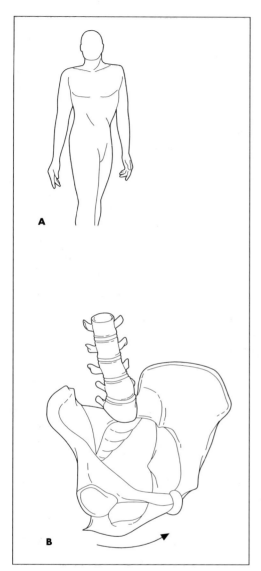

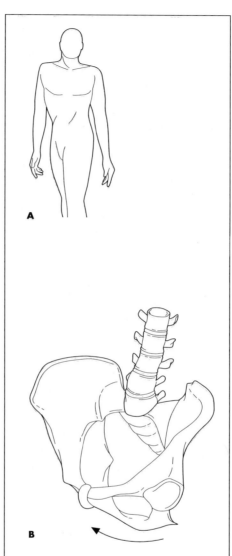

FIGURE 9-3 (*A & B*) Forward rotation of the right side of the pelvis.

FIGURE 9-4 (*A & B*) Backward rotation of the right side of the pelvis.

   Movements of the pelvis in standing are accompanied by compatible movements of the spine. Elevation and depression of the pelvis occur with lateral flexion of the spine. When the pelvis elevates, it produces spinal lateral flexion with the concavity of the curve on the same side. Pelvic depression is accompanied by spinal lateral flexion with the convexity of the curve on that side. Since movement of one side of the pelvis affects the opposite side, when one side is lengthened the other side is shortened. The movement of pelvic elevation results in a trunk that appears shorter on that side. Conversely, pelvic depression contributes to a trunk position that looks lengthened on that side. Since movement of one side of the pelvis affects the opposite side, when one side is lengthened the other side is shortened.

Changes in pelvic tilt also affect the position of the spine. As the pelvis tilts anteriorly, the lumbar spine extends. As posterior tilting movements of the pelvis occur, the spine flexes. However, in patients who move with atypical patterns, anterior and posterior pelvic tilts do not always produce compatible spinal patterns. This makes the assessment process more difficult and is a complicating factor in problem solving and treatment planning.

Rotation of the pelvis to the right is accompanied by rotation of the spine to the right, and rotation to the left with spinal rotation to the left. In this book, when describing atypical or excessive rotation of the pelvis in patients with a hemiplegia, we use the terms *pelvic rotation forward* and *backward* to help therapists learn how to correct pelvic asymmetries.

In normal movement, as rotation of the pelvis increases, rotation of the spine begins in the lumbar area and progresses up the spine. In patients with hemiplegia, the rotation of the pelvis may be accompanied by spinal rotation, but in the presence of poor trunk control, the rotation may not advance above the level of the lowest true rib. During the assessment of patients, it is not uncommon to find atypical pelvic rotation in one direction and upper trunk rotation in the opposite direction, as a counterbalance.

Hip Movements

The hip has three planes of movement, which result in combinations of flexion/extension, abduction/adduction, and internal/external rotation. The hip has many large, multijoint muscles. These muscles cross the hip joint and either the pelvis or knee joint, and sometimes both. In patients with hemiplegia, restrictions in hip joint movement or poor hip joint alignment are common and may be different in sitting versus standing. This occurs as a result of poor proximal control and alignment and/or poor distal control and alignment. Muscle shifting and shorting across the hip joint often contributes to the atypical movement patterns and posturing that therapists encounter during treatment.

Knee Movements

The main movements of the knee are flexion and extension. *Extension of the knee* is the term used to describe movements from any position of knee flexion to the reference position, 0 degrees. In patients with hemiplegia, abnormal alignment or control of the proximal and/or distal joints creates a situation in which the knee is placed in 5 to 15 degrees of true extension. In this book, we refer to this position as *knee hyperextension or recurvatum* (Fig. 9-5).

In hemiplegia, knee recurvatum results from loss of ankle range or control, loss of hip range or control, a combination of loss of ankle and hip control, poor joint alignment caused by muscle shortening or shifting, unbalanced muscle firing patterns, or by combinations of these factors.

Ankle and Foot Movements

Movements of the ankle joint occur in only one plane, the sagittal plane, and are described as dorsiflexion and plantarflexion. These ankle movements are accompanied by parallel rearfoot movements at the ends of the ranges. Dorsiflexion occurs with calcaneal flexion, and plantarflexion occurs with calcaneal extension (equinus).

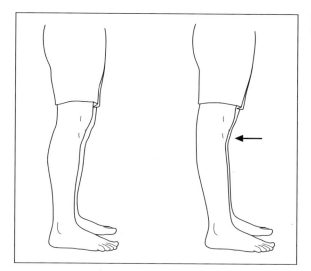

FIGURE 9-5 (*A & B*) Knee hyperextension (recurvatum).

There are many joints of the foot and analysis of their movements is complex. For the scope of this book, we will refer to the movements of the functional segments of the foot: the *rearfoot*, the *midfoot*, and the *forefoot*.

The joints of the foot move in three planes. Movements of adduction, abduction, supination (medial), pronation (lateral), flexion, and extension are possible in each of the three foot segments. These movements of the foot do not occur in isolation, but in patterns. The non-weight bearing pattern of adduction and supination occurs with a small amount of extension. This produces the functional pattern of *inversion* (Fig. 9-6). The non-weight bearing pattern of abduction, pronation, and flexion is described functionally as *eversion* (Fig. 9-7).[2]

During lateral weight shifts of the body in standing, the foot remains in contact with the floor, and the femur and lower leg move over the foot. As the body moves over the stable foot, the relative position of the foot to the lower leg changes. If the foot remains in contact with the floor, lateral movements over one foot result in a relative foot position of eversion (Fig. 9-8), while medial weight shifts away from that foot result in a relative foot position of inversion.

Movements of the body forward and backward over the foot result in relative ankle dorsiflexion and plantarflexion.

Lower Extremity Movements

CONCEPTS AND PRINCIPLES

This section of the chapter analyzes non-weight bearing movements of the leg in standing. To move one leg, we align and control the upper trunk over the lower trunk and have enough strength and control in the standing leg to adjust, yet remain balanced. To allow the muscles of the moving leg to fire and produce movement, we also need to increase lower trunk and pelvic stability. As we move a leg in standing, the foot and ankle muscles must fire to allow the foot to clear the floor. The foot is active during the initiation of functional leg movements. The foot moves on and off the ground (floor, stair-step) in the most efficient way for the desired task. Some tasks require that the heel make contact first, as in walking forwards. Other tasks require

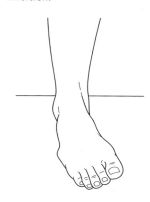

FIGURE 9-6 Foot and ankle inversion.

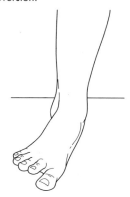

FIGURE 9-7 Foot and ankle eversion.

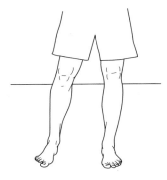

FIGURE 9-8 If the foot remains in contact with the floor, lateral movements over left foot result in a relative left foot position of eversion.

that the toes make contact first, as in walking backwards, walking sideways as the leg reaches out, and stepping downstairs. Still other tasks require the foot be placed down sole first so that the whole foot contacts the floor simultaneously.

In non-weight bearing movements of the leg, the spine, pelvis, and femur move together in more complex patterns as the task becomes more difficult or when balance is challenged. These non-weight bearing movements of the leg and trunk need to be taught and coordinated so that the body has a variety of initiation patterns, appropriate functional sequencing of muscles, and combinations of complex extremity and trunk patterns. If balance is challenged, the arm enters the movement sequence as part of the equilibrium response.

LOWER EXTREMITY MOVEMENT COMPONENTS

The following section identifies the leg movement patterns that are most important for function in standing. Each of these patterns is used functionally for mobility and also for task performance. It is important to remember that as one leg is moving, the other leg is supporting body weight and the trunk remains upright and stable, yet adaptable.

Hip Movements

Hip Flexion with Knee Flexion—Forward Lift

In standing, as the hip moves into the first 45 degrees of flexion with the knee bent, the pelvis remains relatively still. As hip flexion approaches 90 degrees, the pelvis tilts posteriorly and the lumbar spine begins to flex. If the hip flexes more than 90 degrees, spinal flexion progresses up through the thoracic spine. Simultaneous hip and knee flexion may be combined with either ankle dorsiflexion or plantarflexion. Since the pelvic and spinal movements influence both sides of the body, muscle activity in the weight bearing leg is necessary to maintain balance (Fig. 9-9).

Functional Examples

We use this movement with ankle dorsiflexion to lift a leg to place it on a stair-step or curb.

FIGURE 9-9 (*A*) Hip flexion to 45 degrees/no change in pelvis. (*B*) Hip flexion to 90 degrees pelvis moves posteriorly and weight shifts back. (*C*) Hip flexion more than 90 degrees/ spine flexes more.

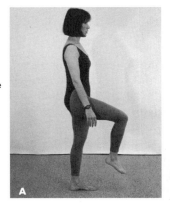
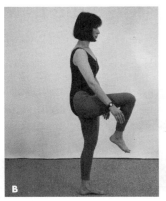
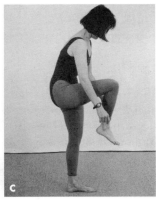

Hip Flexion with Knee Extension—Forward Reach

If the hip flexes with an extended knee, flexion in the pelvis and spine occurs earlier than with forward lift. With the knee extended, the lever arm of the leg is longer, and the body shifts weight back to recruit trunk flexors to maintain balance (Fig. 9-10).

Functional Examples

Hip flexion with knee extension and ankle dorsiflexion is used in late swing and early stance phase of gait. It is also used with ankle plantar flexion to move or kick an object out of the way with your foot.

Hip Extension with Knee Extension—Backward Reach

The movement of the leg and foot backward occurs with hip and knee extension. The foot dorsiflexes initially to clear the floor and then plantarflexes as it makes contact with the floor. The range of hip extension is small, 0 to 10 degrees. The accompanying anterior pelvic tilt and spinal extension are evident early (Fig. 9-11A).

Functional Examples

This movement is used in midstance phase of walking backward. It is also used to prepare for kicking the leg forward.

Hip Extension with Knee Flexion—Backward Lift

The movement of the leg back into an extended position or extended to neutral with the knee in 45 to 90 degrees of flexion is initiated by strong ankle and toe dorsiflexion to clear the foot from the floor (Fig. 9-11B).

Functional Examples

This movement is used to initiate walking backward. It is also used to bring the foot up behind the body for adjusting clothing.

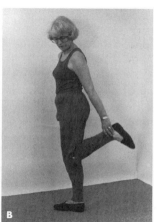
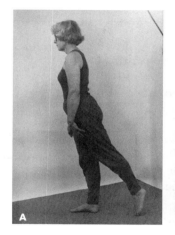

FIGURE 9-10 Forward reach; hip flexion with knee extension.

FIGURE 9-11 (*A*) Backward reach: hip extension with knee extension. (*B*) Backward lift: hip extension with knee flexion.

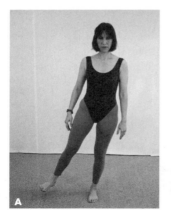 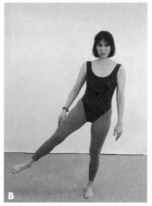 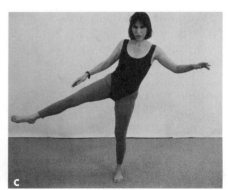

FIGURE 9-12 (A) Abduction to 30 degrees/pelvis level. (B) Abduction to 45 degrees/pelvic elevation. (C) Increased lift of leg/trunk lateral flexion with concavity on the right.

Abduction with Knee Extension—Sideways Lift or Reach

In standing, as the left hip initiates abduction with an extended knee, the first 30 degrees of movement occur in the hip joint. If hip abduction continues, the right side of the pelvis elevates and the spine moves into a lateral curve with the concavity on the right (Fig. 9-12). To lower the leg to the floor, the left hip abductors control the movement of the hip, and the ankle and foot dorsiflex to allow the foot to be placed back on the floor. If the task requires that the leg reach laterally and be placed on the floor in an abducted stance position, the left leg lifts up in abduction and is held there as the lower body initiates a lateral weight shift to the left. The left ankle plantarflexes to reach the foot to the floor. The trunk and pelvis move laterally to the left until the left foot rests on the floor.

Functional Examples

We use this movement to move our leg out to the side to walk sideways, to walk around an obstacle, or to widen our stance.

Adduction with Knee Extension—Reach to Body/Across Body

The non-weight bearing movement of hip adduction in standing has a very small range. We can adduct the leg with either knee flexion or extension (Fig. 9-13A–C). To cross the left leg in front of the right leg, we use a combination of left hip adduction with pelvic rotation to the right (Fig. 9-13D). To cross the left leg behind the right leg, we use a combination of left hip adduction with pelvic rotation to the left.

When we are in an abducted stance we wish to bring the right leg in closer to the left leg. As weight shifts off the right leg, the right pelvis depresses and the right hip remains abducted. The ankle plantarflexes to allow the toes to stay on the floor to assist. With the trunk balanced over the left leg, the right hip adducts to neutral

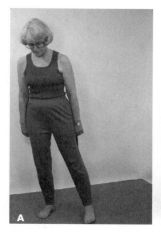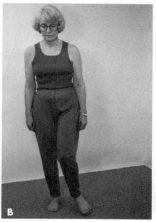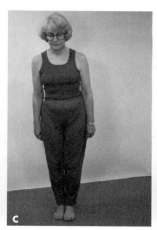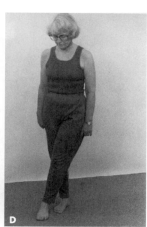

FIGURE 9-13 (A–C) Reach from abducted stance. adduction with knee flexion. (D) Reach across body; adduction with knee extension and pelvic rotation right.

with knee extension and the ankle dorsiflexes, the pelvis returns to a level position, and the foot moves under the body and contacts the floor.

Functional Examples

We use this movement in sideways walking, cross walking, and in changing the size of our stance.

Ankle Movements

Ankle Dorsiflexion

Ankle dorsiflexion control is critical for foot clearance during lower extremity movements in standing. Toe extension often occurs with ankle dorsiflexion activity to help reinforce the ankle movement and contribute to lateral control of the foot. Ankle dorsiflexion occurs with combinations of hip and knee flexion and extension (Fig. 9-14A & B).

Functional Example

We use ankle dorsiflexion to clear the foot as we step upstairs.

Ankle Plantarflexion

Ankle plantarflexion allows us to make contact with the floor as we reach and extend our leg behind or in front of the body. It is used with varying combinations of hip and knee movements (Fig. 9-14C & D).

Functional Example

We use ankle plantarflexion to touch the step as we walk downstairs or to touch the ground as we walk downhill.

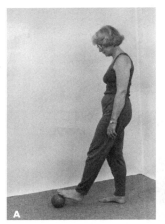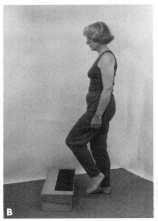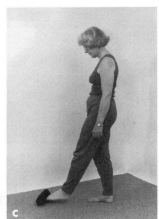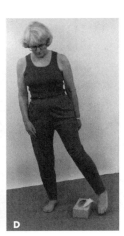

FIGURE 9-14 (A) Ankle dorsiflexion with hip flexion and knee extension. (B) Ankle dorsi-flexion with hip and knee flexion. (C) Ankle plantarflexion with hip flexion and knee extension. (D) Ankle plantarflexion with hip abduction and knee extension.

SIGNIFICANT IMPAIRMENTS THAT INTERFERE WITH PERFORMANCE

Loss of Trunk Control and Alignment

To move the left leg in standing, we shift weight to the right leg while the upper trunk stays aligned over the lower trunk. This establishes the starting position for non-weight bearing movements of the left leg. The control of the upper trunk over the lower trunk and the shift over, but not past, the standing leg are extremely diffi-cult for patients with hemiplegia. Poor trunk control results in an inability to main-tain the position of the upper and lower trunk during the weight shift and over-shifting or compensatory shifting of the trunk to the standing side (Fig. 9-15).

FIGURE 9-15 (A) Normal trunk position during forward lift of the left leg. (B) Patient with left hemiplegia lifting her left leg. She overshifts to the right. Lateral asymmetry is present. The left pelvis rotates backward.

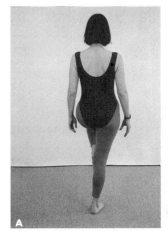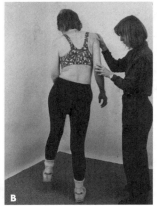

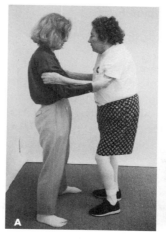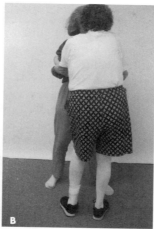

FIGURE 9-16 (A) Patient with a left hemiplegia, who cannot stand independently, attempting to lift her left leg. (B) She tries to shift weight to her right side by moving her right hip laterally, but her trunk does not shift over the right leg. Her upper body is leaning to the left, even with support.

When trunk control is lost because of weakness, it is nearly impossible for patients to lift their hemiplegic leg, even when the trunk and standing leg are supported. These patients do not become independent ambulators. With trunk weakness, the spine is laterally flexed, with the convexity on the hemiplegic side. The pelvis on the convex side of the curve is depressed, and the associated leg pattern is one of flexion (Fig. 9-16).

Weakness results in another possible trunk asymmetry. These trunk patterns are similar to those described in sitting (see Ch. 5), but compounded by the need to combine trunk and leg movement patterns. If the trunk and leg are weak, the pelvis elevates and rotates backward on the hemiplegic side, while the trunk laterally flexes with the concavity to that side (Fig. 9-17). In treatment, the therapist must correct the trunk asymmetries while reeducating the trunk movements in standing. The size of the adult body makes this task difficult and often requires that therapists rely on external supports to help with the goal of providing an assist to upper trunk alignment. The use of a table or countertop for upper extremity forearm weight bearing provides a symmetric supportive surface so the therapist can begin to correct lower trunk and pelvic asymmetries in standing (Fig. 9-18).

If the patient relies on a cane to stand, the overshifting is evident even before the weight shift. Loss of trunk control, reliance on a cane, and the resultant overshifting compounds the trunk weakness and asymmetry (Fig. 9-19).

Patients have difficulty moving the hemiplegic leg if trunk control has not been retrained in the standing position with compatible leg movements. It is not sufficient to train only trunk control in sitting and expect carryover into standing. Trunk movements in standing must be reeducated in conjunction with the related leg patterns with both feet on the ground before the reeducation of non-weight bearing control. (See the section Lower Extremity Weight Bearing Movements in Standing, p.284.) When leg movements in space are retrained, the therapist must combine the appropriate trunk response for the range and pattern of leg motion.

FIGURE 9-17 Patient lifting right leg, with trunk overshifting and pelvic elevation and rotation backwards.

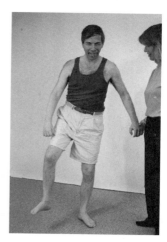

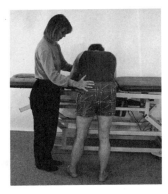

FIGURE 9-18 Use of standing forearm weight bearing to realign and reeducate trunk and pelvic movements in standing in preparation for lifting the left leg.

Weakness and Improper Initiation Patterns

We use one of two initiation patterns to move a leg: some functional movements are initiated distally by the lower leg while other movements are initiated proximally with variations of hip and knee flexion. Patients with primary weakness problems have difficulty with both of these two initiation patterns. They compensate for the proximal leg weakness by initiating leg movements with atypical trunk movements or by extreme reliance on a stable, external aid such as a hemiwalker or quad cane (Fig. 9-20A & B). Some patients, with more muscle return, but still weak, learn to initiate leg movements from the lower trunk and pelvis. They use pelvic elevation, pelvic elevation with rotation, or a posterior pelvic tilt (Fig. 9-20C–E). Over time, pelvic elevation compensations are associated with knee extension, while pelvic posterior tilting is accompanied by slight knee flexion.

In treatment, therapists must teach the patient a variety of leg initiation patterns and reeducate trunk control to provide stability for the leg movements. Patients have the greatest difficulty initiating distal patterns to clear the foot from the floor (Fig. 9-21A). While both proximal and distal initiation pattern must be reeducated, the distal pattern must be taught during all leg movements, especially in early treatment (Fig. 9-21B).

Treatment includes incorporation of distal movements and timing of firing patterns and helps the patient learn to lift the leg up and to place it back down on the floor (Fig. 9-22). In treatment, the therapist often feels the foot pushing down as it comes toward the floor and the knee extends. This push of the foot occurs when the hip and lower leg muscles stop firing and when the tight two-joint muscles of the hip and knee become stretched to their limit as the knee extends. If the gastrocnemius is shortened, the foot pushes into plantarflexion as the knee extends. If the lateral thigh muscles and the posterior calf muscles are both shortened, the tibia externally rotates as the knee extends and the foot inverts with ankle plantarflexion.

FIGURE 9-19 Patient with a left hemiplegia trying to lift her left leg. Her upper trunk has over-shifted to the right as she lifts her leg with pelvic elevation.

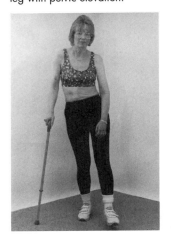

Hypertonicity

Hypertonicity during leg movements in standing is a common problem, although it is not the primary cause for the inability to move and function. Hypertonicity in the leg during movements results in difficulty moving the leg in a wide variety of functional patterns. The leg with extensor hypertonicity feels stiff and awkward, and the patient complains of an inability to lift it off the floor and position it easily or properly in standing. During standing movements, the patterns of extensor hypertonicity in the leg include components of pelvic rotation, knee extension, ankle plantarflexion and foot inversion.

Hypertonicity in the leg during standing movements may be the result of insufficient trunk control, poor alignment of the leg because of muscle shortening, or weakness and loss of initiation patterns. These problems are discussed separately below.

Insufficient Trunk Control

When trunk alignment and control is poor and the patient tries to lift his hemiplegic leg, the pelvis rotates, the upper trunk flexes forward, the hip flexes and abducts,

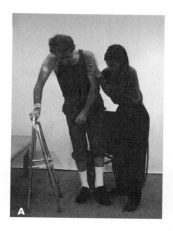
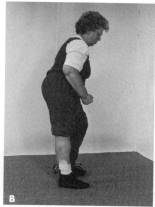
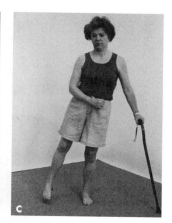

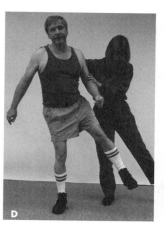
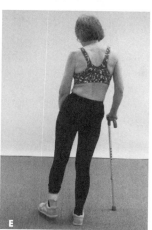

FIGURE 9-20 (*A*) Patient with left hemiplegia and no active leg movements in standing. His upper trunk flexes, and the left upper trunk rotates forward and shears to the right. The left pelvis is rotated back and cannot be passively moved forward to neutral. To lift his left leg, he shifts to the right onto a hemiwalker until the left leg unweights. He cannot lift it actively. His left ankle plantarflexes passively. (*B*) Patient with a right hemiplegia unsuccessfully trying to lift her right leg. She rotates her right pelvis and lower trunk backward to unweight the right leg. (*C*) Patient trying to lift her hemiplegic right leg to the side. She leans far to the left onto her cane to substitute for right hip abduction. Her ankle plantarflexes and the foot inverts. (*D*) Patient trying to abduct left hemiplegic leg. He uses pelvic rotation backward to initiate the movement. (*E*) Patient with left hemiplegia trying to lift up the left leg. She uses pelvic elevation with shearing of trunk to the right.

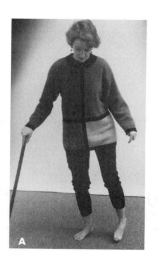
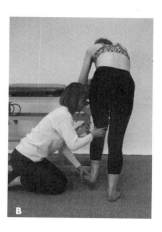

FIGURE 9-21 (*A*) Patient attempting to lift foot off floor. Her anterior tibialis muscle fires, but her ankle plantarflexes. (*B*) Treatment in forearm weight bearing. Therapist's right hand assists hip and knee flexion while her left hand reeducates ankle and forefoot dorsiflexion.

FIGURE 9-22 (*A & B*) Therapist teaches patient to lift leg up and place it down with appropriate distal pattern.

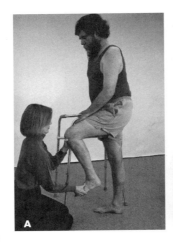
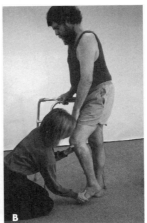

the knee extends, and the ankle plantarflexes with foot inversion. The lift off the floor is accomplished by overshifting to the uninvolved side. With more trunk control but leg weakness, the patient elevates the pelvis and shears the upper trunk to the uninvolved side. The leg lift occurs with active pelvic elevation and active hip flexion with knee extension. The foot pushes strongly and, in most cases, ankle joint dorsiflexion range is limited. In some cases, strong extensor hypertonicity, with the foot inverting and pushing into the floor, makes it difficult or impossible for the patient to initiate a lift off the floor. With more muscle return in the leg, the patient elevates and rotates the pelvis backward with active hip and knee flexion. The foot activity is strong and reinforces the leg pattern (Fig. 9-23A). When these patients move their legs back down, knee extension and ankle plantarflexion and inversion become even stronger. This makes placing the foot flat on the floor difficult and standing balance precarious (Fig. 9-23C).

FIGURE 9-23 (*A*) Patient with right hemiplegia, who cannot stand and balance independently, trying to lift her leg off the floor. The leg has extensor hypertonicity and pushes into the floor as she tries to lift it up. (*B*) Patient with a right hemiplegia with the ability to stand and balance, but with leg weakness. She lifts her right leg with upper trunk shearing to the left, strong pelvic elevation, hip flexion with knee extension, and ankle plantarflexion. (*C*) Patient placing right foot on floor with strong ankle plantarflexion and foot inversion. This makes it difficult to balance on the leg.

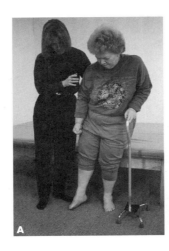
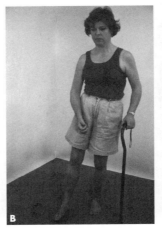
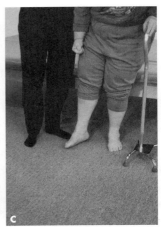

Muscle Shortening and Tightness

Muscle tightness, if present, must be identified and treated first in sitting and then in standing with upper body support (see the section Lower Extremity Weight Bearing Movements [p. 284] and Ch. 8). Patients with strong extensor hypertonicity who cannot lift their leg up in standing can often move the hip and knee in sitting. When they stand, the loss of trunk control and tightness of two-joint muscles are more significant and result in an increase of extensor tension in the leg. Changes in alignment of the ankle joint caused by gastrocnemius muscle shortening can result in ankle plantarflexion and foot inversion when the knee is extended. Patients who display this type of hypertonicity can move their ankle into dorsiflexion when sitting (i.e., when the knee is flexed). The "push" of their foot into the floor comes when the knee extends, thus stretching the shortened gastrocnemius at its insertion. Since this muscle inverts the calcaneus, the foot inverts and plantarflexes. Over time, return in both the anterior and posterior tibialis muscles results in strong inversion. Patients who lift their leg with a strong flexor pattern have more obvious foot inversion, because the knee is not as extended. Weak toe extensors (lateral foot muscles) if present, have a very difficult time balancing this inversion (Fig. 9-24).

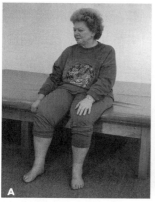
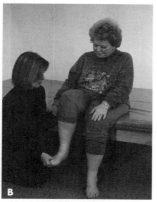
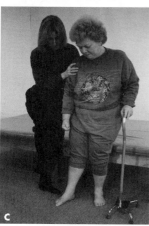
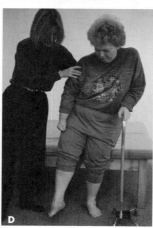
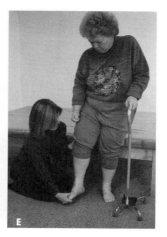

FIGURE 9-24 (*A & B*) In sitting, patient with right hemiplegia can assist the therapist move the hip, knee, and ankle. (*C*) Patient in standing with strong extensor hypertonicity in right leg. (*D*) Patient struggles to lift up right leg. She overshifts to the left to clear the plantarflexing foot from the floor. (*E*) Therapist meets strong resistance and is unable to pick up the patient's leg or stop the push of the foot.

Weakness and Loss of Initiation Patterns

When the leg moves in space, the pattern produced may appear hypertonic but may be the result of weakness and/or loss of the ability to initiate for the desired pattern. While the weakness and loss of initiation pattern may be the primary cause of the pattern, other causes may overlap. The strong knee extension pattern during leg movements is often thought to be "spasticity," but may be the unbalanced use of the quadriceps muscle to lift the leg. If the function requires hip and knee flexion (forward lift) but the patient initiates with a pattern of pelvic elevation, the hip may not flex, but the quadriceps may fire and produce hip flexion with knee extension (forward reach). Reestablishment of trunk control and reeducation of various hip and knee patterns will diminish the patient's need to rely on only this knee extensor pattern to lift the leg.

Flexor Hypertonicity

In the standing position, flexor hypertonicity results in the leg lifting off the floor during attempts at standing. The flexor pattern is one of pelvic elevation or rotation backwards, partial hip flexion with external rotation, knee flexion, ankle plantarflexion, and foot inversion. If the leg cannot make contact with the floor because of this pattern, the patient cannot learn to stand safely. These patients need treatment that focuses on reestablishing the ability to place weight on their leg before they concentrate on learning to move the leg (see p. 284). However, patients may also use this mass flexion pattern when moving the leg. The cause of this flexor hypertonicity is a result of poor trunk control and unbalanced, but active, muscle activation patterns. These patients recruit hip flexor muscles as the pelvis rotates backward and lateral two-joint hip and knee muscles flex the knee (Fig. 9-25).

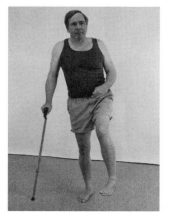

FIGURE 9-25 Patient with a left hemiplegia, with the ability to stand and balance without support, lifting his left leg. His leg is stiff and heavy as he lifts with pelvic elevation and rotation backward. The hip and knee flex, and he lifts the foot with strong inversion and ankle plantarflexion.

Careful assessment, as noted in the first part of this chapter, allows the therapist to plan treatment to address the cause of the hypertonicity as well as the reeducation needs of the patient.

ASSESSMENT GUIDELINES

Assessment of leg movements in standing should include trunk control during unilateral stance, trunk control during assisted movements of the leg, control of distal and proximal initiation patterns, and strength and control of the leg patterns themselves, both as the leg moves off the floor and back onto the floor.

I. Describe the starting position of the trunk and stance leg. Describe the pattern of weight shift onto the stance leg.

II. Describe the distal and proximal initiation patterns as the leg moves off the floor.

III. Assess the strength and variety of leg movement patterns. Identify the movements that are performed with repeated atypical patterns.

IV. Use your hands on the patient's trunk and pelvis to correct alignment and to assist with proximal control.

    What leg movements appear or improve when you assist?

    What problems do not change immediately with handling and will require further treatment to change the movement components?

V. What pattern does the patient use as he places the foot down on the floor?

    Use your hands to assist the trunk and/or pelvis. Does the leg movement pattern change? What movements appear or improve when you assist?

    What patterns/problems do not change immediately with handling and will require further treatment?

VI. Provide support to the trunk and use your hands proximally and distally on the leg to assist the movements. What improves or changes? Identify the muscle groups that are active during functional movements.

VII. List the major trunk control problems during leg movements.

VIII. List the major proximal impairments in the leg that are interfering with movement.

IX. List the major distal impairments in the leg that are interfering with movement.

THERAPY GOALS

Functional Goals

The functional goals for the leg during non-weight bearing movements in standing are to move the affected leg in standing for comfort, to position the leg, to perform functional activities, and to use as part of a balance response.

Treatment Goals and Techniques

Treatment Goal: Correct trunk alignment and reestablish trunk control during weight shift to stance leg.

Treatment Techniques: Forearm and extended-arm weight bearing to provide symmetry to upper trunk while therapist realigns trunk in preparation for leg movements (Fig. 9-26).

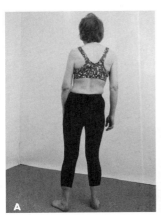
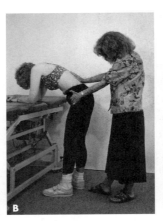
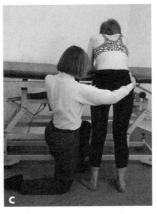
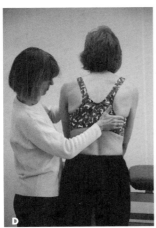
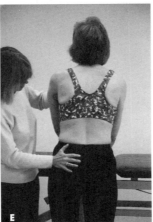

FIGURE 9-26 (*A*) Patient's trunk is sheared to the right. (*B*) A left hemiplegic patient is in forearm weight bearing; therapist realigns upper trunk over lower trunk as patient performs anteroposterior weight shifts. (*C*) Therapist's hands correct pelvis as patient shifts weight laterally. (*D*) Patient moves to extended-arm weight bearing, placing hips in extension. Therapist's left hand corrects lateral trunk position by lifting upper trunk up and back while her right hand helps patient learn to shift the upper body back over the pelvis. The therapist's body is against the patient's left hip to remind her not to hang laterally on the left hip. (*E*) Therapist moves her right hand to the pelvis to teach lower-extremity-initiated weight shifts to the right in preparation for practicing movements of the left leg.

Treatment Technique: Reeducate trunk and leg initiation patterns (Fig. 9-27).

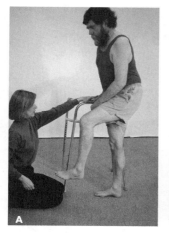
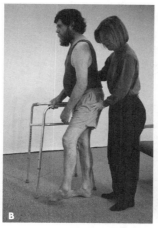
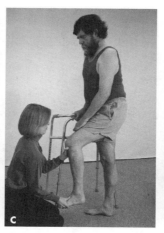
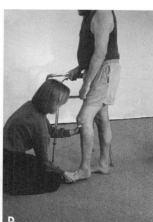

FIGURE 9-27 (*A*) Patient with a left hemiplegia lifting his left leg. His trunk leans forward and his pelvis rotates back as he lifts his leg. (*B*) Therapist corrects trunk and pelvis and asks patient to practice lifting his left leg. (*C*) Patient practices trunk pattern with verbal reminders as therapist assists the initiation pattern of the foot and hip as the leg lifts up. (*D*) Therapist helps patient practice moving leg back down without the ankle or foot pushing.

Treatment Goal: Train trunk and leg movement patterns in standing.

Treatment Technique: Teach sideways reach with arm support (Fig. 9-28).

FIGURE 9-28 (*A*) Patient with a right hemiplegia. Therapist holds her right ankle and foot and assists the sideways reach pattern. (*B*) As the patient abducts through more range, the therapist reminds the patient to elevate her pelvis. (*C*) The therapist reminds the patient to shift more to her left as the leg abducts and the trunk laterally flexes. (*D*) While the patient practices moving the leg independently, the therapist encourages appropriate pelvis and trunk patterns.

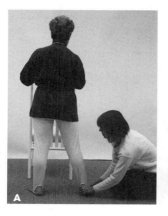
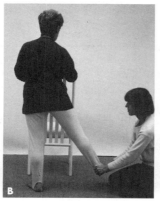
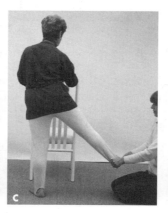
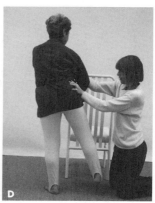

Treatment Goal: Retrain and strengthen initiation patterns and incorporate lower extremity movements into functional activities.

Treatment Technique: Practicing leg movements with distal activation patterns with use of unilateral support. Practicing the leg movements in function (Fig. 9-29).

FIGURE 9-29 (*A*) Patient with a left hemiplegia practicing lifting her leg in a sideways reach pattern. The therapist's left hand encourages ankle dorsiflexion while her right hand helps the patient abduct the left leg without rotating the pelvis backward. (*B*) Patient practices hip, knee, and ankle dorsiflexion without excessive pelvic elevation. (*C–E*) Patient uses less support, a straight cane, as she practices using the same initiation pattern to lift her left foot onto a step.

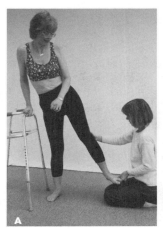
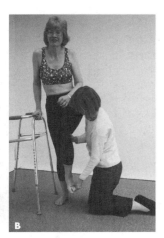
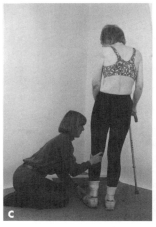
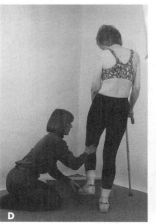
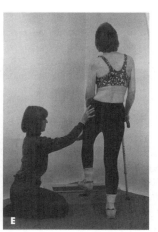

Treatment Goal: Reeducation of ankle and foot muscles. Incoporation of movement reeducation with functional activity.

Treatment Technique: Correcting alignment, practicing initiation pattern, and reeducating ankle and foot muscles with leg behind the body (Fig. 9-30A–C).

Treatment Technique: Reeducation of distal movements with the leg in front of the body and incorporating the movements into function (Fig. 9-30D–J).

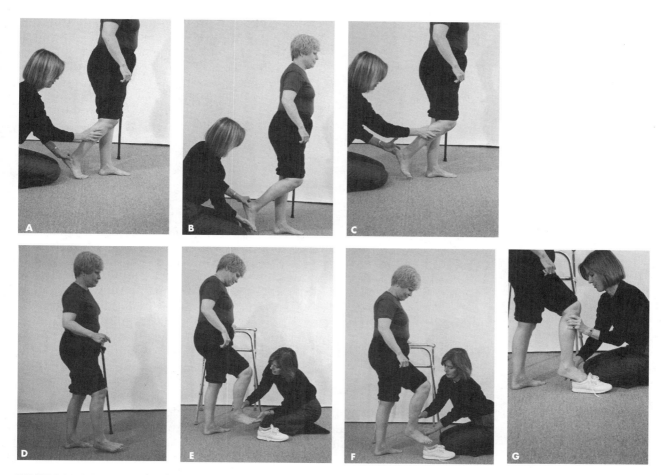

FIGURE 9-30 (*A*) Patient with right hemiplegia holds her forefoot on the floor. Therapist's hands correct alignment of the tibia and rearfoot: her right hand internally rotates the tibia to neutral while her left hand keeps the calcaneus from inverting and directs a downward pressure into the ball of the foot. If muscle tightness exists, she can use this position to lengthen shortened tissue before reeducation starts. (*B*) With the knee held in flexion, the patient practices moving the ankle and toes. The therapist stabilizes the rearfoot and provides minimal assistance to the forefoot. (*C*) As the patient gains the ability to move the ankle and foot with less assistance, the therapist moves her right hand back to the lower leg to correct and assist the tibial position. (*D*) Patient lifts her leg in front of her body. The ankle remains plantarflexed and the foot inverts with toe curling. (*E*) Therapist's right hand internally rotates the tibia to neutral and assists the lift of the leg to allow the patient to practice ankle and foot movements. Her left hand is under the toes to assist while the patient lifts her ankle and foot. (*F*) Therapist continues to assist the lift of the leg and helps the patient practice plantarflexing the ankle with the goal of having her toes touch the shoe. (*G*) The therapist moves her hand so her left hand helps the leg move down as the patient plantarflexes her ankle and places the front of her foot into the shoe. The foot inverts as it enters the shoe. (*Figure continues.*)

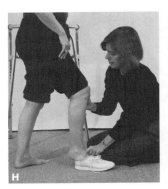
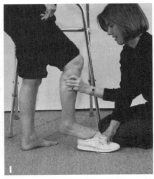
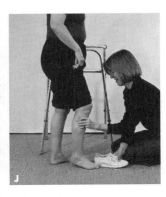

FIGURE 9-30 (*Continued*) (*H*) Therapist moves her right hand to the midfoot and assists as the patient tries to lower her leg and move her plantarflexed foot further into the shoe. (*I*) The therapist holds the shoe as the patient flexes her knee to move the foot back out of the shoe. The therapist uses her left hand to correct excessive tibial external rotation that is accompanying the foot inversion and to assist the knee flexion. (*J*) Therapist helps the patient control the movement of the leg and foot back down to the floor.

Lower Extremity Weight Bearing Movements

CONCEPTS AND PRINCIPLES

The starting position for our analysis of weight bearing movements of the legs is standing with the upper trunk aligned over the lower trunk. The pelvis and hips are in a neutral position and the knees, while straight, are not stiff or locked in a rigid position. The feet are placed comfortably 5 to 8 inches apart and form the base of support for the movements. The base of support includes the space defined by the contours of the feet and the area between them. The ankles are in a neutral position with the sole of the foot perpendicular to the axis of the leg. The ankle joint is the fulcrum of leg movements in standing when the hip and knee remain in a position of neutral extension. This section will describe movement components in the leg in response to *weight shifts initiated by the legs* and to *weight shifts initiated by the upper body.*

LOWER EXTREMITY WEIGHT BEARING MOVEMENT COMPONENTS

Lower-Extremity-Initiated Movements

The weight bearing movement components of the leg that are described in this section occur as a result of lower-extremity-initiated movements that shift body weight between the feet. These movements will be analyzed with the feet in three different positions. During functional activities, we shift body weight when our feet are *parallel;* when our feet are parallel and wide apart in *abducted stance;* and when our feet are in an uneven stepped position, *(step/stance).* When the right foot is ahead of the left foot, the position is called *right step/stance,* and if the left foot is ahead of the right, the position is *left step/stance.*

During standing weight shifts, the trunk remains upright and adjusts its posture to the lower-extremity-initiated movements. This means that the upper trunk remains aligned with the lower trunk and moves with the legs over the feet. The fulcrum of these movements is the ankle joint. To stay within the base of support during these lower body weight shifts, the range of trunk movements is relatively small. When lower-extremity-initiated weight shifts are larger, they move the center of gravity of the body past the border of the feet. If this occurs, an equilibrium response is recruited and the resultant trunk and leg components may not be the same as those when the trunk moves within the base of support. The movement components that are part of balance control in standing are described at the end of this section.

Feet Parallel (see Table 9-1, p. 287)

Anterior Weight Shift—Increased Ankle Dorsiflexion

In standing, when an anterior weight shift is initiated by the legs, the spine remains extended. The trunk moves forward with the pelvis, thighs, and lower legs, resulting in ankle dorsiflexion. Weight is transferred from the heel of the foot to the front of the foot, and the hips move into more extension. The pelvis does not move into an anterior tilt, but the spine may move into more extension as the center of gravity comes close to the anterior edge of the base of support (Fig. 9-31A & B).

Functional Examples

This movement is used during forward reach with the arms and as a counterbalance to arm movements behind the body.

Posterior Weight Shift—Increased Ankle Plantarflexion

As a posterior weight shift is initiated by the lower body, the ankles plantarflex and the pelvis and thighs move back toward the heels. The hips flex a small amount, and the upper body shifts forward. This movement is small because the line of gravity falls close to the heels. The amount of change in movement at the hip joint and in the spine is relative to the amount of weight shift (Fig. 9-31C).

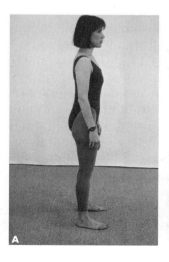 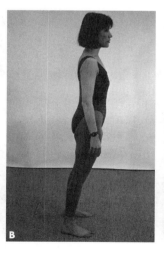 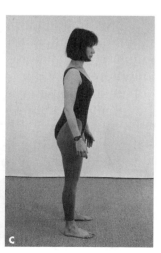

FIGURE 9-31 (A) Neutral standing position. (B) Lower-extremity-initiated anterior weight shift. (C) Lower-extremity-initiated posterior weight shift.

Functional Examples

This movement is used on the weight bearing side as we step or walk backwards. It is also used during dressing activities, when we move our arms to our thighs or knees.

Lateral Weight Shift—Increased Abduction/Adduction

When a lateral weight shift to the right is initiated by the lower extremities, the upper trunk remains erect and stable over the lower trunk and follows the movement of the pelvis. As the weight is shifted over the right foot, the right hip is in relative adduction and the left hip is abducted in relationship to the pelvis. The right hip and shoulder are over the right foot. The soles of the feet remain on the floor while body weight is shifted to the lateral border of the right foot and to the medial border of the left foot (Fig. 9-32).

Functional Examples

This movement is used to shift weight to one leg before stepping. It also accompanies lateral arm movements on the same side of the body.

Rotational Weight Shifts

When rotational movements are initiated by the lower extremities in standing, the upper and lower trunk remain stable and aligned over each other and follow the leg movements. During rotation to the right in standing, the body remains centered between the two feet, the left side of the pelvis moves anterior to the right side of the pelvis. The left hip internally rotates and the right hip externally rotates. The spine rotates to the right; the upper trunk either follows the movement of the lower trunk or the upper trunk remains stable while the lower trunk follows the movement of the legs and rotates to the right. If the knees remain extended, the movement translates down into the feet. The lower legs follow the rotation of the thighs,

FIGURE 9-32 (*A*) Neutral starting position. (*B*) Lower-extremity-initiated lateral weight shift to the right. (*C & D*) Lower-extremity-initiated lateral weight shift to the left.

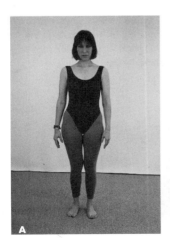
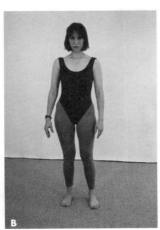
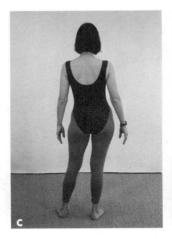
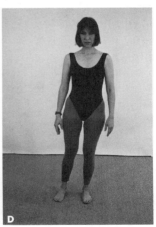

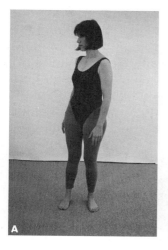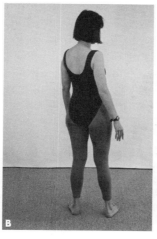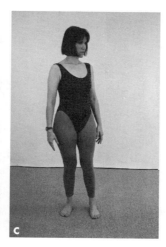

FIGURE 9-33 (*A & B*) Lower-extremity-initiated rotation to the right. (*C*) Lower-extremity-initiated rotation to the left.

TABLE 9-1 Movement Summary: Lower Extremity
Weight Bearing Movement Components*a*

WEIGHT SHIFT	TRUNK	PELVIS/HIP	ANKLE/FOOT
Anterior	Remains aligned	Hip extension	Dorsiflexion
Posterior	Remains aligned	Hip flexion	Slight plantarflexion
Lateral on weight bearing side	Stable and aligned over pelvis	Hip adduction	Weight on lateral border
Lateral on non-weight bearing side	Stable and aligned over pelvis	Hip abduction	Weight on medial border

a Feet parallel, shifting within the base of support; leg-initiated movements.

and weight is shifted to the outside of the right foot and to the inside of the left foot. If the movement continues to its limit, the right foot will invert, and the left foot will evert (Fig. 9-33).

Functional Examples

This movement is used to turn and during leisure activities, such as sports or dancing.

Abducted Stance (see Table 9-2)

Lateral Weight Shift

When a lateral weight shift to the right is initiated by the lower extremities with the feet abducted to shoulder width, the upper and lower trunks remain aligned and adjust to the movement of the legs. However, the movement of the pelvis and hips becomes more obvious than lateral weight shift movements with the feet in a narrower parallel position. As the center of gravity moves over the right foot, the right side of the pelvis moves laterally and elevates and the right femur adducts in relationship to the pelvis. At the same time, the left side of the pelvis moves medially and drops as the left femur abducts relative to the pelvis. Body

FIGURE 9-34 (*A*) Abducted stance. (*B*) Lower-extremity-initiated lateral weight shift to the right in abducted stance. (*C*) Lower-extremity-initiated lateral weight shift to the left in abducted stance.

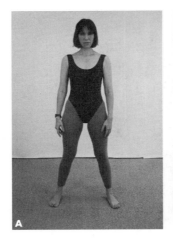 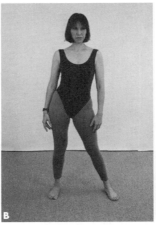 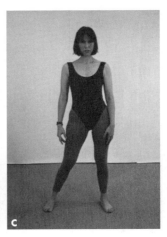

TABLE 9-2 Movement Summary: Lower Extremity Weight Bearing Components in Abducted Stance

WEIGHT SHIFT	PELVIS	HIP	ANKLE
Lateral, on weight bearing side	Lists up (elevation)	Adduction	Weight to lateral side of foot
Lateral, on non-weight bearing side	Lists down (depression)	Abduction	Weight to medial side of foot

weight is shifted to the lateral border of the right foot and to the medial border of the left foot. If the entire foot remains in contact with the floor, the right calcaneus everts relative to the ankle and the left calcaneus is relatively inverted (Fig. 9-34).

This position is a useful treatment activity that allows reeducation of hip abduction and adduction control, and hip extension control in standing.

Functional Examples

This movement is used as we step sideways. Abducted stance is also used to provide increased balance by widening the base of support during abducted reach of the arm.

Step/Stance Position (see Table 9-3, p. 290)

Anterior Weight Shift

When we step the right foot in front of the left foot and keep the pelvis, lower trunk, and upper body aligned, the legs are in a right step/stance position. The trunk is erect over the feet, and equal weight is supported on each foot. In this position, the right hip is in flexion with knee extension and ankle plantarflexion. The starting position for the left leg is hip extension, knee extension, and slight ankle dorsiflexion. The shoulders face forward. Since the position of the legs results in pelvic rotation to the left, the hips rotate relative to the pelvis: the right hip externally rotated, the left hip internally rotated (Fig. 9-35A).

To analyze this movement, it is important to remember that the feet do not come off the floor. As weight shifts anteriorly, the upper trunk remains aligned over the lower trunk and follows the anterior movement of the lower extremities. The right hip remains in flexion but moves toward extension; the right ankle moves towards dorsiflexion. The left hip moves into more extension and the left ankle moves into more dorsiflexion (Fig. 9-35B).

Functional Examples

This movement is used in the double support phase of gait. It is also used in arm functions, such as opening a door or reaching up into a shelf, where one foot moves forward to assist the stability of the body by widening the base of support.

Posterior Weight Shift

As we initiate a posterior weight shift from the lower extremities with the legs in a right step/stance position, the upper trunk is aligned over the lower trunk and the shoulders face forward. As the pelvis moves back, the right hip moves into more flexion, and the ankle moves into more plantarflexion. The left hip moves into flexion, and the ankle moves from dorsiflexion toward neutral or plantarflexion (Fig. 9-35C).

Functional Examples

This movement occurs during backward walking. It is also used to shift the body away from a door before pulling it toward you.

FIGURE 9-35 (A) Right step/stance position. (B) Lower-extremity-initiated anterior weight shift in right step/stance position. (C) Lower-extremity-initiated posterior weight shift in right step/stance position.

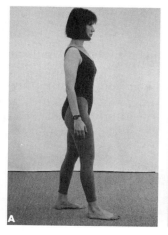
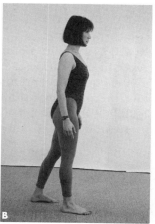
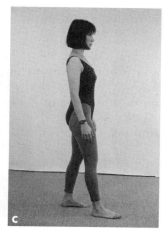

TABLE 9-3 Movement Summary: Lower Extremity
Weight Bearing Movement Components in Step/Stance[a]

WEIGHT SHIFT	HIP		ANKLE
Anterior	Forward leg	More extension	More dorsiflexion
	Back leg	More extension	More dorsiflexion
Posterior	Forward leg	More flexion	Plantarflexion
	Back leg	Less extension	Less dorsiflexion

[a] Pelvis in frontal plane, no rotation, feet slightly apart.

Upper-Trunk-Initiated Movements

During upper-trunk-initiated movements, the trunk and arms move outside the base of support. These upper trunk movements result in weight shifts and position changes in the legs to maintain stability and balance (see Table 9-4, p. 293).

Anterior Weight Shift

When an anterior weight shift is initiated from the upper body in standing, the spine flexes forward from the head and neck and continues through the upper thoracic spine. In response to this anterior weight shift of the upper body, the hips flex and the lower trunk and pelvis shift backward toward the heels. This results in increased ankle joint plantarflexion, if the knees remain in extension (Fig. 9-36A).

When an anterior weight shift is initiated from the upper body in standing, and the task requires reaching all the way to the floor, we may respond with an alternate pattern: knee flexion and ankle dorsiflexion to lower the body and arm to the floor (Fig. 9-36B). To return to the standing position, we initiate the movement with extension of the trunk and legs. The movement is complete when the upper and lower trunk are upright over the hip joints.

Functional Examples

This movement is used to reach an arm forward and down to a table, to touch the knee or lower leg, or to pick up an object off the floor.

Posterior Weight Shift

Upper-trunk-initiated posterior weight shifts are not frequently used in functional tasks. When they occur, they result in the arms or the head extending to reach or look up. As the cervical and thoracic spine extend, the lower body adjusts to provide a balance assist. To do this, the pelvis moves forward, the hips extend, the ankles dorsiflex, and weight is shifted forwards toward the balls of the feet. This adjustment usually occurs with a slight increase in knee flexion (Fig. 9-36C).

Functional Example

This movement is used to reach up with the arms or to look at something overhead.

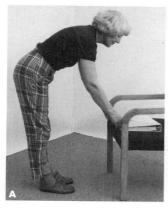
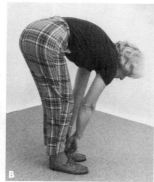
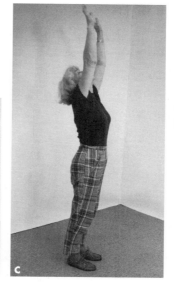

FIGURE 9-36 (A) Upper trunk initiated anterior weight shift resulting in increased hip flexion, knee extension and ankle plantar flexion. (B) Upper trunk initiated anterior weight shift resulting in increased hip and knee flexion. (C) Upper trunk initiated posterior weight shift.

Lateral Weight Shift

When a lateral weight shift to the left is initiated from the upper body in standing, the head, right shoulder, and arm move laterally and down, resulting in a lateral flexion of the spine, with the concavity on the left (Fig. 9-37). To remain balanced and to stay up, one of two lower body patterns is used: either the lower body moves the center of gravity over the right foot, or more weight is placed on the left leg. If the lower body shifts to the right, it is a harder balance task and is used less frequently . Increased body weight is felt on the medial border of the left foot and on the lateral border of the right foot. To return to erect standing, the shoulders move medially to the right, until they are aligned over the pelvis and legs. As the upper body moves up and to the right, the center of gravity moves medially to lie between both feet.

Functional Examples

This movement is used to reach an arm sideways and down to manipulate an object that is lateral to the body.

Flexion Rotation Weight Shift

When the upper body initiates a weight shift that combines anterior and lateral movements on a forward diagonal to the left, down toward the floor, the spine moves into flexion with vertebral rotation to the left (Fig. 9-38A). The right shoulder girdle is anterior to the left, and the right rib cage is elongated relative to the left rib cage. As this occurs, the lower body shifts the center of gravity closer to the right foot to maintain balance. Since, by definition, the movement is occurring in the upper body, the lower body and lower extremity movement is minimal. As the pelvis shifts back and to the right, the hips move into more flexion; the left hip externally rotates, and the right hip internally rotates. The left foot inverts, and the right foot everts.

FIGURE 9-37 Upper-trunk-initiated lateral weight shift to the left.

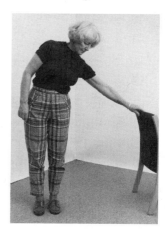

FIGURE 9-38 (*A*) Upper-trunk-initiated flexion rotation to the left. (*B*) Upper-trunk-initiated extension rotation to the left.

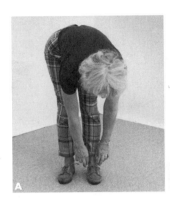 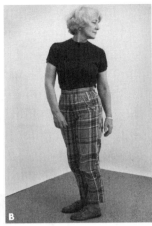

Functional Examples

This movement is used to turn the upper body or reach an arm across midline and down.

Extension Rotation Weight Shift

As the upper body initiates a weight shift that combines posterior and lateral movements on a backward diagonal to the left, the spine moves into extension with vertebral rotation to the left (Fig. 9-38B). The right shoulder girdle moves anterior; the left shoulder girdle and the lower body respond with an anterior movement of the pelvis. As the upper body moves to the left, the lower body adjusts so that weight is distributed evenly on both legs or taken more on the right leg. Since the lower body movement is minimal, there may be no movement of the hips into extension, but more hip extensor muscle activity occurs. As the lower body shifts to the left, more weight is maintained on the lateral border of the right foot and on the medial border of the left foot.

TABLE 9-4 Movement Summary: Upper-Body-Initiated
Lower Extremity Weight Bearing Movement Components

Weight Shift	Trunk	Pelvis/Hip	Ankle/Foot
Anterior	Flexion	Flexion	Plantarflex if knees extend Dorsiflex if knees flex
Posterior	Extension	Extension	Dorsiflex
Lateral left	Concavity left	Neutral	
Flexion rotation left	Flexion rotation left	Flexion	Weight medial on left, lateral on right
Extension rotation left	Extension/ rotation left	Extension	Weight medial on left, lateral on right

Functional Examples

This movement is used frequently as we turn our head and neck to look behind us or to look as we initiate turning to one side. Patients need this movement so they can look behind them to check the position of a seat before they sit down and to begin to retrain the task of turning and changing direction in standing.

MOVEMENT COMPONENTS OF BALANCE CONTROL IN STANDING

Weight Shift, Equilibrium, Protection

While balance control in standing includes areas other than movement control, we are limiting our analysis to the movement components of balance. *Balance control in standing* is the ability to perform movement components that combine trunk and leg patterns, to perform these components in functional sequences, and to combine trunk, leg, and arm movement patterns in balance responses. All these parts of balance control are on a continuum that is identical to the components of balance control in sitting (see Ch. 5).

As we shift our weight in standing, but remain within our base of support, whether it is both feet on the ground or one foot on the ground (with or without arm support) predictable patterns of trunk and leg muscle activity occur, as we described earlier (Fig. 9-39A & B). As we continue moving and shift our center of gravity outside the base of support, we recruit additional trunk movement patterns or increased leg strength to keep ourselves from falling. The arms respond to assist the trunk and leg, if needed.

FIGURE 9-39 (A) Starting position. (B) Therapist shifts subject's body backward within base of support. She has facilitated a lower-extremity-initiated posterior weight shift: hips begin to flex and ankle moves into less dorsiflexion. (C) As therapist continues to shift the subject backward, her trunk works harder, her ankles dorsiflex, and her arms move forward to keep the body from falling backward. These movements, opposite to the weight shift, are movements of an equilibrium response. (D) Therapist moves the subject backward suddenly, and the subject steps back with one leg. This is a protective response to keep from falling when she can no longer balance over her current base of support.

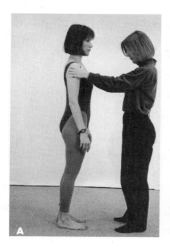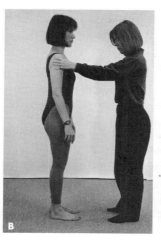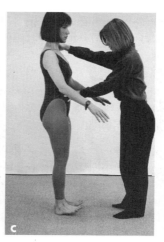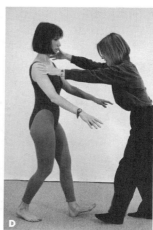

The patterns that we use are opposite the perturbation in order to keep the body from falling. This is known as an equilibrium response (Fig. 9-39C). As the weight shift continues or is quickly imposed and our body no longer has the strength or strategies to keep it upright, we prevent ourselves from falling by moving our arms or legs to increase our base of support. This is known as a protective response (Fig. 9-39D). In treatment, therapists can reeducate and retrain the movement components of the trunk and legs in response to weight shifts and thereby contribute to standing balance control.

SIGNIFICANT IMPAIRMENTS THAT INTERFERE WITH PERFORMANCE

Loss of Trunk Control

Trunk control in standing is a prerequisite for these weight bearing movements of the legs in standing. Loss of trunk control results in difficulty standing and in trunk asymmetries. Altered trunk alignment changes the position of the pelvis and hip. Asymmetries of the pelvis and hip change the tension in and the line of pull of hip and knee muscles. Trunk asymmetries, translated down into the leg, make it harder to reeducate control of weak leg muscles.

Loss of trunk control also leads to a loss of the ability to transfer weight over the legs. This inability to shift weight between the two legs is devastating to patients with hemiplegia because it results in loss of balance control. When the trunk is unstable and unable to move between the two legs, it is difficult or impossible for the patient to lift one leg off the ground without severe compensations.

Loss of trunk control in standing results in atypical alignment patterns. Three common patterns occur: loss of extension control, loss of lateral control, and loss of rotational control.

Loss of Extension Control

Loss of extension control of the trunk in standing results in excessive upper trunk flexion with increased hip flexion. This problem is compounded if there is weakness in the upper extremity. A weak upper extremity is heavy and reinforces the tendency for the upper trunk to flex forward (Fig. 9-40A & B). As the upper trunk flexes forward, the lower trunk and pelvis rotate backward as a counterbalance. Knee recurvatum exists as the pelvis rotates backward because the line of gravity moves in front of the knee joint (Fig. 9-40C & D).

Loss of Lateral and Rotational Control

The upper trunk may also move into lateral flexion with the concavity of the spine on the affected side. With the concavity of the spine on the affected side, the hemiplegic side of the pelvis may elevate. The pelvic elevation lifts the leg and the patient's ankle plantarflexes to keep part of the foot in contact with the floor (Fig. 9-40E & F). Sometimes the hemiplegic side of the trunk is both laterally flexed and forward flexed. If the upper trunk flexes and rotates forward, the pelvis on this side elevates and rotates backward. Since these two opposite rotational movements are used as counterbalances for standing, the patient's body may look shortened but not rotated. The therapist may not be able to identify the rotations until one portion of the trunk asymmetry is corrected (Fig. 9-40G & H).

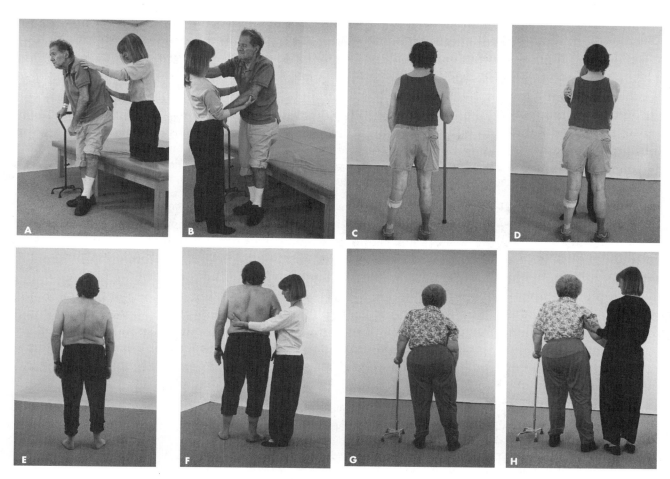

FIGURE 9-40 (A) Patient with severe left hemiplegia and weakness of the trunk, arm, and leg. As he stands, his upper trunk falls forward, and because the arm is weak and heavy, the left upper trunk rotates forward. His left hip is in flexion, there is no weight on the leg, and he relies heavily on a cane. (B) Therapist asks patient to put his right arm on her left shoulder to assist with the correction of the forward trunk position. As she lifts his left arm as much as possible without pain, she assists trunk extension, and his hip moves into less flexion. Her left hand is on his right lower rib cage directing weight on a diagonal toward his left hip to encourage weight on both feet. (C) Patient with left hemiplegia and left upper trunk forward flexion. (D) Therapist, in front of patient, lifts both arms in a symmetric grip. Her right hand supports the right glenohumeral joint and extends the upper trunk back to a symmetric position. (E) Patient with right hemiplegia and increased lateral trunk flexion, concavity on the right. His right shoulder is low and forward. (F) Therapist corrects trunk position; with her right hand she lifts the upper trunk up and back, and with her left hand on his left rib cage directs a downward diagonal message to shift weight onto his right leg. (G) Patient with right hemiplegia. Her upper trunk is rotated and flexed forward while her right pelvis is elevated and rotated backward. (H) Therapist corrects the upper trunk forward rotational position with a unilateral grip. The backward rotation of the pelvis and lower trunk is now more obvious.

The upper trunk may also be laterally flexed with the convexity of the spine on the affected side. With this trunk pattern, the pelvis on the hemiplegic side is usually depressed. Pelvic depression is accompanied by femoral adduction and/or knee flexion. If the arm is weak the upper trunk rotates forward. When the pelvis is depressed and the knee flexed, the pelvis and lower trunk may rotate forward with the upper trunk.

Trunk movement components in standing are similar to trunk movement components in sitting, except that control of the trunk in standing is dependent more on and influenced by lower extremity control. Patients with good trunk control in sitting may be able to perform all the sitting trunk movements but be unable to perform some trunk patterns in standing because of weakness and lack of control in the leg. The lack of control in the leg influences the position of the pelvis and trunk, and conversely, lack of control in the trunk influences the position and control of the legs.

In treatment, therapists must retrain control of the trunk in standing as early as possible. Because of the large size of the body and the number of joints that require support or control, this is one of the most difficult and frustrating tasks in early treatment. Trunk control in standing is a treatment priority. Early treatment goals must include maintaining symmetric trunk alignment as the patient initiates active weight shifts with both the upper trunk and the lower extremities. Extension control of the upper trunk over the lower trunk provides the prerequisite alignment and control necessary to allow hip extension strength and control to develop (Fig. 9-41A–C) As control and strength in trunk movements increases, the therapist moves her manual guidance from just the trunk, to the trunk and leg.

Before standing trunk control is well established, upper extremity weight bearing can be used in standing treatment to stabilize upper trunk position and to provide extra stability to the body. This stability to the upper trunk allows the therapist

FIGURE 9-41 (A) Patient with left hemiplegia and poor trunk control. He cannot stand without assistance and support. The overshifting to the support and the loss of trunk control result in the left heel being off the floor. (B) Therapist uses her hands to correct trunk asymmetries and to encourage use of the left leg. (C) Therapist uses standing against a wall as an assist to help the patient learn to realign his body and extend his trunk. This position can be used to begin active leg initiated movements; the patient can move up and down, left and right. (D) Therapist uses upper extremity forearm weight bearing in standing to support the trunk as she helps the patient learn to initiate weight shifts from his hemiplegic leg.

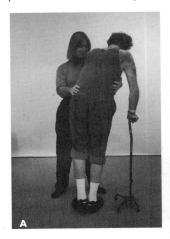
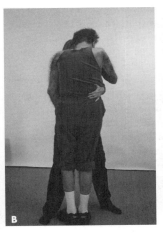
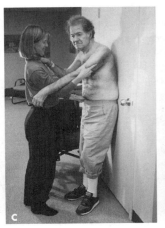
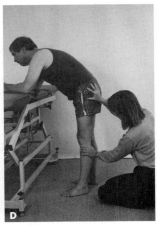

to focus on lower extremity treatment goals without concern for the patient's safety. As the patient regains control of the upper and lower trunk, the therapist continues to move her manual guidance more distally, to the thigh, knee, lower leg, or foot (Fig. 9-41D).

Lower Extremity Weakness

In standing, the position of the leg is maintained by muscle activity in the pelvis, hip, knee, ankle, and foot. The muscles of the hip and knee must contract to stabilize these joints for erect standing. The ankle and foot are the fulcrum of lower body movements in standing, so strength and control of ankle movements are critical to allow adjustments of body position. In addition, activity in leg muscles keep the foot in contact with the floor.

When the involved leg is weak, the patient is unable to produce some or all of these important movement components. Patients with leg weakness have difficulty balancing the contraction of muscles to keep the foot in contact with the floor and the knee extended as body weight is distributed over both legs. When the knee is not controlled as the patient attempts to move onto the leg, the knee buckles and the patient may become fearful of falling. This discourages him from practicing placing weight on the weaker leg so that he can move the opposite leg. Knee flexion because of weakness is accompanied by hip flexion. When retraining control of the knee, the therapist must remember to include simultaneous treatment of the hip. In standing, knee extension to neutral occurs with hip extension. Patients with hemiplegia may try to extend the affected knee without changing the hip position. If the hip remains in flexion, attempts at straightening the knee result in knee recurvatum.

In treatment, the therapist must help the patient learn how to sequence muscle contraction and strengthen the hip and knee muscles to allow knee extension with appropriate pelvic and hip movements. Standing forearm or extended-arm weight bearing positions help in treatment of leg weakness, because the position provides stability to the upper body as the therapist helps the patient learn to strengthen and control lower extremity movements. If the patient has learned to stabilize the knee by locking or pushing into recurvatum with plantarflexion of the ankle joint, reeducation of knee control in standing must include treatment of the ankle and foot. Knee control problems are accompanied by hip and ankle control problems. Therapists must assess and prioritize treatment of all three areas to retrain control of the knee successfully in standing.

Weakness of lateral hip musculature results in an inability to control lateral weight shifts. This movement is one of the most difficult to train in patients with hemiplegia, because patients have a tendency to initiate the movement from the pelvis without appropriate trunk or hip control. As a result, they overshift laterally and "hang" on their lateral hip ligaments for stability. This excessive lateral sway results in internal hip rotation and knee recurvatum. In treatment, they need to be taught to initiate from the leg and keep the trunk and pelvis aligned within the base of support (Fig. 9-42). Patients need lateral hip stability to perform unilateral stance on the hemiplegic side and to progress forward during walking. Correct training in standing will prepare for this phase of walking (Fig. 9-43).

Leg weakness and asymmetries contribute to the loss of trunk alignment and control. If the leg is weak, the patient usually supports body weight on the uninvolved leg. The weak leg is positioned in hip and knee flexion and ankle plan-

FIGURE 9-42 (A) Subject standing on left leg with trunk and pelvis aligned over foot. (B) Patient with a left hemiplegia overshifting laterally with loss of trunk alignment and left lateral hip control.

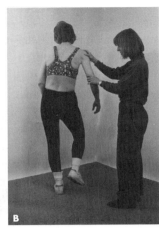
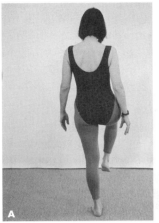

FIGURE 9-43 (A) Patient with a left hemiplegia in standing. (B) Patient using excessive lateral pelvic sway to shift laterally. The left knee hyperextends. (C) Therapist training lower-extremity-initiated lateral weight shift. She teaches the patient to stop the excessive lateral movement and to initiate the movement lower in the leg. (D) She holds the left knee out of recurvatum, while guiding lateral weight shifts. (E) The patient shifts over his left leg with minimal assistance from the therapist.

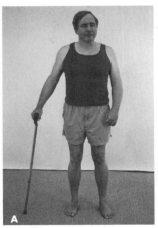
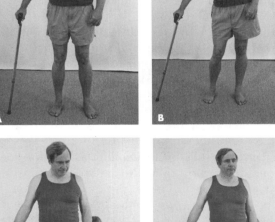
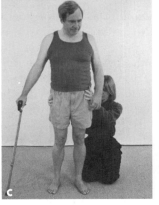
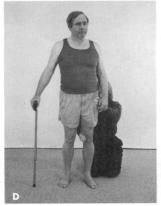
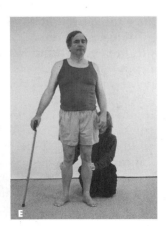

tarflexion. With a flexed weak leg, the pelvis depresses and the spine laterally flexes with the convexity on the hemiplegic side. With severe, prolonged weakness of the lower extremity and poor trunk alignment and control, patients cannot stand safely. Attempts at standing are precarious and usually assisted with a brace and a quad cane. The quad cane becomes a substitute for the weak leg.

Therefore, reeducation of leg movement patterns must occur with either appropriate trunk patterns or with trunk support. The combination of a trunk treatment goal with a leg treatment goal will lead to earlier carryover of both strength and function.

Loss of Lower Extremity Alignment

Postural deviations in the trunk and weakness in the leg muscles influence the position of the pelvis, femur, lower leg and foot. Although these asymmetries are initially present because of loss of muscle activity and control, they eventually result in muscle and soft tissue tightness. Once muscle and soft tissue tightness are present it is more difficult to reeducate weak or missing musculature.

Upper Trunk Influences on Lower Trunk and Pelvis

Trunk symmetries caused by loss of upper trunk control and weakness set up the following lower trunk and pelvic asymmetries. Therapists must not forget how greatly the loss of arm control and alignment influences the upper trunk.

1. Rib cage rotation backward with pelvic rotation forward as a counterbalance

2. Rib cage rotation forward with pelvic rotation backward as a counterbalance

3. Lateral flexion of the spine (convexity on the same side) with pelvic depression

4. Upper trunk overshifting/shearing to the opposite side with pelvic elevation

5. Upper trunk flexion in patients with severe weakness, with a posterior pelvic tilt and lower trunk flexion.

6. Upper trunk flexion (kyphosis) with anterior pelvic tilt and lower trunk extension.

Lower Trunk and Pelvic Influences on Hip and Knee

These pelvic and trunk asymmetries influence the position of the hemiplegic hip and knee.

1. Forward inclination of the trunk, either with spinal rotation or lateral flexion cause hip flexion and knee extension.

2. When the patient cannot support body weight on the weak leg, pelvic forward rotation on the hemiplegic side occurs with hip internal rotation; pelvic elevation and backward rotation occurs with external rotation.

3. Pelvic elevation occurs with hip abduction; pelvic depression occurs with hip adduction.

Hip and Knee Influences on the Ankle

Ankle asymmetries and tissue tightness are related to hip and knee alignment problems.

1. Hip flexion/knee hyperextension pattern leads to ankle plantarflexion. As the knee moves into hyperextension, the proximal portion of the tibia moves back with the knee, while the distal portion of the tibia stays forward.

2. Excessive knee flexion during standing or walking as a method of preventing knee recurvatum with ankle dorsiflexion. Excessive ankle dorsiflexion also is present if the midfoot collapses in eversion/pronation during weight bearing.

Before treating lower extremity weakness, the therapist must remember to assess the influences of the trunk and proximal joints on lower extremity asymmetries. Lower extremity asymmetries must be corrected before reeducation strategies are effective and lasting. For example, if knee control in standing is a goal, treatment must address alignment and control problems of both the hip and ankle. This may be done in a position of extended-arm weight bearing. First, the therapist corrects pelvic and femoral alignment while asking the patient to initiate lower extremity weight shifts. Then the therapist realigns the lower leg and ankle joint and asks the patient to perform lower-extremity-initiated movements. Finally, the therapist can monitor the ankle position and the hip position, while asking the patient either to perform knee flexion and extension or to initiate anteroposterior weight shifts to reeducate knee control.

Lower Extremity Hypertonicity

Lower extremity hypertonicity may cause the leg to assume a position of excessive extension or excessive flexion. Extensor hypertonicity of the leg in standing is more prevalent than flexor hypertonicity, but flexor hypertonicity is more devastating because its presence makes it impossible to function in standing.

Extensor hypertonicity places the knee in excessive extension or *recurvatum* and changes the position of the remaining joints of the leg. When the leg is held stiffly and the knee extends, the ankle plantarflexes and the foot pushes into the floor. With ankle plantarflexion, the heel comes off the floor, the calcaneus moves into equinus, and the foot inverts. If the ankle and foot patterns are severe, the distal tibia externally rotates. Strong ankle plantarflexion with knee recurvatum shifts weight backward and puts the hip in flexion. Pelvic position depends on the amount and pattern of trunk control present. Sometimes the pelvis rotates backward and the hip externally rotates; if the pelvis rotates forward, the hip internally rotates. This "spastic" extensor pattern makes it difficult for the patient to stand because the entire foot is not in contact with the floor. The extensor hypertonicity in the leg produces a change in trunk position. An abnormal position of the trunk and leg make weight support and balance difficult.

We describe three possible causes for hypertonicity: hypertonicity from poor trunk or hip control, hypertonicity as a result of muscle shortening and loss of joint alignment, and hypertonicity from unbalanced muscle contraction.

Hypertonicity from Poor Trunk or Hip Control

Hypertonicity can result from poor trunk control or hip control in standing. Patients may have enough trunk control in sitting to allow isolated movements of the hip, knee, and ankle, but as they move to standing, the leg develops extensor hypertonicity, and isolated movements are impossible. This hypertonicity is due to insufficient trunk and hip control in standing. The patient recruits excessive muscle activity in the leg to compensate for proximal instability. Trunk stability and control is a precursor for lower extremity movement control in standing. If the patient does not develop trunk control in standing, and the patient is not taught to accept weight on the leg, the leg muscles and soft tissue become tight and restricted. These legs cannot be moved passively because the joints are stiff and range is limited in all positions (Fig. 9-44A & B). If extensor hypertonicity is due to poor trunk or hip control and the leg has mobility, the extensor hypertonicity will lessen or disappear, when the therapist manually supports and or stabilizes the trunk, pelvis, and hip joint.

Hypertonicity from Muscle Shortening and Loss of Joint Alignment

In patients with weakness, muscle shortening and loss of joint alignment can cause extensor hypertonicity. As hip and knee position change, muscles shorten and their line of pull may shift. For example, in patients with poor trunk and leg control, standing is limited. Muscles shorten and joint alignment changes as compensatory strategies are used to attempt to stand. If the hip flexors shorten and the pelvis rotates forward, the hip internally rotates. The tensor fascia lata muscle, moving more anteriorly with hip flexion and internal rotation, if shortened and tight, acts as a strong knee extensor. This passive knee recurvatum is often labeled *extensor*

FIGURE 9-44 (A & B) Patient with poor trunk control who has not had training in standing to reeducate movement patterns. His left leg is in a position of pelvic rotation backward, hip flexion, abduction, knee extension, lower leg external rotation, and ankle plantarflexion. The joints are stiff, and his leg position is difficult to change. (C) Patient with a left hemiplegia standing with left knee recurvatum. (D) Therapist corrects knee recurvatum by moving the pelvis backward to neutral with her left hand while her right hand corrects ankle joint plantarflexion and holds the tibia in a neutral position over the foot.

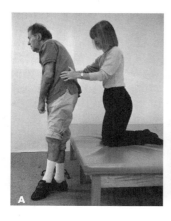
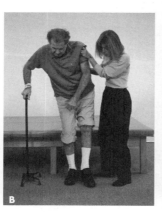
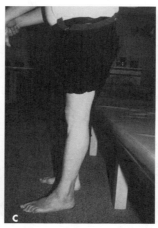
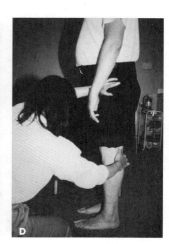

hypertonicity. Therapists must remember that shortened muscles can act on poor aligned limb segments in unexpected ways. The line of muscle pull is altered by changes in alignment, and in hemiplegia, this change in limb alignment is both proximal and distal to the shortened muscle (Fig. 9-44 C & D).

Shortened lower leg muscles result in ankle plantarflexion and knee recurvatum during standing. Knee extension places a stretch on a shortened gastrocnemius and pulls the ankle into plantarflexion and the foot into inversion. Likewise, a shortened gastrocnemius muscle limits ankle dorsiflexion range. The position of ankle plantarflexion and foot inversion makes it difficult to place the foot down in a position to support the leg. The therapist must assess ankle range in sitting to determine if loss of ankle joint range is causing the knee recurvatum. If the ankle cannot be moved to 0 degrees or 10 degrees in sitting, this loss of range will cause knee recurvatum. When the patient stands, the ankle remains plantarflexed, and the therapist cannot correct it (Fig. 9-45). Treatment must systematically lengthen the shortened muscles to allow more normal alignment of both distal and proximal leg segments. This must be followed by muscle reeducation to allow functional carryover. The shortened or shifted muscles most frequently involved in leg extensor hypertonicity are the tensor fascia lata (hip flexion, tibial external rotation), hamstrings (medial, internal rotation), gastrocnemius (knee extension, ankle plantarflexion, calcaneal equinus and supination), anterior and posterior tibialis (inversion foot). If the ankle can be held in 0 degrees to 10 degrees in standing, but the knee still is in recurvatum, then the therapist must further assess leg control.

FIGURE 9-45 (*A*) Patient with a right hemiplegia in sitting. Her right ankle is plantarflexed, and the heel is not on the floor. (*B*) Therapist cannot dorsiflex the ankle to neutral. (*C*) Patient stands with strong knee recurvatum and extensor hypertonicity. (*D*) Therapist corrects strong foot inversion by internally rotating tibia to neutral. Ankle remains plantarflexed. (*E*) Therapist cannot correct ankle joint position in standing.

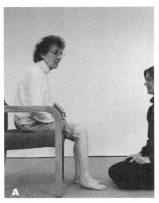
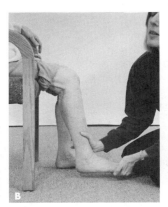
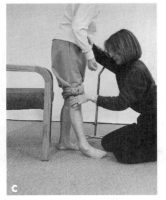
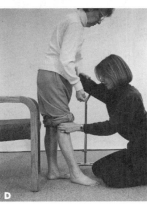
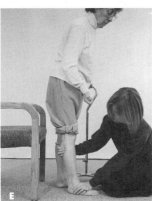

Hypertonicity from Unbalanced Muscle Contraction

In other cases, unbalanced muscle contraction is the cause of extensor hypertonicity. Strong, unbalanced contraction of leg muscles occurs when the patient attempts to stand and balance. This may occur because treatment did not address these movement problems or because there is insufficient return of strength and control in all the muscles of the trunk and leg that are necessary for normal control in standing. With these patients, the therapists must reeducate initiation, duration, and appropriate cessation of muscle firing to decrease the extensor hypertonicity.

Treatment Planning

Some patients have extensor hypertonicity in the leg because of all three causes. In treatment, the therapist must carefully assess the control and alignment of the trunk, hip, and ankle/foot and plan treatment that is specific to each problem (Fig. 9-46).

With each patient, the therapist must assess the cause of the hypertonicity and as the first part of treatment, address the cause of the extensor posturing before beginning to reeducate lower extremity movement components. If the hypertonicity is from poor trunk and hip control, the therapist will assess and treat the alignment and control problems of the trunk and hip in standing. When hypertonicity is related to muscle tightness and shortening resulting in poor alignment, treatment must gradually and systematically lengthen muscles during functional movement sequences to provide enough length and control to eliminate the posturing. While lengthening muscles, the therapist must always remember to reeducate strength and control in weak or missing musculature to allow permanent changes to occur.

Flexor spasticity in the leg occurs less frequently, but is an alarming symptom, because it signals the potential loss of the ability to stand. The flexor pattern in the leg is one of hip flexion with external rotation or abduction, knee flexion, tibial

FIGURE 9-46 (*A*) Patient with a left hemiplegia and extensor hypertonicity. (*B*) Therapist assesses and corrects trunk and pelvic position. As she rotates the pelvis forward to neutral, the knee is less extended, but the foot supinates more. (*C & D*) Therapist stands patient with his brace on to control some of the ankle/foot problems and then rotates his left pelvis forward. The leg is now in more neutral alignment, but the correction of the leg reveals more clearly the upper trunk rotational asymmetry.

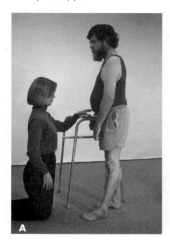
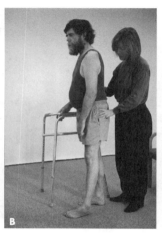
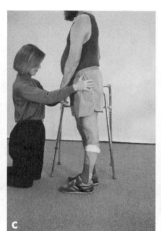
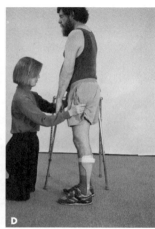

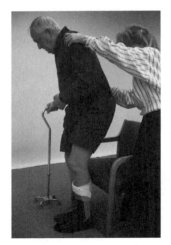

FIGURE 9-47 Patient standing with his left leg in a pattern of flexor hypertonicity. He cannot place it on the floor.

external rotation, ankle plantarflexion and strong supination of the foot. Activity in the anterior and posterior tibialis muscles produces strong supination, but because of changes in foot and ankle alignment and shifting of muscle tendons, the movement of supination occurs with ankle plantarflexion.

The treatment of patients with flexor hypertonicity must include modified standing to place weight on the legs. The therapist may have to allow some trunk asymmetries in the initial treatment sessions so she can teach the patient to keep the foot in contact with the floor while body weight is shifted onto the leg. Trunk movements in sitting can be used to decrease alignment problems in the trunk and reeducate trunk control and hip control (see Chs. 5 and 8). This is combined with appropriate handling to decrease muscle shortness, to correct alignment, proximally at the pelvis and hip and distally at the ankle and foot. Forearm upper extremity weight bearing in standing is a useful technique with these patients. The position supports the trunk symmetrically and allows the therapist to focus on the problems of the leg. Weight bearing on the foot can be introduced in supine and sitting to decrease withdrawal from sensory stimulation. If flexor spasticity is allowed to dominate during the stand, the patient will soon lose the ability to stand in any fashion (Fig. 9-47).

ASSESSMENT GUIDELINES

Assessment of lower extremity movement patterns (weight bearing patterns) in response to either lower-extremity-initiated movements or upper-trunk-initiated movements should include an assessment using verbal commands, an assessment with control provided to the upper body, and an assessment with control or improved alignment provided to the lower extremity. This information will be useful in determining the major problem that is interfering with movement and postural control in the standing position.

I. Position the patient in standing and describe any problems that interfere with placing the involved leg in weight bearing. Describe the position of the trunk with the legs in different positions (feet parallel, abducted stance, step/stance).

II. Assess the control of the hemiplegic leg as the patient initiates upper body and lower extremity movements in standing. Identify the movements that are performed with repeated atypical patterns.

III. Use your hands on the patient's trunk and leg to correct the alignment and assist the movements.

> What improves when you put your hands on the patient to correct asymmetries or to assist the movements?

> What problems do not change immediately with handling and will require further treatment to change the movement components.

IV. List the major impairments in the trunk that are interfering with standing weight shifts.

V. List the major impairments in the leg that are interfering with standing weight shifts. Identify both proximal and distal impairments.

THERAPY GOALS

Functional Goals

Treatment of the trunk and lower extremity in standing is used to decrease the secondary problems that are interfering with movement control and to reeducate normal patterns of functional movement. The training of weight bearing movement patterns in standing is necessary to meet the following functional goal: To support body weight, on both legs or one leg, and safely stand and balance while moving for comfort or during functional tasks.

Treatment Goals and Techniques

Treatment Goal: Correct trunk alignment and reeducate trunk and leg control during lower-extremity-initiated movements.

Treatment Technique: Maintain trunk alignment during lower-extremity-initiated anterior/posterior weight shifts with feet parallel and in right step/stance. Muscle tightness between the pelvis and legs and insufficient trunk control make this movement difficult (Fig. 9-48).

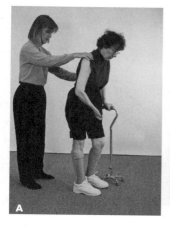 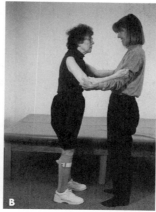 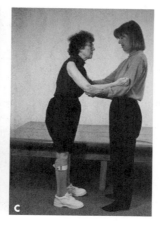

FIGURE 9-48 (*A*) Patient with a right hemiplegia in standing. Upper trunk is flexed forward; the right pelvis and lower trunk are rotated backward. Her right hip is flexed, and the right knee is hyperextended. (*B*) Therapist uses a bilateral symmetric arm grip to help the patient correct the trunk position in standing. The therapist's left arm holds the distal humerus and cradles the patient's forearm and hand against her forearm and humerus. The therapist uses both her hands to help move the patient's upper trunk back into an upright position. (*C*) Patient practices shifting her weight posteriorly. As she moves back and places more weight on her heels, the therapist helps her move the trunk forward. *(Figure Continues)*

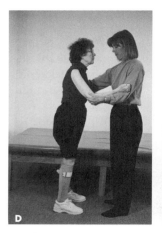 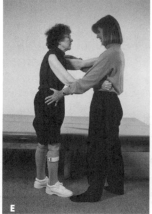 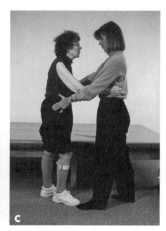

Figure 9-48 *(Continued)* (D) When the patient practices moving her body forward to place more weight on the balls of her feet, the therapist places her right hand on the lateral aspect of the rib cage to assist the movement forward. (E & F) Patient, in right step/stance, practices lower-extremity-initiated anterior/posterior weight shifts. The therapist moves her left hand to the patient's right pelvis while continuing to support the patient's arm and upper trunk. She uses her forearm to hold the patient's lower arm against her body. The patient performs the leg-initiated forward and backward movements while the therapist helps the trunk portion of the task.

Treatment Goal: Provide trunk support while reeducating lower extremity movement components during lower-extremity-initiated weight shifts in standing.

Treatment Technique: Forearm weight bearing in standing during lower-extremity-initiated weight bearing movements (Fig. 9-49A–D).

Treatment Goal: Lengthen tight leg muscles.

Treatment Technique: Lower-extremity-initiated weight shifts in standing forearm weight bearing. Following the sequence above, the therapist moves behind the patient (Fig. 9-49E–H).

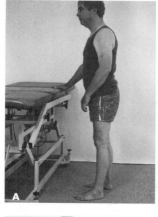

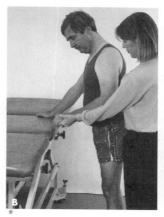

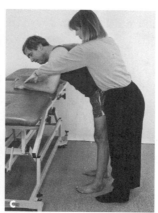

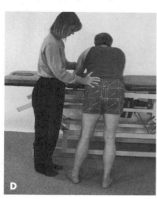

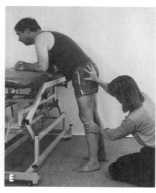

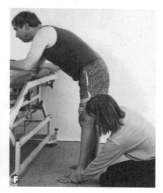

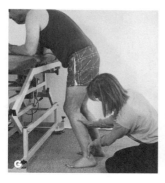

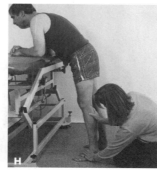

FIGURE 9-49 (*A–C*) Therapist helps patient with a left hemiplegia place his arms in forearm weight bearing by asking for an upper-trunk-initiated anterior movement. The arm must be prepared for this weight bearing position before leg treatment starts. (*D*) Therapist aligns trunk and pelvis as patient begins to shift anteriorly. She places her left hand under his axilla, with the back of her hand on his rib cage. Her right hand corrects pelvic rotation. Both hands help him move his trunk and pelvis to a mid-position over the feet. Patient practices anterior/posterior and lateral weight shifts with the trunk in a more symmetric position. (*E*) The therapist keeps her right hand on the pelvis and moves her left hand to the proximal tibia. Her left hand directs a downward pressure into the foot and corrects tibial rotation. With her hands in this position, she asks the patient to shift forward and back and keeps the thigh and lower leg in good alignment. The weight shift backward lengthens tight hamstring muscles, and a weight shift forward lengthens a tight gastrocnemius muscle when the therapist maintains alignment. If the movement goes beyond muscle length and causes an unwanted asymmetry, she asks the patient to stop and back off the movement to allow the muscle to slowly lengthen. (*F*) Alternate hand grips to maintain appropriate leg interrelationships. (*G & H*) Therapist moves her right hand to the proximal aspect of the back of the lower leg. This hand corrects tibial asymmetries and keeps pressure down into the heel as the patient practices knee bends.

Treatment Technique: Extended-arm weight bearing in standing during lower-extremity-initiated weight bearing movements (Fig. 9-50).

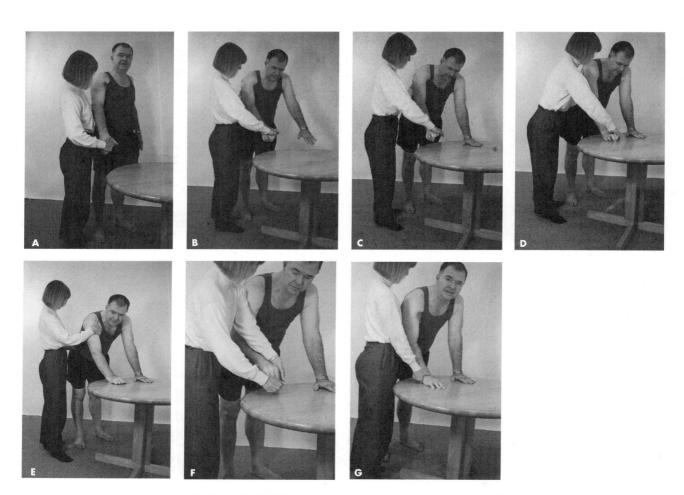

FIGURE 9-50 (*A–D*) Therapist uses axillary/hand shake grip (see Ch. 7) to prepare the arm to move down to the table. The upper trunk initiates an anterior weight shift, and the therapist places the patient's fisted hand on the table. The therapist is assisting the depression of the arm as the patient moves. It is this arm weight bearing reeducation that makes it possible for the patient to keep his arm actively supporting him in Figures H and L. (*E–G*) Patient moves forward and back. As the wrist and finger muscles lengthen, the therapist stops, opens the right hand, and places it back on the table. (*Figure continues*)

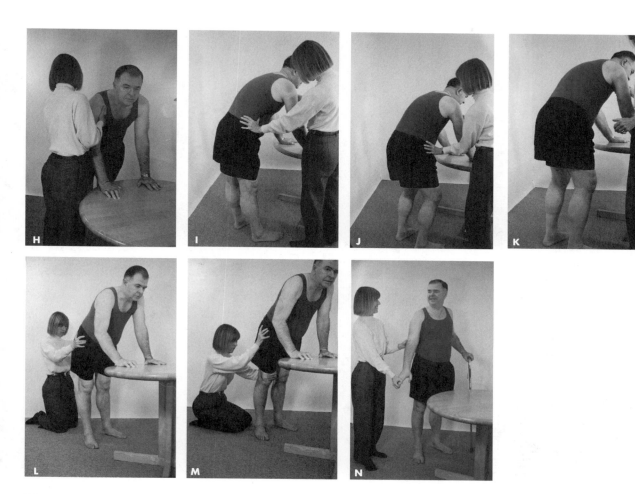

FIGURE 9-50 (*Continued*) (*H–K*) Therapist switches hands and places her right hand under the patient's axilla to continue to support the upper body. She places her left hand on the lower trunk/pelvis to continue to maintain trunk alignment as the patient practices anterior/posterior weight shifts and knee bends. (*L & M*) Therapist moves behind the patient and uses her hands to correct leg alignment as he continues to practice lower-extremity-initiated movements. (*N*) At the end of the practice period, the therapist helps him move his upper body into extension.

Treatment Goal: Correct leg alignment and practice leg components of lower-extremity-initiated weight bearing movement in standing.

Treatment Technique: Standing weight shifts with feet parallel, in set/stance and in abduction, no arm support (Fig. 9-51).

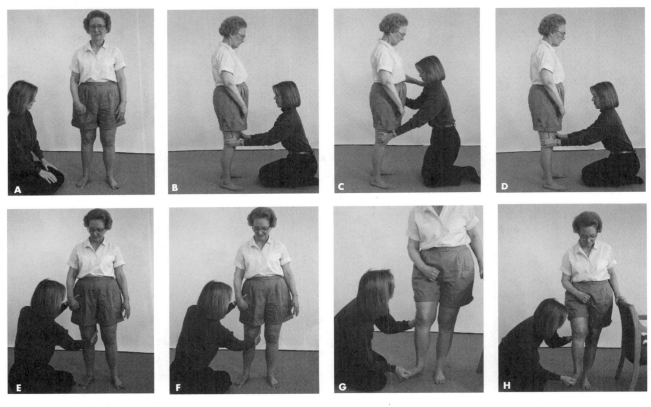

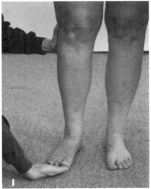

FIGURE 9-51 (*A & B*) Starting position, patient with a right hemiplegia. She walks independently with a brace and cane and complains of leg posturing and tightness. (*C & D*) Therapist uses bilateral leg grips to eliminate right knee recurvatum and assist as the patient shifts anteriorly and posteriorly. (*E*) The therapist's left hand is on the lateral aspect of the right hip while her right hand is on the medial aspect of the knee during lateral movements. As the patient shifts to her right, the therapist's left hand prevents her from overshifting and her right hand corrects femoral rotation and knee recurvatum. (*F*) As the patient shifts to her left, the therapist's hands help the right leg move into relative abduction. The patient's toes have curled under during this lateral movement. (*G–I*) Therapist stops the weight bearing movements and asks the patient to lift her leg up actively. This active movement into flexion stops/balances the standing firing patterns, and the therapist lengthens tight foot and ankle muscles. The patient controls the movement of the leg back onto the floor, and the therapist corrects the forefoot. (*Figure continues*)

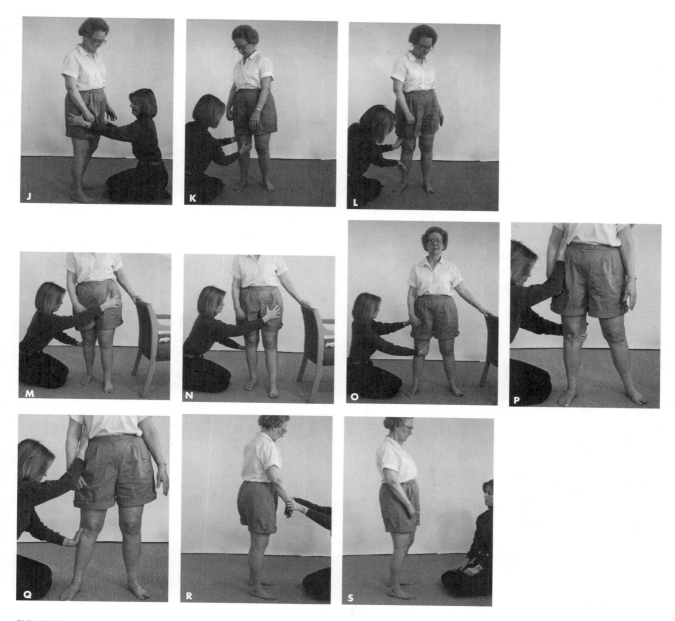

FIGURE 9-51 *(Continued)* *(J–L)* Therapist assists as patient practices rotational leg patterns. *(M & N)* Therapist corrects pelvic rotation and keeps the right foot on the floor as patient practices anterior/posterior weight shifts in left step/stance. *(O–Q)* In abducted stance, patient initiates lateral weight shifts, and therapist corrects hip/lower leg alignment as she assists the weight shift across the right foot. *(R & S)* Patient practices with less assistance and alone.

Treatment Goal: Teach upper-trunk-initiated movements in standing.

Treatment Technique: Correct trunk alignment and assist the leg movement components (Fig. 9-52).

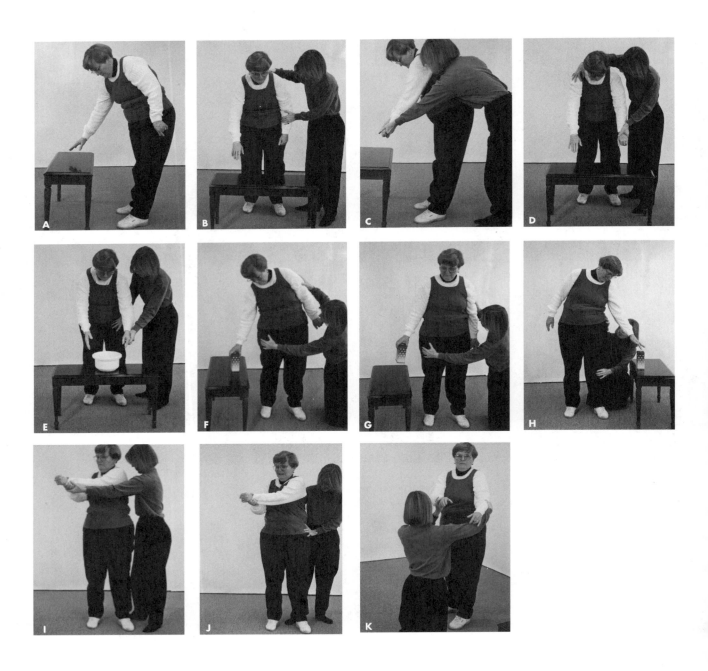

FIGURE 9-52 (*A*) Patient with a left hemiplegia trying to reach both arms down to the bench.) (*B–D*) Therapist assists arm and trunk components of an upper-trunk-initiated anterior weight shift. (*E*) Therapist helps remind patient to keep weight on both legs as hips flex and shift back. (*F–H*) As patient initiates an upper trunk lateral weight shift, the therapist helps her with the leg weight shift. (*I–K*) Upper trunk rotational movements require the most assistance for this patient. She tries to rotate her upper trunk without excessive movement from the leg. The therapist moves her hands either to correct alignment or assist the movement.

Treatment Goal: Combine and reeducate trunk and leg components of unilateral stance on the affected side.

Treatment Technique: Forearm weight bearing in standing to allow therapist to correct trunk alignment while patient practices the leg movements (Fig. 9-53).

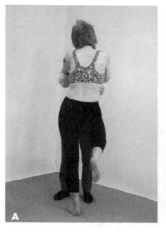 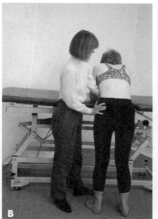 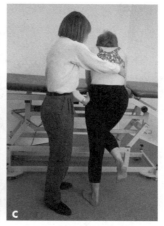

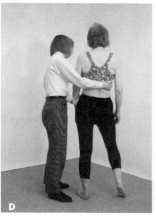 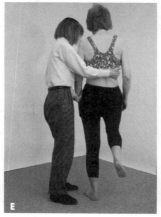 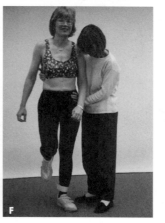

FIGURE 9-53 (*A*) Patient with a left hemiplegia standing on her left leg with support but not correction from the therapist. Her upper trunk is sheared to the right. (*B*) Patient is in forearm weight bearing. Therapist uses her hands to correct the trunk position. Her left hand reaches around the front of the body to the lateral aspect of the right rib cage and her left forearm rests on the lower ribs. She uses her right hand on the patient's left pelvis as counterpressure as she rotates and moves the rib cage back over the pelvis. (*C*) Alternate hand placements to correct upper trunk shearing to the right. With the trunk corrected, the patient practices shifting onto the left leg and lifting the right leg. (*D–F*) Patient stands without support; therapist corrects trunk alignment and asks patient to practice standing on her left leg.

Treatment Technique: Correcting leg alignment and practicing unilateral standing balance without support (Fig. 9-54).

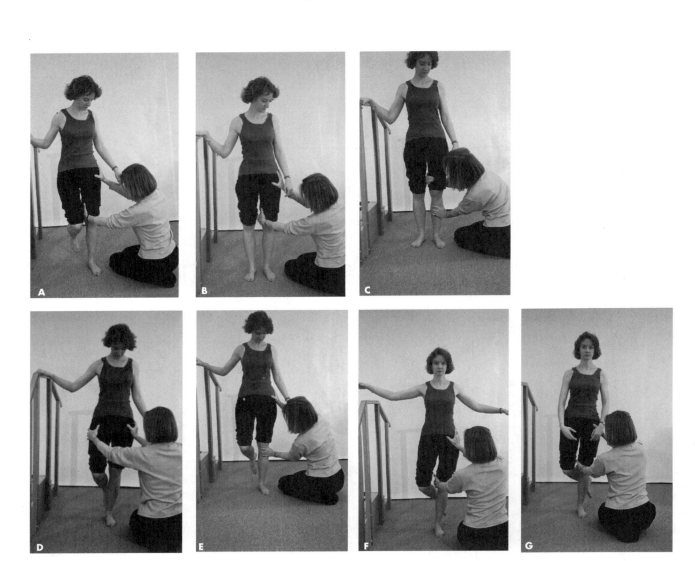

FIGURE 9-54 (*A*) Patient with a left hemiplegia standing on her left leg. Therapist is assessing the movement pattern of the pelvis, hip, and knee. As the patient lifts her right leg, her left pelvis rotates backward, the hip internally rotates, and the knee hyperextends. (*B & C*) Therapist teaches patient the desired position of the pelvis and hip/hip and knee. (*D–E*) Patient lifts her right leg as the therapist helps her practice correcting the pelvis and knee. (*F & G*) Patient practices without support but with reminders from the therapist's hands.

Treatment Goal: Facilitate automatic leg responses to upper body movements.

Treatment technique: Use of distal arm grip to facilitate leg weight shifts and equilibrium responses in standing (Fig. 9-55).

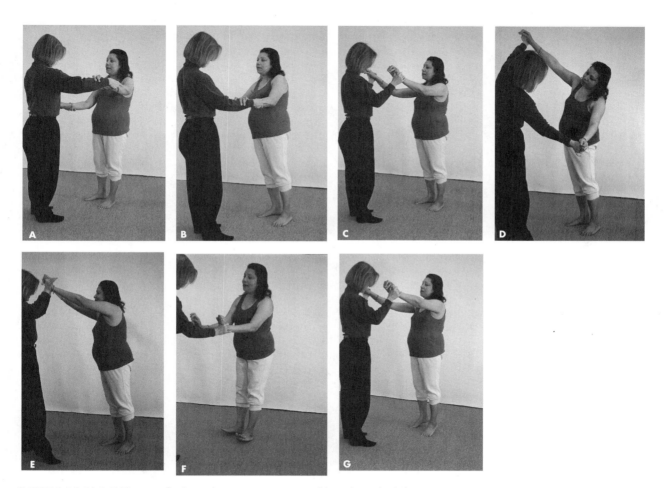

FIGURE 9-55 (*A & B*) Therapist facilitates lower-extremity-initiated lateral weight shift. (*C*) Therapist facilitates lower-extremity-initiated anterior weight shift. (*D*) Therapist facilitates upper-body-initiated lateral weight shift. (*E*) Therapist facilitates lower-extremity-initiated extension rotation. (*F & G*) Therapist facilitates equilibrium response to lower-extremity-initiated movement.

REFERENCES

1. Soderberg G: Kinesiology: Application of Pathological Motion. Williams & Wilkins, Baltimore, 1986

2. Kapandji IA: Physiology of the Joints. Vol 2: Lower Limb. 5th Ed. Churchill Livingstone, New York, 1982

ADDITIONAL READING

Klein-Vogelbash S: Functional Kinetics. Springer-Verlag, New York, 1990

Calais-Germain B: Anatomy of Movement. Eastland Press, Seattle, 1991

10

Trunk and Extremity Movements in Supine

CONCEPTS AND PRINCIPLES

While the supine position is more commonly associated with rest than function, specific movements of the trunk and extremities in supine are necessary for comfort, independence, and safety. To sleep or rest in supine, we use our arms to adjust the blankets or pillows, to put our glasses on the bedside table, and to move our arms, legs, and trunk to get comfortably and safely positioned. We must be able to lift our arms, legs, and trunk away from the surface of the bed and to use the support of the bed as a base for movement. When these movements are not automatically available, as is common with the acute neurologic patient, settling into bed requires assistance, and the patient may find himself precariously close to the side of the bed, wedged up against the foot of the bed, or lying with the hemiplegic arm trapped beneath him as the night goes on. Thus, therapists must work in supine to help the patient develop trunk and extremity movement patterns that contribute to bed mobility skills and functional supine movement patterns.

Since acute care patients have poor endurance in sitting and may require treatment at bedside, a large proportion of early treatment often is done in supine. The time spent in this position is a very valuable part of movement reeducation. In supine, the patient's trunk and extremities are supported by the bed. This total support eliminates the need for the patient to balance himself in the upright position and makes it easier for the therapist to establish a symmetric body position and reeducate movements of the hemiplegic trunk, arm, and leg. Supine position is often the first place where the patient is able to move his involved arm or leg independently. It may also be the first place he is able to activate compatible trunk and extremity movements. Although movement control may not automatically transfer from supine to sitting or standing, where the body's relationship to gravity is different, supine treatment provides the patient with a sensory and motor memory of movement that will be used again in sitting and standing. As the patient's endurance increases, the amount of treatment time that must be spent in supine decreases. However, therapists continue to return to the position in later stages of rehabilitation for treatment of the arm and leg and to prepare the patient to function more efficiently in bed.

Supine is also a useful treatment position for addressing primary and secondary impairments in the trunk and extremities. Supine is the position of choice for treatment of shoulder pain, severe spasticity in the arm or leg, and problems of muscle shortening that restrict range of motion. For patients with these impairments, stabilizing the trunk in supine can make assessment of extremity joint and muscle/tissue problems easier. The stability of the trunk in supine is also very useful during treatment, as it allows the therapist to be very precise with extremity mechanics when moving a painful limb and to more easily lengthen tight or hypertonic muscles between the trunk and extremities without loss of trunk alignment. The changes in muscle length and joint mobility gained in supine make the task of movement reeducation in the upright positions easier and pain free.

MOVEMENT COMPONENTS

The movement components of the trunk, arm, and leg that are used for function in supine have already been identified in previous chapters. The important difference in supine is that the entire back surface of the body is in contact with the bed, where it becomes the body's base of support. The force that gravity exerts on the supine body encourages extension in the trunk, and all movements away from the bed oppose the pull of gravity. The length of the arm is supported on the bed, so that there is no distracting force on the shoulder joint. In the lower extremities, the thigh and calf are supported by the bed, but the feet are plantarflexed and the back of the heel is the only part of the foot in contact with the bed. Movement of the legs in bed usually occurs with foot contact, but most movements of the arms in bed require that the hand move in space (i.e., the leg functions in weight bearing to push or lift the lower body, while the hand functions for grasp and manipulation).

Movements of the Trunk

Because the starting position of the trunk is in extension, movements of the upper or lower body away from the bed in a straight plane introduce flexion into the spine. Movements of the upper or lower body on a diagonal plane will introduce either flexion or extension rotation.

Movements Initiated from the Upper Body

When the head and upper trunk move forward symmetrically away from the bed, the upper spine flexes and the scapulas abduct. As the head, shoulders, and upper trunk leave the bed, the area of the body that is in contact with the surface is decreased (Fig. 10-1).

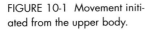

FIGURE 10-1 Movement initiated from the upper body.

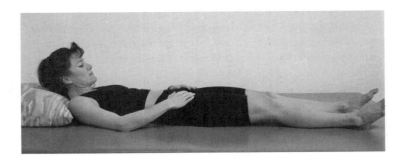

Functional Example

This movement is used to move from supine to long sitting or to lift your head off the pillow.

Upper Body Rotation

When the same movement is initiated so that the head and only the left arm and left side of the trunk move anteriorly, the forward diagonal movement of the upper trunk results in a pattern of flexion rotation to the right. As the left arm reaches forward, the scapula abducts and upwardly rotates and the left rib cage moves forward away from the bed, while the left side of the pelvis and left leg remain in contact with the bed. The right arm and rib cage also remain in contact with the bed and assume increased weight. For this pattern of flexion rotation to be produced, the head must leave the bed and rotate to the left. If the head stays back on the pillow, the flexors of the neck and trunk do not become active, and the arm moves into horizontal adduction without trunk rotation (Fig. 10-2).

Functional Example

This flexion rotation pattern is used to initiate rolling or to reach for something on the bedside table.

Movements Initiated from the Lower Body

When the lower extremities flex at the hips and knees so that the femurs move toward the chest and the feet leave the bed, flexor muscle activity is increased in the lower trunk. Most lower extremity movements in supine are initiated with hip and knee flexion rather than hip flexion and knee extension. Flexion at the hips and knees is the preferred way of lifting the legs off the bed, because it makes it easier for the body to control the weight of the legs by reducing the length of the lever

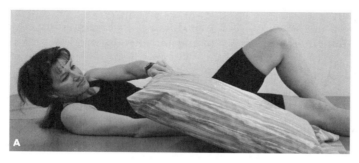

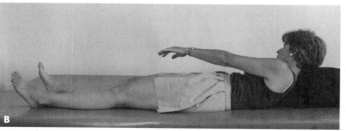

FIGURE 10-2 (*A & B*) Upper body-initiated flexion rotation.

FIGURE 10-3 (*A & B*) Movement initiated from the lower body.

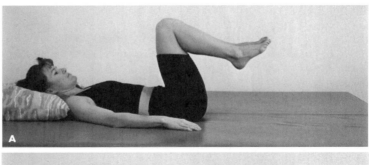

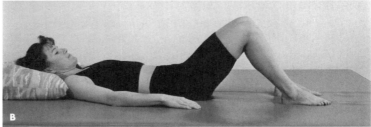

arm. It also reduces the stress that straight leg movements place on the spine and the abdominal muscles. If the flexion continues through the full range of available hip and knee motion, the thighs come to rest near the chest, and the feet are in the air. Hip flexion above 90 degrees is accompanied by posterior pelvic tilting and flexion of the lumbar spine. The head, upper spine, and rib cage, and the scapulas and arms remain in contact with the bed with the upper spine in extension (Fig. 10-3A).

Partial flexion of the hips and knees with the feet in contact with the bed is used more frequently for function in supine. In this movement pattern, the lordosis of lumbar spine decreases and the pelvis moves into a slight posterior tilt as the hips flex (Fig. 10-3B).

Functional Example

The movement of full hip flexion has no important function uses but is a common component of many stretching and exercise programs because of the way it lengthens the low back extensors. The flexor movement that places the foot on the bed for weight bearing is used to position the foot to push for rolling or bridging.

Lower Body Rotation

When only the left leg is flexed, the lordosis of the lumbar spine and anterior tilt of the pelvis decrease, but the pelvis and the sacrum remain in contact with the bed. If the flexed left leg moves into horizontal adduction and the pelvis rotates to the right so that the left side of the pelvis and lower trunk leave the bed, the trunk is placed in extension rotation to the right. The same pattern of extension rotation occurs whether the left foot is weight bearing on the bed or in the air (Fig. 10-4).

Functional Example

These leg movements are used to initiate rolling or to lift one side of the pelvis off the bed.

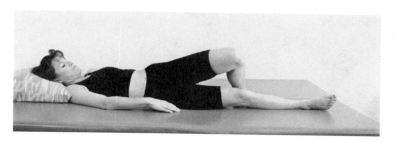

FIGURE 10-4 Lower-body-initiated extension rotation.

Functional Movements of the Upper Extremity

The section below describes general categories of arm movements that are important for function in supine. More detailed information about the normal components of arm movements in space and during weight bearing are contained in Chapters 6 and 7.

Movements to Bring the Hand off the Bed

From a starting position of extension by the side of the body, arm movements that combine elbow flexion with shoulder flexion and humeral abduction or adduction will bring the hand to the face and head, chest, or opposite arm or move it overhead. When the hand is moving to the body, the upper trunk stays supported on the bed. The patterns of scapulohumeral rhythm that occur in sitting and standing with the humerus above 60 degrees of elevation must also occur in supine. Neck flexion or rotation is used when necessary to keep the hands in the visual field (Fig. 10-5).

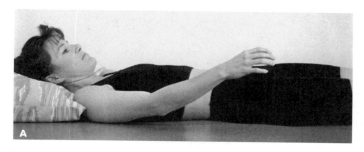

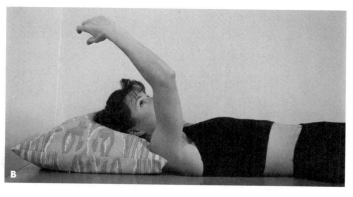

FIGURE 10-5 (*A & B*) Movements to bring the hand off the bed.

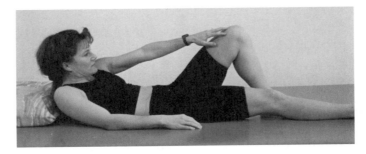

FIGURE 10-6 Upper trunk flexion with shoulder flexion and elbow extension.

To bring the hands forward to the legs or to adjust the blankets, a pattern that combines upper trunk flexion with shoulder flexion and elbow extension is necessary (Fig. 10-6). To reach across the body, trunk flexion rotation occurs in combination with adduction of the arm.

Positioning the Arm for Comfort

While sleeping or resting in bed, the arms may be positioned on the body, over the head, behind the head, or out to the side (Fig. 10-7). These patterns require full mobility at the shoulder joint and available muscle length between the scapula and rib cage.

FIGURE 10-7 (*A*) Position of rest by the side of the body. (*B*) Resting the arm overhead.

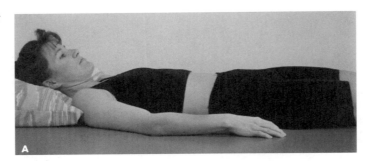

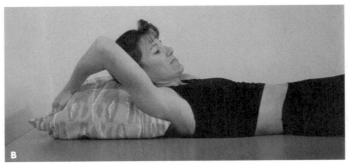

Weight Bearing on Forearms

Symmetric upper extremity weight bearing in supine is used to lift the spine and rib cage off the bed in preparation for moving them to a new position or to place the head in an upright position. To assume the position, the elbows push into the bed as the upper trunk flexes away from the bed (Fig. 10-8A).

Weight bearing on one forearm occurs when the opposite arm reaches across the body with simultaneous flexion rotation in the upper trunk (refer back to Fig 10-2A). The amount of weight that is transferred to the forearm depends on the amount of flexion in the spine. The more the upper trunk flexes and moves away from the bed, the more weight is shifted to the weight bearing forearm (Fig. 10-8B & C).

As the left arm reaches across, forward, and up, the left shoulder girdle rotates forward and to the right. The right shoulder girdle also moves forward but rotates back.

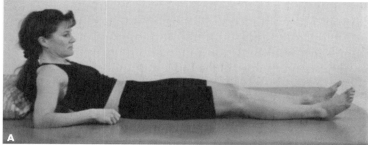

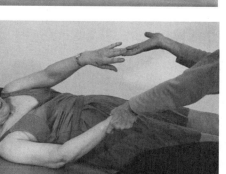

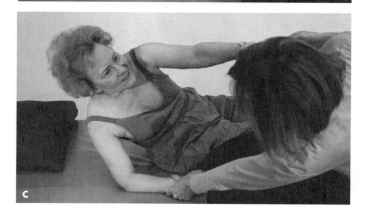

FIGURE 10-8 (*A*) The elbows push into the bed as the upper trunk flexes away from the bed. (*B*) When the head and shoulder girdles are close to the bed and the upper trunk is in only slight flexion, weight is supported on the humerus of the right arm. (*C*) When the head and shoulders move farther from the bed, the right forearm becomes the weight bearing surface of the arm.

Functional Movements of the Lower Extremity

Movements on the Surface of the Bed

The legs have functional movements along the surface of the bed in the planes of abduction/adduction. These movements determine how close together the feet are to each other and to the edge of the bed. Abduction to the edge of the bed is often used before sitting up. Adduction of the extended leg with slight flexion of the hip will bring the leg across the other leg for rest in this position.

Moving the Leg off the Bed or Back on

Function in supine also requires the ability to move the leg from the dangling position over the edge onto the bed to complete the process of lying down. When the foot dangles off the edge of the bed, the hip is extended, the knee flexed, and the ankle plantarflexed. To lift the leg to the bed, the ankle dorsiflexes and the hip flexes, while the position of the knee remains flexed. Often the foot is placed on the bed with the hip and knee still flexed. The foot then slides down the bed as the leg moves from flexion to extension.

Weight Bearing Patterns of the Leg

Weight bearing on the feet in supine is used to lift the weight of the pelvis off the bed or to assist the movement of the lower trunk and pelvis to a new position. Weight bearing may occur on both legs simultaneously, or on just one leg.

Moving the Leg into Weight Bearing Position

While it is possible to use the extended leg in weight bearing by pressing the heel into the bed, the lower extremity weight bearing pattern that is most important for treatment occurs with the hips and knees in flexion and the foot placed flat on the bed. To move from extension to this flexed, weight bearing position, the leg must actively flex at the hip, knee, and ankle joints. Flexion occurs at all three joints simultaneously, and the heel slides up the bed toward the hips. When the desired amount of leg flexion has been achieved, the foot rests flat on the bed. When flexion of both legs is desired, the legs perform the flexion movements one at a time or simultaneously (Fig. 10-9).

Bilateral Weight Bearing: Bridging

In supine, weight bearing on both feet is used to lift the pelvis off the bed. In this pattern, the heels of the feet push into the bed, the knees move forward over the feet, and the hips move into extension as the pelvis and lower spine leave the bed (Fig. 10-10). This movement is used to place a bed pan under the body or to adjust the position of the hips for comfort. It is also commonly used in treatment to activate hip extensors with abdominals.

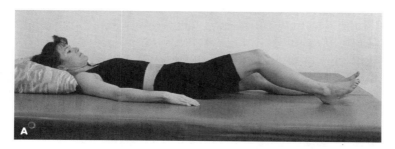

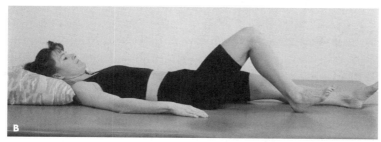

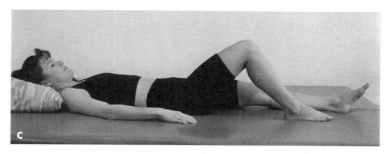

FIGURE 10-9 (A–C) Moving the leg into weight bearing position.

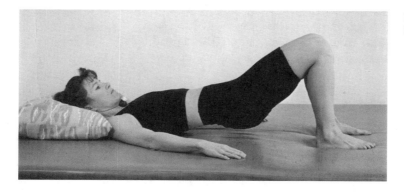

FIGURE 10-10 Bilateral weight bearing: bridging.

FIGURE 10-11 Bilateral weight bearing with lower trunk rotation.

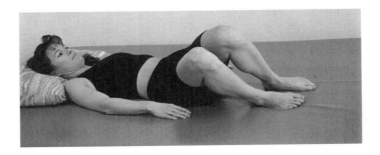

Bilateral Weight Bearing with Lower Trunk Rotation

Bilateral weight bearing can also be combined with rotation of the lower trunk. If both knees move together to the right, extension rotation to the right occurs in the trunk. In the first part of the movement, the left femur adducts and moves to the midline of the body and the right femur abducts and moves away from the midline so that the distance between the two femurs stays consistent and the pelvis remains on the bed. As the left femur moves across the midline of the body, the left hip and pelvis lift off the bed and rotate to the right. At the same time, the right side of the pelvis moves back into the bed, and body weight shifts to the right hip. During the initial stage of pelvic rotation, the lumbar spine is extended and rotated, but the left rib cage stays close to the bed. As pelvic rotation continues further to the right, extension will travel higher in the spine, and the left side of the rib cage will rotate forward to the right (Fig. 10-11). The left shoulder girdle and arm remain in contact with the bed during the movement. This results in a lengthening of the left side of the rib cage and in the muscles that connect the left shoulder, rib cage, and pelvis.

This movement can be used to initiate rolling. It is also a common treatment activity used to improve alignment and mobility and lengthen tight muscles in the hemiplegic side.

Unilateral Bridging (Half Bridging)

Half bridging occurs when only one leg is placed in a flexed weight bearing position and only one side of the pelvis is actively lifted and moved. When the left leg is placed in weight bearing and initiates the movement of bridging by pushing into the bed, the left side of the pelvis lifts off the bed, and the left hip extends. As the left hip moves toward extension, the pelvis rotates toward the right, placing the spine in extension rotation to the right (Fig. 10-12). This movement is used to initiate rolling to the left or to adjust the position of the lower body in bed.

FIGURE 10-12 Unilateral bridging (half bridging).

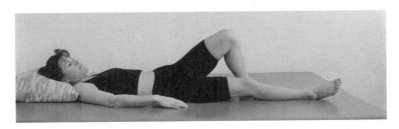

Bed Mobility

Changes in the position of the body in bed can be accomplished through rolling, which will be described in Chapter 11, or by shifting the body closer to the top, bottom, or side edges of the bed while remaining in a more or less constant supine position. The task of sliding in bed while remaining in supine is similar to scooting in sitting, in that it is used to make small positional adjustments in body position relative to the support, rather than move the body to a new position. Sliding in bed is accomplished by alternating upper and lower extremity weight bearing movements and rotational movements in the trunk. The weight bearing movements are used to clear the hips and the upper spine from the bed and move them to a new position. To start the movements, both legs are flexed, with the feet flat on the bed near the pelvis. The arms are in an extended position close to the hips, with forearms pronated and hands resting on the bed.

Sliding Up in Bed

Sliding up is accomplished in two stages. To initiate the movement, the feet and forearms actively depress into the bed so that the spine extends, the hips extend, and the pelvis and spine/rib cage are lifted high off the bed. The feet and arms then push backwards but remain in contact with the bed, causing the knees to partially extend and the body to slide toward the head. At the end of the upward slide, the body returns to rest on the bed. If more movement is needed, the feet step up closer to the hips, the hands slide up away from the hips, and the process is repeated (Fig. 10-13).

FIGURE 10-13 (*A & B*) Sliding up in bed.

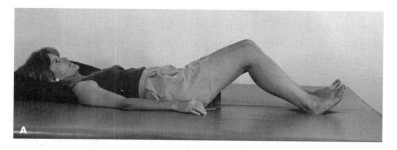

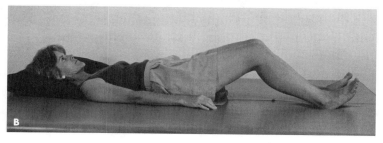

FIGURE 10-14 (*A & B*) Sliding down in bed.

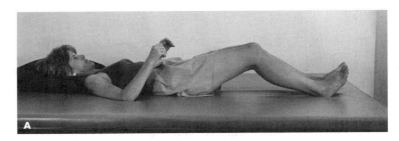

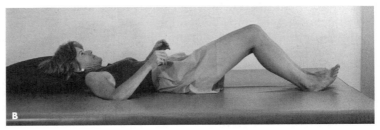

Sliding Down in Bed

Sliding down movements are initiated in the same pattern of spinal and hip extension used to slide up in bed. When the spine, shoulders, and hips have left the bed, the feet actively dorsiflex and the knees actively flex to move the pelvis down toward the heels. At the same time, active elbow flexion pulls the shoulder girdle down toward the elbow. When the movement has been completed, the spine, shoulders, and hips return to rest on the bed. To repeat the movement, the feet first step down away from the hips, and the process is repeated (Fig. 10-14).

Sliding Sideways in Bed

Sideways movements in bed are performed in two stages. To move to the right, the pelvis is first lifted then moved laterally to the right. This places the lower body further to the right than the upper body (Fig. 10-15A). Next, the left elbow and hand push to move the upper spine and rib cage to the right. This movement lifts the upper trunk off the bed and results in slight rotation of the shoulders to the left (Fig. 10-15B). As the body returns to the bed, the center of the body is aligned with the legs.

FIGURE 10-15 (*A & B*) Sliding sideways in bed.

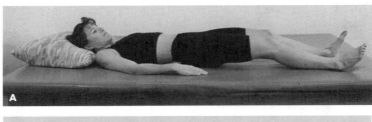

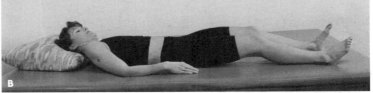

SIGNIFICANT IMPAIRMENTS THAT INTERFERE WITH PERFORMANCE

Weakness/Movement Deficits in the Trunk and Extremities

Weakness in the muscles of the trunk and extremities is the major cause of loss of function in supine. In supine, the force of gravity acts to pull the whole body back into the bed. Most functional movements in this position require the trunk, arm, and leg to move away from the support of the bed. This requires sufficient muscle strength to lift the weight of the body against the force of gravity. Severe muscle weakness or paralysis in the hemiplegic side often interferes with functional movements of the arm, leg, and trunk and exaggerates the affects of gravity on body posture. Severe weakness on the hemiplegic side causes the head, rib cage, pelvis, and leg to be pulled closer to the bed, resulting in obvious asymmetry between the two sides of the body and abnormal resting positions (Fig. 10-16A). Patients with this problem are unable to move their hemiplegic arm or leg, to use them to support body weight, or to independently position them in safe, comfortable resting positions.

Muscle weakness in the trunk may affect the flexor and extensor muscles of the involved side. When the flexors of the upper trunk are weak, upper-body-initiated movements away from the surface of the bed cannot be performed. This loss of upper trunk flexor control makes it difficult to lift the head and shoulders off the pillow, to roll, or to sit up. It also interferes with arm function in movements such as reaching across midline or supporting body weight on one forearm. Similarly, loss of strength in the lower trunk flexors and extensors affects performance of lower extremity movements and trunk movements that initiate from the lower body.

Trunk muscle weakness most frequently occurs in combination with flaccid paralysis of the arm and leg. In supine, most functional arm movements require coordination of scapula and shoulder muscles with elbow flexors. When these shoulder and elbow muscles cannot actively contract, the hemiplegic arm is unable to move away from the bed to reach for bedclothes or items on the bedside table, to assist in rolling, or to accept weight (Fig. 10-16B). In the leg, strength in the flexors of the hip, knee, and ankle are needed to lift the leg from extension on the bed into a flexed position and to weight bear on the flexed leg for activities such as bridging, bed mobility, and rolling. Weak leg flexors prevent the leg from moving into the flexed position and from participating in these supine functions.

When muscle weakness of the trunk or extremities is the cause for loss of function, treatment can improve performance through careful reeducation of the normal movement patterns and repeated practice of these patterns to build strength and independence. In supine, this process of reeducation involves several parts. First, the therapist should retrain functional movement patterns in the arm or leg while the trunk is supported on the bed (Fig. 10-16C). She must also retrain movement patterns of the trunk in supine. During this part of treatment, she supports the hemiplegic arm and/or leg in an appropriate position for the task. When the patient is able to assist with the extremity and trunk movements, the therapist begins to introduce movement patterns that combine trunk movements with those of an arm and leg (Fig. 10-16D). Specific treatment activities for these stages are presented in the treatment section of this chapter and in the chapter on rolling. In addition, the patient with persistent muscle weakness must be taught compensatory

FIGURE 10-16 (*A*) Severe muscle weakness on the hemiplegic
right side, resulting in postural
asymmetries between the two
sides of the body. Note the tilting
of the head toward the hemiplegic shoulder and the extreme
external rotation of the hemiplegic leg. (*B*) Muscle weakness
in the hemiplegic right arm interferes with movement away from
the bed during upper-trunk-initiated rotation. This arm weakness
results in an incompatible
trunk/arm relationship. (*C*) The
therapist maintains normal alignment in the hemiplegic right arm
by supporting the shoulder and
the distal forearm and hand. She
is teaching the arm to lift off the
bed in an extended arm reach
pattern. (*D*) The patient initiates
upper trunk flexion rotation
toward his hemiplegic side. The
therapist's hands are supporting
the shoulder joint as he accepts
weight on his hemiplegic arm.

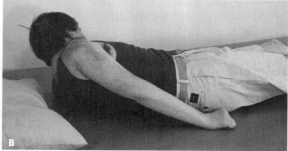
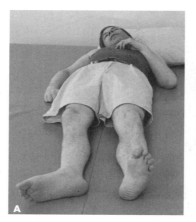
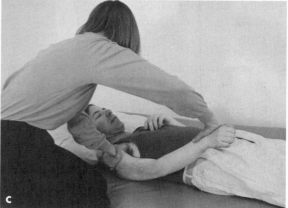
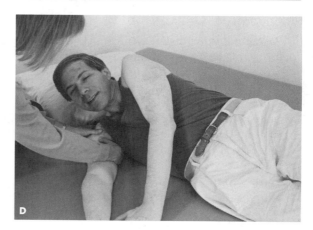

strategies for positioning the involved arm and leg and incorporating them into
rolling and bed mobility so he regains functional independence in supine with the
best movement patterns possible.

Extremity Hypertonicity

Hypertonicity in the affected arm and/or leg is a common problem that may interfere with comfort and function in supine. Flexor hypertonicity in the arm prevents
the arm from lying extended by the side of the body and blocks use of the arm for

reach or weight bearing. A flexed position of the arm also makes it difficult to lie on the involved side or to roll completely to the uninvolved side. Extensor hypertonicity in the leg prevents the leg from flexing or being passively positioned in flexion and maintains the leg in a stiff, extended position during rolling or bed mobility activities (Fig. 10-17A). Severe extensor spasticity associated with brain injury may cause the heel of the foot to press into the bed or the ball of the foot into the footboard.

The extent and severity of problems associated with hypertonicity in supine varies widely among patients. Patients whose muscle tone fluctuates between low tone at rest and hypertonicity during walking or difficult activities often experience a rapid and dramatic decrease in tone in the hemiplegic arm and leg as soon as they lie down. This state of low muscle tone generally persists in supine as long as they are resting. Muscle tone in the hemiplegic arm and/or leg generally increases again when these patients attempt to move the involved extremities or change position in bed. Patients with constant hypertonicity in their affected arm and leg may not demonstrate any noticeable decrease in muscle tone in supine. However, supine treatment may be used very effectively with these patients to decrease abnormal muscle tension and reeducate normal movements.

Hypertonicity in the affected trunk, arm, and leg must be decreased and the normal position of the limb restored as part of the process of movement reeducation. Abnormal muscle tension in the arm and leg is frequently related to changes in resting alignment between the proximal and distal limb segments or to changes in position of the trunk that result in altered lines of muscle pull and changes in length/tension relationships. Supine treatment activities offer a very effective means to restore alignment between the limb segments and increase symmetry in the trunk, which results in decreased muscle hypertonicity. Treatment techniques such as scapula mobilization and trunk rotation lengthen hypertonic muscles and lead to a marked decrease in muscle tension in the extremities. For example, extensor spasticity in the leg is decreased by specific handling techniques that allow the therapist to flex the hip and knee and place the foot in weight bearing on the mat. This can be followed by rotation of the lower trunk on the upper trunk to lengthen hypertonic muscles that connect the trunk, arm, and leg and further decrease abnormal muscle tension (Fig. 10-17B & C).

As abnormal muscle tension decreases, the therapist can change the resting position of the trunk and limbs and restore normal alignment to the hemiplegic side. The steps for decreasing hypertonicity in the arm and leg in supine are described in Figures 10-20 and 10-22.

Hypertonicity in supine may also be associated with abnormal patterns of muscle activation. When this is true, muscle tone in the hemiplegic arm and/or leg increases dramatically as the patient attempts to move his hemiplegic side. This pattern of hypertonicity becomes less frequent as control of normal movement components in the hemiplegic trunk and extremities increases. The therapist should reeducate normal movements of the hemiplegic arm and leg and movement patterns that combine the trunk and extremities, to prepare the patient to use his hemiplegic side in supine without hypertonicity and atypical movements. These techniques are also described in the treatment section of this chapter.

Reducing hypertonic muscle tone is a very important part of treatment for both patient and therapist, and supine is one of the best treatment positions for decreasing hypertonicity in the hemiplegic trunk and limbs. Most patients enjoy supine

FIGURE 10-17 (*A*) Flexor hypertonicity in the right arm and extensor hypertonicity in the right leg in supine. (*B*) The therapist bends the leg at the hip and knee and places the foot in weight bearing on the bed. She holds this position until the extension tension gradually relaxes. Note the slight relaxation in flexor tone that is occurring in the hemiplegic arm as she controls the leg. (*C*) When muscle tension in the leg is decreased, the therapist manually assists lower trunk rotation to the left. This movement will result in further changes in upper extremity hypertonicity.

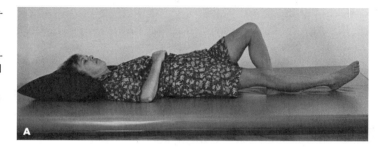

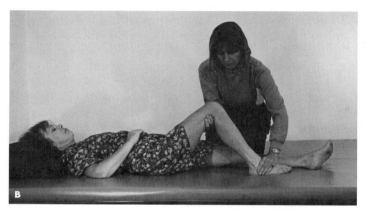

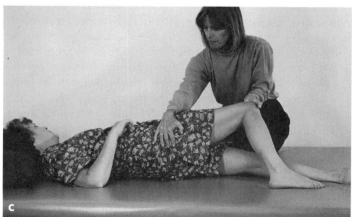

treatment activities that relax tight muscles and loosen stiffness in the trunk, because these activities increase comfort, ease of movement, and range of motion. When abnormal muscle tension in the arm or leg is decreased, the patient is able to experience the feel of effortless movement in the hemiplegic arm or leg. This allows him to participate more actively in the process of movement reeducation and often results in improved kinesthetic memory for normal movement that can be used again in other positions.

Changes in muscle tension associated with supine treatment are very important for the therapist as well. Since these changes are an important precursor to movement reeducation, therapists often use supine treatment activities to decrease muscle tone and change abnormal patterns of muscle activation. Once hypertonicity has been reduced, the therapist switches her treatment emphasis to movement reeducation in supine or in sitting or standing. While the changes in tone obtained in supine may not automatically carry over into upright postures, the skilled therapist is usually able to maintain the improvements in muscle tone as the patient moves from supine to other positions.

Changes in Alignment

Supine is often the best place to assess and identify changes in alignment in the trunk and extremities. It is easy to identify changes in trunk posture and postural asymmetries in supine, because the two sides of the body lie against the bed differently when these problems exist. The patient's body may be in an asymmetric position in supine because of muscle weakness or paralysis on the involved side. These changes in alignment also occur when hypertonicity and unbalanced muscle firing pull bones and joints into new resting positions. Changes in alignment associated with either weakness or hypertonicity gradually become deformities, if secondary problems of joint stiffness and/or muscle shortening are allowed to develop. Deformities are obvious changes in body position that are difficult to correct. Supine treatment activities can be used to lengthen tight muscles, loosen stiff joints and alignment, and gradually restore alignment.

The alignment changes that are most significant in supine include both changes in trunk position and in extremity position. In the trunk, excessive trunk flexion, excessive trunk extension, and rotational asymmetry in the spine, rib cage, and pelvis are the most common problems. Severe flexion of the upper trunk is most common in very elderly patients. This problem makes it difficult for the patient to lie comfortably in supine without multiple pillows to support the head and upper body. It often creates problems in the hemiplegic shoulder girdle, because the anterior position of the scapula causes the hemiplegic shoulder to rest in hyperextension. Excessive lumbar extension is common in both stroke and brain-injured patients. It is often associated with extensor hypertonicity in the hemiplegic leg. Spinal rotation brings one side of the rib cage away from the bed, so that its contour is higher and more prominent than the rib cage on the other side. Both rotation toward the hemiplegic side and away from the hemiplegic side are common (Fig. 10-18A). Asymmetries between the two sides of the pelvis are associated with spinal rotations in the lumbar spine that bring the affected side of the pelvis forward or back relative to the other side. It is important to note that all these trunk problems exist when the patient moves from supine to sitting or standing. The reader should refer to Chapters 5 and 9 for more information on how these problems affect movement and function.

Alignment problems in the hemiplegic arm and leg may be related to problems in the trunk or develop independently. Often, an abnormal resting position of the hemiplegic extremities in supine contributes to abnormal trunk alignment. For example, when the hemiplegic leg is weak, it lies in excessive abduction and external rotation in comparison with the position of the other leg. This leg position may rotate the pelvis and lower trunk backward on the hemiplegic side. Similarly, a

FIGURE 10-18 (*A*) The right side of the rib cage and the iliac crest of the pelvis are more prominent and farther forward than the left side, indicating that the trunk is rotated to the left. The therapist's hands are marking the bony landmarks. Note the extension in the lumbar spine. (*B*) The therapist's hands on the rib cage are rotating the hemiplegic side back and the left side forward to restore symmetry to the trunk and rib cage. (*C*) The therapist is unable to move the hemiplegic leg into the position of flexion/adduction/ neutral rotation that would match the right leg. (*Figure continues*)

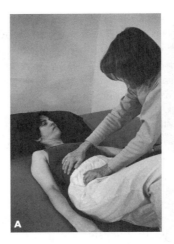
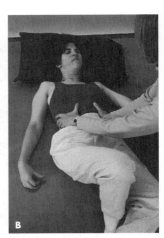
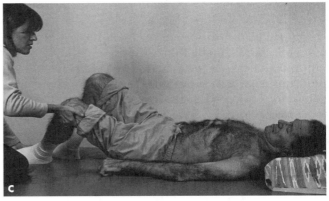

flexed hypertonic arm is often associated with elevation of the scapula and internal rotation of the humerus. This arm position may pull the hemiplegic side of the upper trunk into flexion and contribute to rotation forward of the rib cage on the hemiplegic side. In other cases, trunk problems affect the position of the hemiplegic arm and leg by changing the position of the scapula and pelvis.

Once the therapist has identified how the patient is aligned in supine, she begins to attempt to correct alignment. Severe asymmetries in trunk position should be corrected by hand placements on the rib cage, pelvis, or shoulders (Fig. 10-18B). Extremity alignment is corrected through hand placements on the proximal and distal extremity. The response of the patient's body to these corrections will vary according to the types of impairments that have caused them. If the alignment changes are due to muscle weakness, the therapist feels the weight of the weak body segment but no resistance to the correction in muscles and joints. If the therapist cannot easily correct the position of the trunk or limbs, the asymmetric position is being maintained by muscle tension or joint stiffness or a combination of both (Fig. 10-18C). Further manual assessment is needed to determine the particular muscles that have shortened and the joint movements that are blocked by hypomobility. These secondary impairments of muscle and joint will have to be addressed in treatment to reestablish normal alignment in the trunk, arm, and leg.

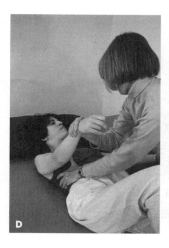
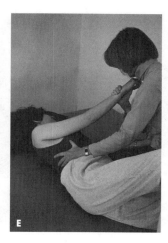

FIGURE 10-18 (*Continued*) (*D*) Active assistive movements of the arm while the rib cage is stabilized against the bed are used to lengthen tight muscles between the scapula/arm and trunk. (*E*) Upper-body-initiated rotation toward the uninvolved side. The therapist is stabilizing the patient's lower trunk and pelvis with her left hand and using the patient's right arm to help her combine trunk and arm movements. This movement will lengthen tight muscles between the rib cage and pelvis.

Supine activities to restore alignment should precede active movement reeducation or training of bed mobility, whenever problems of joint hypomobility and muscle shortening interfere with normal positioning. This is done by systematically lengthening tight muscles and selecting movement patterns to increase joint movement and mobility. For example, since the trunk is stabilized by the bed, extremity movements in supine lengthen the muscles that connect the arm or leg to the trunk (Fig. 10-18D). Rotation of the upper trunk on a stable lower trunk or vise versa will lengthen muscles in the trunk and help correct asymmetric trunk or limb postures (Fig. 10-18E).

The alignment changes that are gained in supine will prepare for movement reeducation and in supine. These changes will also carry over into other positions, assisting the task of movement reeducation. This treatment must be followed by reeducation of movement, including active-assistive or active exercise, so that changes in muscle length and tension or corrections in alignment lead to improved patterns of movement and function.

UNDESIRABLE COMPENSATORY PATTERNS

Undesirable compensations in supine occur during attempts to perform functional movements such as sliding in bed, rolling, or reaching. In supine, as in the other positions discussed in this book, most undesirable compensations involve use of the intact arm and leg to move the body, without normal muscle activity and participation of the hemiplegic side of the body. Many one-sided compensations result in increased hypertonicity and extremity posturing in the hemiplegic arm and leg. Figure 10-19 illustrates a typical one-sided movement pattern during the task of sliding up in bed. The patient accomplishes the task by pushing with her left leg. She is unable to bend her right leg up to assist in the movement. As she pushes with her left leg, her hemiplegic right leg pushes strongly into extension and lifts off the bed. When the patient's hemiplegic extremities are weak, undesirable one-sided compensations result in the hemiplegic arm or leg being left behind or placed in an incompatible position relative to the trunk. (Refer back to Fig. 10-16B for an example of this problem.)

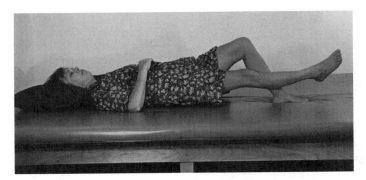

FIGURE 10-19 One-sided movement pattern during sliding up in bed, (an undesirable compensatory pattern).

ASSESSMENT GUIDELINES

Assessment in supine is necessary when the patient has functional limitations in bed mobility and positioning, when support of the trunk will make assessment of primary and secondary impairments easier, and when it will be used as a major treatment position. If the patient's problems do not place him in one of these categories, it may not be necessary to devote treatment time to assessment and treatment in supine.

I. *Movement components.* Assessment in supine can be used to identify patterns of movement and existing movement components in the trunk, arm, and leg. The goal of this area of assessment is to identify the movement components in the trunk, arm, and leg that can be performed normally, specific movement deficits, and atypical or compensatory patterns of movement. Supine is often the position of choice for assessing movement control in the arm and leg when the extremity muscles are weak and hypotonic. It is also very useful for assessing hypertonic arms because of the general reduction of flexor tone that occurs when the patient lies down.

II. *Bed mobility skills.* This area of assessment looks at the patient's ability to use his hemiplegic side to perform functional tasks in the supine position. The goal is to identify functional limitations and to plan treatment activities to address this limitation through movement reeducation or compensatory training.

III. *Secondary impairments.* The use of supine to identify impairments was discussed earlier in the chapter. The purpose of this part of the assessment is to gather information about problems and their interrelationships and to plan a treatment strategy for intervention in supine or in other positions.

THERAPY GOALS

Functional Goals

The supine treatment techniques included in the following section are used to help the patient meet the following functional goals:

1. To be able to perform functional movements of the trunk, arm, and leg with the hemiplegic side in supine.

2. To be able to combine trunk and extremity movements for mobility and comfort in supine.

3. To be able to change the position of the body in bed.

Treatment Goals and Techniques

Treatment Goal: Maintain/restore normal resting alignment and tissue mobility in the arm to ensure painfree movements.

Treatment Technique: Scapula mobilization in supine. This technique is used to maintain or restore shoulder girdle alignment and mobility in supine in preparation for movement reeducation. It is used with patients with hypotonicity and weakness to maintain scapula/humeral rhythm and muscle tissue length and mobility. It is also used with patients with hypertonicity in the arm to decrease muscle tension and restore alignment and mobility to the shoulder, arm, and hand. Scapula mobilization is also very useful for treatment of shoulder/arm pain from any cause, because it allows the therapist to move the scapula and avoid painful movements of the shoulder joint. Scapula mobilization in supine should be performed on all patients before movement reeducation, to ensure that the arm can be moved into flexion, abduction, and external rotation without pain and to determine the passive range of motion that is available in the arm.

The treatment series shown in Figure 10-20A–O is demonstrated on a patient with flexor hypertonicity in her right arm.

Treatment Technique: Scapula mobilization in sidelying is shown in Figure 10-20P–R.

Treatment Technique: Soft tissue tightness and hypertonicity in the forearm, wrist, and hand may not be eliminated by scapula mobilization. Specific treatment of the distal arm and hand may be necessary to restore normal alignment to the forearm, wrist, and hand and decrease tension in the wrist and finger flexors (Fig. 10-20S–X).

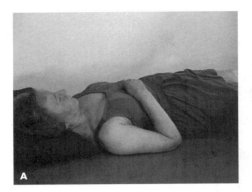

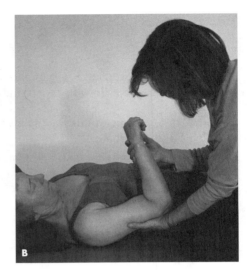

FIGURE 10-20 (*A*) The patient before treatment, right hemi-plegia. (*B*) The therapist kneels on the mat close to the patient's hemiplegic hip. The kneeling position is used so that the therapist can move easily between sitting and kneeling during the treatment, thus keeping a consistent distance between her body and the hemiplegic arm. The therapist grasps the hemiplegic arm at the distal humerus and distal forearm. She uses her right hand to move the patient's hand and forearm away from the chest, while her left hand supports the humerus away from the bed. As she moves the forearm to line up with the shoulder, her left hand rolls the humerus in the direction of external rotation. Ideally, the therapist should be able to bring the forearm completely in line with the shoulder joint and externally rotate the shoulder joint to neutral. If this is not possible, she stops when muscle tightness blocks further correction. Note how the therapist has allowed the elbow joint to remain flexed, but has pronated the forearm. Pronation of the forearm helps to release tension in the biceps. The therapist does not attempt to extend the elbow until the axis of the forearm is in line with the axis of the humerus, the humerus is as close to neutral rotation as muscle tightness will permit, and the forearm is in pronation. (*C*) The therapist maintains the humerus in a stable position with her left hand. With her right hand, she holds the forearm in pronation while gradually bringing the elbow into extension. The therapist does not pull against the tight biceps muscle to obtain elbow extension. Rather, she waits to feel a release in tension, then exerts pressure along the top of the forearm and wrist to bring the hand down. When the elbow can be brought into at least partial extension, the therapist is ready to begin to move the scapula. These scapula movements will result in further reduction of muscle tension in the shoulder, elbow, and forearm. (*D*) The therapist needs to switch hand placements for the next part of the technique. She moves her left hand to the distal arm so that she can place her right hand under the humerus. (*Figure continues*)

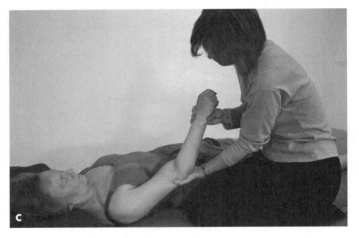

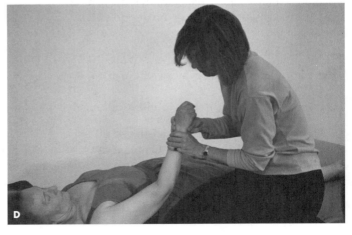

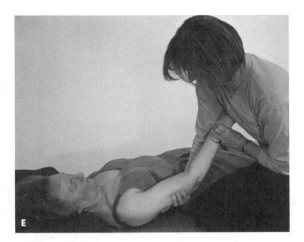

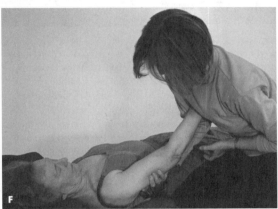

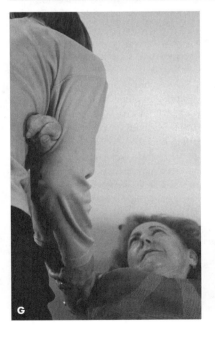

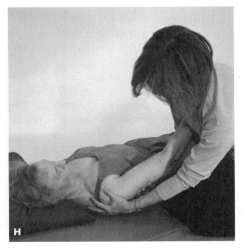

FIGURE 10-20 (*Continued*)   (*E*) The therapist bends closer to the hemiplegic arm and places the distal forearm and hand between her right humerus and her rib cage. Her right hand supports the humerus and holds the shoulder joint in external rotation. (*F & G*) She then cradles the arm between her humerus and rib cage, so that the arm position is stabilized through its full length without use of her left hand. (*H*) The therapist places her left hand over the top of the shoulder joint. She then uses pressure from her hands to move the scapula into elevation and depression and slight abduction/adduction. (*Figure continues*)

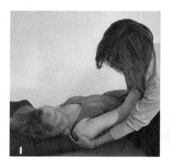 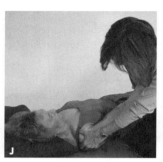 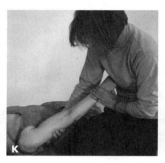 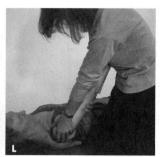

FIGURE 10-20 (*Continued*) (*I*) To elevate the shoulder girdle, the therapist pushes up along the shaft of the humerus. The therapist's left hand supports the glenohumeral joint and ensures that the shoulder moves up. Scapula elevation has a big range in the normal shoulder joint. The therapist stops her upward pressure when she encounters tissue resistance. (*J*) The therapist moves the shoulder girdle down from its elevated position to its starting position and slightly beyond this into depression. This activity is one of the best for bringing an elevated shoulder back to normal resting position. The therapist's hand on the top of the shoulder delivers a push into depression. The hand under the humerus moves down at the same rate and the same distance so that the position of the shoulder joint is unchanged. Note that the scapula rests close to the bed and that the humerus is maintained in a constant amount of flexion during this movement. The therapist should repeat this pattern until muscle resistance to the movement has decreased. Once the shoulder girdle is moving freely in elevation/depression, the therapist can exert gentle pressure with the palm of her left hand against the front of the shoulder to move the scapula back toward the bed in adduction. She follows this with pressure from her left fingertips to move the scapula away from the bed in the plane of abduction. (*K*) If the therapist feels a relaxation in elbow flexion or shoulder internal rotation from the scapula movements, she should stop, reposition the arm in increased elbow extension and humeral external rotation, and repeat the scapula mobilization. (*L*) When the scapula is moving freely in elevation/depression and slight abduction/adduction with the arm by the side of the body, the therapist brings the humerus into 60 degrees of flexion, using the same two-handed grip to control the position of the hemiplegic arm. As the humerus comes into increased elevation, the therapist has to extend her hips and move out of sitting to kneeling so that the hemiplegic arm remains in constant contact with her body. In 60 degrees of humeral flexion, the mobility of the scapula in abduction/upward rotation can be influenced. The therapist's two hands bring the shoulder girdle away from the bed in a movement that follows ths shaft of the humerus. The therapist can use the fingers of her left hand to guide the movement of the scapula into abduction and upward rotation. Her left thumb and index finger stabilize the head of the humerus in the joint and also prevent the shoulder from elevating during the reaching movement. The therapist's hands then bring the shoulder girdle back toward the bed, moving the scapula in the direction of adduction with upward rotation. The humerus is maintained in a constant position of flexion while the therapist moves the scapula on the rib cage. (*Figure continues*)

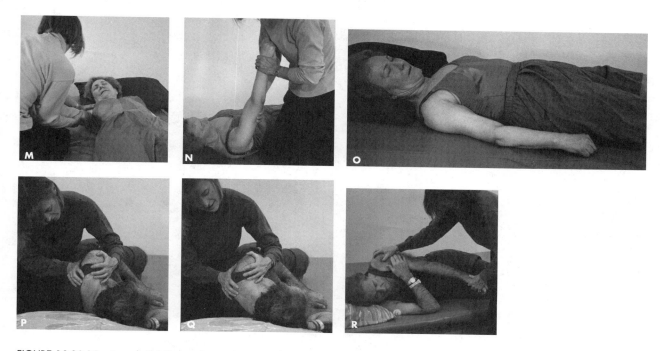

FIGURE 10-20 (*Continued*) (*M*) To lengthen tight pectoral muscles and increase the mobility of the shoulder in scapula adduction with humeral external rotation, the therapist moves the arm into horizontal abduction and repeats the scapula glides. Adduction of the scapula should be emphasized with the arm in this position. (*N*) The therapist gradually brings the shoulder joint into greater degrees of flexion. When the arm approaches 90 degrees of flexion, the therapist will need to change hand placements again. At this time, she moves her left hand from the top of the hemiplegic shoulder to the wrist and hand. This grip allows continued movement of the scapula. The therapist may continue scapula movements and gradually increase the range of shoulder elevation, as long as the scapula movements are available and appropriate. Note how the elbow is now fully extended and the forearm is in full pronation. (*O*) After treatment, the arm is relaxed and extended by the side of the body. The hand remains flexed. (*P*) Scapula mobilization in sidelying may be used when the patient cannot tolerate treatment in supine. It is also very useful when the patient has a painful shoulder, because the therapist is able to place her hands right over the scapula and to see as well as feel its mobility. The therapist's other hand is placed over the front of the shoulder, where it stabilizes the shoulder joint and holds the humerus in a stable position on the patient's hip or in front of his body. The therapist elevates the shoulder girdle by pushing up with both hands. (*Q*) A downward pressure is used to depress the shoulder girdle. Scapula glides into abduction/adduction are also possible in this position. To adduct the scapula, the therapist exerts a gentle backward pressure against the front of the shoulder and clavicle. At the same time, her hand over the scapula moves the scapula back toward the spine. For scapula abduction, the hand on the scapula moves the whole shoulder blade forward away from the spine, while the hand on the anterior shoulder stabilizes the position of the humerus and shoulder joint and allows the scapula to move. (*R*) The therapist has changed the position of the patient's arm and her hand placements. In this figure, the therapist has placed the patient's arm in 30 degrees of flexion. Her right hand is placed over the shoulder joint, with the thumb against the head of the humerus anteriorly and her fingers over the scapula. In this position, she can also mobilize the scapula in elevation depression and abduction/adduction. She will have to flex the shoulder another 30 degrees before rotation of the scapula is added. (*Figure continues*)

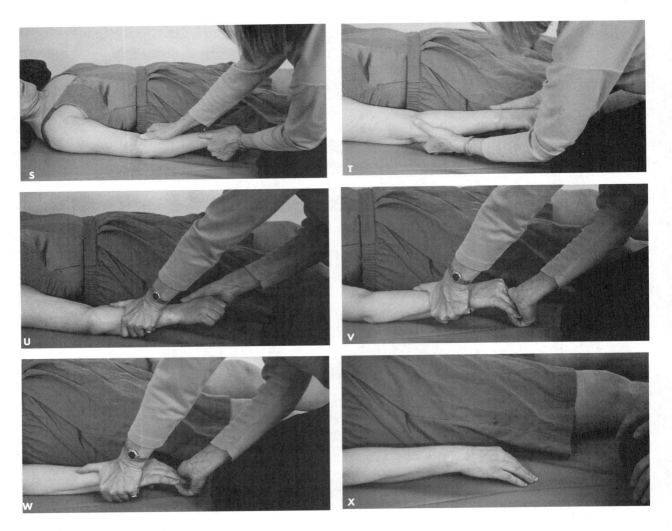

FIGURE 10-20 (*Continued*) (*S*) Soft tissue work on the extensor surface of the forearm. The therapist has placed the patient's arm in elbow extension with forearm pronation, with the axes of the humerus and forearm in line with each other. The therapist's left hand is stabilizing the position of the forearm, while she uses the thumb and fingers of her right hand to roll and massage the muscles on the top of the forearm. There is a diagonal force between the therapist's two hands that is lengthening both flexors and extensors of the wrist and fingers. Her right hand is rolling the proximal forearm tissues toward the thumb side of the hand in this picture. (*T*) The therapist has switched the position of her two hands so that her left hand can work on the tissues of the flexor surface of the proximal forearm. With this grip, the therapist's left thumb may roll the forearm muscles toward the ulnar side of the hand, or her left fingers may roll the flexor muscles on the underside of the forearm toward the ulnar side of the arm. (*U*) To lengthen tight wrist and finger flexors and open a tight hand, the therapist uses her left hand to maintain the forearm in pronation. Her right hand aligns the axis of the hand with that of the forearm and lifts the hand and wrist out of flexion. She holds this position until the pull of the wrist into flexion subsides. The patient's fingers are tightly flexed as she extends the wrist to neutral, showing an exaggerated tendodesis response. (*V*) The therapist moves her left hand to the distal forearm and holds the wrist in the neutral position described in the last figure. The therapist's right fingers go into the palm under the patient's fingertips. She cups the fingertips between her fingertips and her palm and extends the fingertips as much as possible. She then holds this position. As the pull into flexion decreases, she brings the patient's fingertips out of flexion into interphalangeal extension with the metacarpal phalangeal joints in flexion. (*W*) As tension across the metacarpophalangeal joint decreases, the therapist slowly extends this joint also so that the fingers are fully extended with the wrist in neutral. The therapist maintains the wrist and fingers in this position until all the resistance in the wrist and finger muscles has vanished. (*X*) The hand rests in a natural relaxed position after treatment.

Treatment Goal: To reeducate the patterns of movement in the hemiplegic arm that are important for function in supine.

The technique of scapula mobilization described above is always performed before movement reeducation of the arm. This is necessary to ensure that the arm can be moved through 90 degrees or greater of shoulder elevation without pain and that excessive muscle tone or abnormal activation will not interfere with the quality of movement. The patient in the following treatment series has sufficient motor recovery in his hemiplegic arm to allow independent arm movement in supine. However, all the treatment activities presented can be used with weakness and incomplete recovery as well.

Treatment Technique: Use of guided movement and placing to reeducate extended-arm movements (Fig. 10-21).

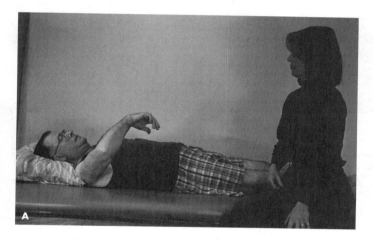

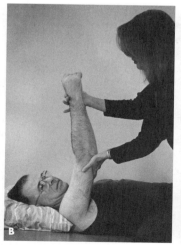
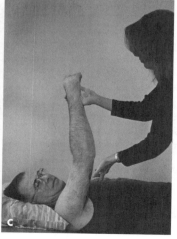

FIGURE 10-21 (*A*) The patient's arm movements in supine before treatment. He is able to lift his arm from the bed using a pattern of humeral abduction and internal rotation, elbow flexion, and wrist flexion. (*B*) The therapist uses techniques of scapula mobilization to bring the shoulder out of abduction and internal rotation and increase extension at the elbow and wrist. Using hand placements on the patient's humerus and wrist that allow her to maintain the arm in an extended position, she moves the patient's arm in small arcs of shoulder movement in the planes of horizontal abduction/adduction or flexion/extension. She asks the patient to feel the movements first, then to assist them. (*C*) When the therapist feels the patient's muscles contracting to assist the movements, she stops moving the arm and asks the patient to try to hold his arm stable in the position in which she has placed it. She lightens her control of the arm briefly to test whether the patient's muscles are contracting with sufficient strength to hold the position. In this picture, the therapist is able to let go completely with both hands while the patient maintains a stable arm position. This Bobath treatment technique is called "placing" because it is based on the normal placing response. While first training the movements, the therapist should not completely remove her control of the arm, as it may fall and injure the shoulder joint. She begins to ask for placing by lightening her touch, then removing one hand at a time. Removing her control from the patient's wrist will tell her whether the patient is able to control elbow and wrist extension and forearm rotation. Removing the hand from the humerus will provide information about control at the shoulder. (*Figure continues*)

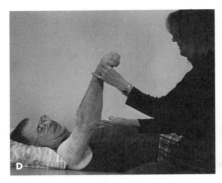
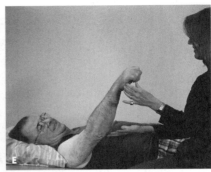

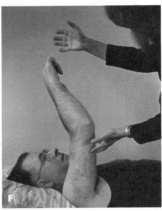
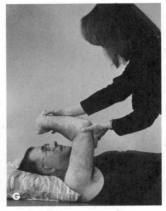
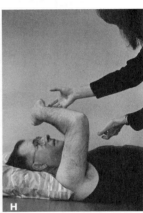

FIGURE 10-21 (*Continued*) (*D & E*) The therapist has lowered the arm slightly and is repeating the process. Placing is easiest when the shoulder is at or above 90 degrees of flexion/abduction, because the muscles that stabilize the shoulder are at their greatest mechanical advantage in this range. For this reason, the therapist begins to ask the patient for shoulder girdle placing with the arm elevated at 90 degrees. When the patient is able to control the arm in this position, she can gradually lower the arm and ask for similar control. The goal of this activity is for the patient to be able to lower his arm from flexion overhead to rest on the bed and to raise it from the bed into elevation. If the patient is unable to maintain the arm stable below 90 degrees, the therapist should prepare for this control with guided movements of the arm toward the mat and back up into elevation. (*F*) The patient may also practice reaching movements with the extended arm. Here, the therapist is asking the patient to reach for her hand, a movement that requires control of horizontal adduction. She may then move her hand into horizontal abduction and ask for reaching. Note the therapist's light contact with the patient's humerus that prevents the arm from falling below 90 degrees of elevation. Reaching should also be practiced toward the mat and back over the head. (*G*) Placing is also used to train elbow flexion and extension movements in supine. With the arm elevated to 90 degrees of flexion, the therapist and patient practice flexing his elbow to bring his hand to his head, then elbow extension to reach his hand back toward the ceiling. (*H*) The patient may also try to maintain his arm in a stable position with his elbow bent, or to bring his hand from the top of his head to his mouth or opposite shoulder in movements that combine elbow flexion with shoulder movement. (*Figure continues*)

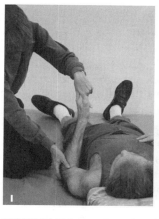
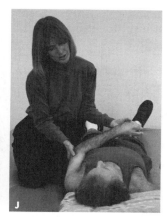
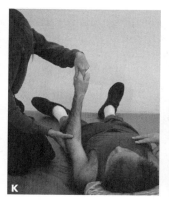
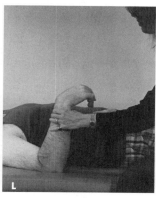
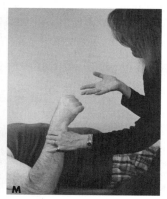

FIGURE 10-21 (*Continued*) (*I*) Movements that combine elbow flexion with shoulder movement can also be introduced from a starting position of extension by the side of the body. Here, the therapist is assisting the movement of elbow flexion with the humerus in extension. (*J*) She can combine elbow flexion with shoulder internal rotation to bring the hand to the chest, and with external rotation to move away from the chest. This movement is very important for positioning the arm for comfort. (*K*) From the starting position of elbow flexion with shoulder extension, the therapist also trains shoulder flexion, the pattern used to bring the hand from the mat to the face or pillow. (*L*) Distal movements of the wrist and fingers are often trained in supine. This may be performed with the arm supported on the bed or with the arm extended overhead. In this series, the therapist asks the patient to extend his wrist from the flexed position, with his elbow in flexion and his humerus supported on the bed. (*M*) The patient is able to extend his wrist independently, although in his arm movements before treatment the wrist was in flexion. For a patient with more distal weakness, the therapist would begin with active assistive movements and placing to regain wrist extension control. Forearm rotation movements can also be easily reeducated with the arm in this position. These movements are also very important to reeducate for arm and hand function in all treatment positions.

Treatment Goal: To maintain or restore normal alignment and tissue length in the hemiplegic leg. In supine, loss of normal resting alignment is common in patients with severe low tone and weakness. When these patients lie supine, the leg is positioned in excessive abduction and external rotation at the hip and lower leg. This abnormal leg position can usually be easily corrected by the therapist because it is not associated with abnormal muscle firing or hypertonicity. However, poor alignment in supine often leads to extensor hypertonicity in the leg. This extensor pattern develops when muscles on the front and back of the leg shorten or shift their line of pull, resulting in resistance to passive flexion in the hemiplegic hip and knee. Extensor hypertonicity that results from poor alignment in supine is positional; the leg muscles are not active. It is corrected by systematically realigning the hip and lower leg and releasing the tight muscles. This same system should be used with patients with hypotonicity to prevent the development of extensor hypertonicity. In patients with severe brain damage and strong total body extension, the extensor tone in the leg is due not only to poor alignment and shortened muscles, but also to true spasticity. The same passive, methodical realignment may also help the therapist move these legs into a more flexed position during treatment, but may not result in lasting reduction of tone or muscle length. It is important to remember that as soon as muscle tension is decreased and alignment corrected, the therapist must begin to reeducate supine leg movements so the patient can learn to control actively flexion/extension of his hemiplegic leg.

Treatment Technique: Decrease extensor hypertonicity in the leg (Fig. 10-22).

FIGURE 10-22 (A) The therapist is trying to bend the patient's hemiplegic leg. The leg cannot be bent because of extensor hypertonicity. (B) The therapist first corrects hip joint and femoral alignment. Her right hand places a downward pressure on the anterior surface of the hip joint, lengthening the anterior hip muscles. Both of her hands slowly roll the femur into external rotation, lengthening the medial hamstrings and the tensor fascia lata. This correction rotates the hip joint to neutral and allows the hip and knee to be passively flexed. (C) The therapist's right hand maintains the correction at the hip/pelvis, while her left hand lifts the knee to increase hip and knee flexion. Flexion of the leg is introduced slowly so that flexion occurs at the same rate at the hip and knee, and the foot remains close to the bed. The therapist stops trying to flex the leg when she feels resistance. As resistance decreases, she moves the leg into more flexion. The therapist is using the fingers of her left hand to apply pressure to the insertion of the iliotibial band and the distal lateral musculature to allow the knee to flex further. Note the obvious supination of the foot and external rotation of the tibia. (D–F) The therapist changes her hand placements. She moves her right hand from the hip to the distal femur and slides her left hand out to move it to the tibia. She holds the femur in its corrected position with her right hand. Her left hand internally rotates the lower leg to neutral. As the rotational components of the femur and lower leg become compatible, the knee is easily flexed and the supination of the foot decreases. As the therapist de-rotates the lower leg, she also directs a downward message into the heel to increase weight bearing on the foot. (G) As the therapist holds the correction at the hip and lower leg, the ankle joint dorsiflexors relax so that the foot moves down to the bed. Her left hand placement allows her to exert pressure on the tendons of the tibialis anterior and extensor hallicus muscles and to increase weight bearing in the foot. Note apparent adduction of the foot on the lower leg. (H) The therapist has moved her left hand to the top of the foot to realign the foot with the lower leg and further lengthen the long tendons of the ankle and toe muscles. Pelvis/hip, femur, knee, lower leg, and foot are now in correct relationship to each other. The therapist will begin the process of movement reeducation with this corrected leg alignment.

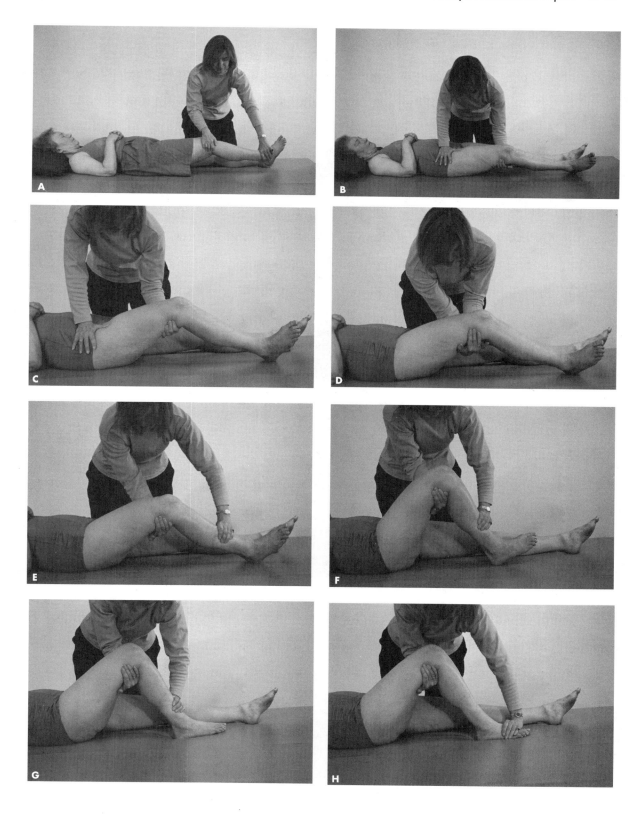

Treatment Goal: To reeducate normal movement patterns in the hemiplegic leg that are important for function in supine. This treatment series is demonstrated on a patient with low tone and weakness. It could also be used with patients who have hypertonicity and unbalanced return, once normal alignment has been restored and hypertonicity reduced.

Treatment Technique: Active assistive movements of weak leg with therapist correcting alignment (Fig. 10-23).

FIGURE 10-23 (A) The patient before treatment, right hemiplegia with weakness. (B) The patient is trying to lift her leg into the flexed position. Lifting the hemiplegic leg into the flexed weight bearing position is one of the most important leg movements in supine. The patient is able to flex her hip using her quadriceps but cannot flex the knee or ankle to bring the foot to the bed. Although the hemiplegic leg extends as she tries to lift it, it is not stiff and hypertonic. (C) The therapist begins movement reeducation by moving the leg into flexed weight bearing. She will ask for control of hip movements in this position, where the hip flexors are shortened, before asking the patient to move the leg into and out of the flexed position. (D) The therapist uses her left hand to stabilize the patient's foot on the mat. Her right hand is placed so that her palm and fingers cover the back of the knee joint (popliteal fossa). Her right thumb can be placed over the distal femur or over the top of the tibia. With the foot in the weight bearing position, the therapist asks the patient to try to use his leg muscles to stabilize the leg in the position in which she places it (*placing*). The therapist's hands control the relationship of the femur to the pelvis and to the foot. During the first efforts at placing the leg, the femur should be in a neutral position in line with the hip joint and foot, rather than abducted or adducted. The therapist may deliver a message backward along the femur to the hip joint to provide proprioceptive input to the hip. If she feels hip muscles contracting but the foot slides, she may use her right hand to deliver a message down the shaft of the tibia to the heel of the foot to increase the sensory message of weight bearing, or she may exert pressure from her left hand into the sole of the foot to plant it more firmly. (E) The patient with severe weakness and hypotonicity may have a difficult time finding hip muscles with the foot on the bed. To make the activity easier, the therapist can lift the foot off the bed and increase flexion at the hip. Note how the therapist holds the patient's ankle in dorsiflexion when the leg is non-weight bearing. The patient attempts to stabilize the femur position in neutral, then to maintain it in horizontal abduction/adduction after the therapist changes the position of the leg. When the patient is able to hold the leg stable in varying hip positions, he may practice actively moving the knee in and out while the therapist supports the weight of the leg. (F) The therapist returns the foot to the bed and repeats the above stages. The patient is now able to maintain her leg in the flexed position. (*Figure continues*)

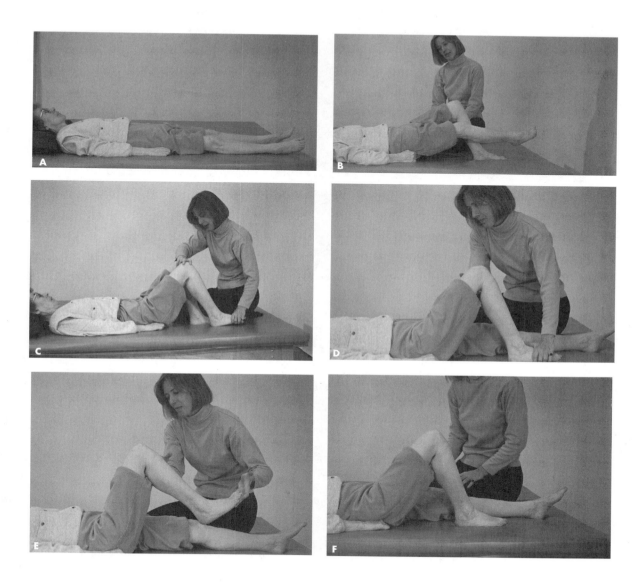

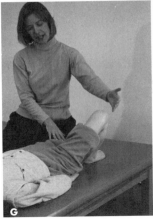
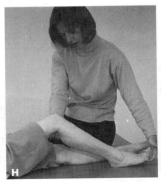
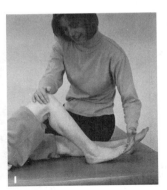

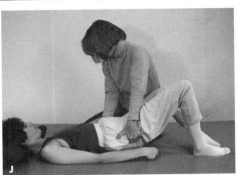
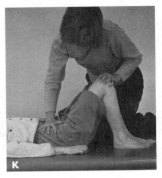
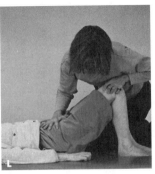

FIGURE 10-23 (*Continued*) (*G*) She practices moving her femur into abduction/adduction while the foot is in weight bearing. (*H*) To increase hip control and strength, the therapist slides the patient's foot down several inches on the bed, decreasing the amount of hip and knee flexion. The patient is asked to hold her leg in this position. Hip abduction/adduction movements can also be practiced. The patient will have a more difficult time controlling the position of the leg as it moves closer to hip and knee extension. (*I*) The therapist helps the patient step her leg back up into more hip and knee flexion. To assist this motion, the therapist supports the front of the foot so that the ankle does not fall into plantarflexion. Her two hands work together to lift the foot slightly off the mat and move it closer to the hip joint. It is important that the foot stay close to the mat during this movement so that the patient uses hip flexors and hamstrings to position the foot, rather than the quadriceps. The therapist repeats this activity, gradually moving the leg closer to full extension before asking the patient to return it to the flexed position. The goal of this activity is to teach the patient to lift the leg off the bed with hip and knee flexion. (*J*) The flexed weight bearing position is also used to train unilateral and bilateral bridging. During bridging, the hip extensors and abdominals contract to lift the pelvis off the bed without excessive lumbar extension. To facilitate the movement, the therapist may use a bilateral hip/pelvis grip. The therapist places her hands over the lateral aspect of the proximal femurs at the level of the hip joints. Her fingertips support the back of the femur, and her thumbs lie close to the ASIS of the pelvis. To assist the bridge, the therapist lifts the pelvis. (*K*) An alternative grip. The therapist's left hand is placed over the hemiplegic knee and her right hand over the front of the pelvis and abdomen. (*L*) As the patient attempts to lift her pelvis, the therapist's left hand guides the knee forward over the heel and delivers a downward message along the shaft of the tibia to the heel to stabilize the foot on the bed. In this picture, the therapist's hand on the pelvis is not assisting the movement of lifting, but is preventing excessive anterior tilting of the pelvis. The therapist could move her right hand to the right hip and pelvis to provide more assistance to hip extension.

Treatment Goal: Restore alignment and symmetry in the trunk.

Treatment Technique: Abnormal alignment in the trunk and pelvis should be corrected before trunk movements are reeducated (Fig. 10-24). It is often necessary to realign the trunk and pelvis before reeducating movements of the arm and leg. Some alignment problems are corrected with the use of firm manual pressure designed to release tight muscles and move the body back into symmetric alignment.

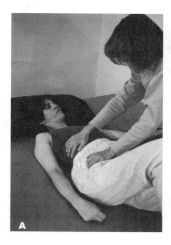
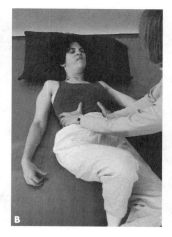
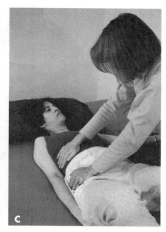

FIGURE 10-24 (A) The patient's right pelvis and rib cage have rotated to the left, and the lumbar spine is in too much extension. The therapist's hands are marking the position of the ribs and pelvis but are not yet correcting their alignment. (B) The therapist uses a symmetric rib cage grip to rotate the right side of the rib cage backwards into the bed. Her thumbs and thenar eminences are placed along the bottom edges of the ribs so that the thumbs face up and the palms and fingers encircle the lower rib cage. The therapist exerts pressure with the heel of her left hand to rotate the patient's right side backwards. At the same time, the fingers of her right hand on the back of the patient's left ribs rotate the left side forward. The therapist goes slowly and makes small corrections in rib cage position as she feels the muscles release to her pressure. As the position of the rib cage becomes more symmetric, the therapist can add a slight pressure back toward the bed to correct the excessive arching of the back and lengthen the low-back extensors. (C) When the asymmetric rib cage rotation has been corrected, the therapist changes her hand position so that she can maintain the rib cage correction and rotate the right side of the pelvis back to line up with the rib cage. The therapist has placed the heel of her left hand over the patient's ASIS and hip joint. She exerts a rotary pressure into the front of the pelvis to move it back and to the right. In this photo, the position of the rib cage and pelvis have responded to manual pressure and the two sides of the body are now symmetric. (*Figure continues*)

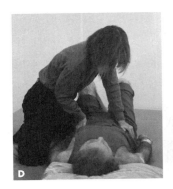

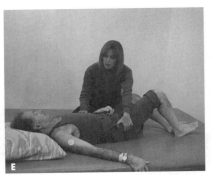

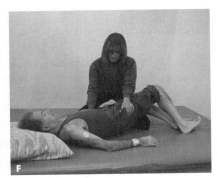

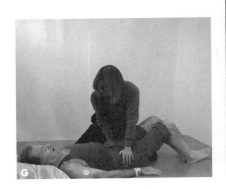

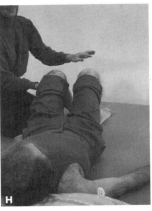

FIGURE 10-24 (*Continued*)   (*D*) A symmetric pelvis grip can also be used to correct rotational asymmetry in the pelvis. Note how the patient's hemiplegic left rib cage and pelvis appear higher and more prominent than on his right side, indicating rotation to the right. The therapist is trying to rotate the left side of the pelvis back with her right hand, while her left fingers bring the patient's right pelvis forward by the same amount. She uses a firm, sustained pressure to obtain a release in the tight muscles. As the muscles release, she will be able to rotate the pelvis to the left. In this treatment session, the therapist initially used rotation to the left and back to the midline to correct alignment, then added rotation to the right to lengthen tight muscles. (*E*) Active assisted lower trunk rotation can also be used to correct rotation asymmetry in the trunk and pelvis. In this activity, the patient is asked to turn his knees to his left so that his right pelvis leaves the bed. The therapist selects this direction for movement because it moves the hemiplegic side of the rib cage and pelvis in the direction that will make the trunk more symmetric. The therapist is using her left arm on the patient's uninvolved side to cue the pelvis to move correctly. Her right arm is stabilizing the hemiplegic rib cage. (*F*) As the patient continues to rotate his lower body to the left, the right side of the pelvis and rib cage rotate back into the bed. (*G*) The patient then reverses the rotation and moves his knees and pelvis back to the midline, or to the right. Rotation of the lower body to the right would move the pelvis in the wrong direction for correction of alignment. However, this movement would be valuable to lengthen tight muscle between the right rib cage and pelvis and improve mobility in the spine and rib cage. (*H*) After the movement has been repeated several times, the position of the patient's pelvis and left leg are in symmetric alignment with the right side. Compare the alignment of the left leg in this figure with its position in Figure D. The improved leg position demonstrates the relationship between trunk/pelvis alignment and position of the leg.

Treatment Goal: To reeducate normal trunk movements in supine.

Treatment Technique: Treatment techniques for reeducation of upper and lower body rotation are included in the chapter on rolling (Ch. 11). Readers should consult this chapter for handling techniques.

Treatment Goal: To train bed mobility.

Treatment Technique: Sliding sideways and up/down in bed (Fig. 10-25A–C) is taught after the techniques of bridging, because the movement patterns are similar. Refer to Figure 10-2 H–J for reeducation of bridging.

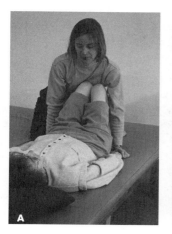
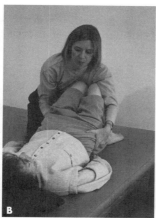
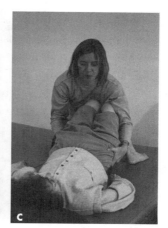

FIGURE 10-25 (*A*) The therapist flexes both legs and cradles the patient's knees between her two arms with her chest close to the knees. (*B*) She places her hands on the patient's hips and assists the pelvis off the bed with hip extension. (*C*) Sideways movements are often easier to train than up and down. As the patient clears the bed, the therapist uses her hands to move the pelvis laterally to one side. In this picture, the patient is moving her pelvis laterally to the left, away from her hemiplegic side. The therapist's left hand is controlling the pelvic movement. To move the pelvis to the right, the therapist would use her right hand to move the pelvis, while her left hand would provide stability to the hemiplegic hip. (*Figure continues*)

Treatment Technique: Sliding up and down in bed is most easily trained using a bilateral knee grip (Fig. 10-25 D & E).

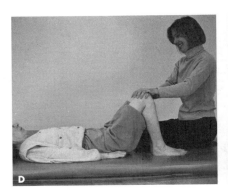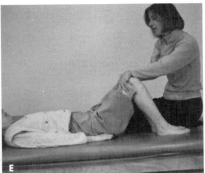

FIGURE 10-25 (*Continued*)   (*D*) To practice sliding up in bed, the patient's legs are flexed so that the heels of the feet rest close to the hips. The therapist's hands are over the tops of the knees. (*E*) The patient lifts her hips off the bed and pushes with her feet to move up toward the pillow. To help the patient move up, the therapist's hands deliver pressure down along the shafts of the tibias into the heels. This pressure prevents the hemiplegic foot from slipping as the patient extends her knees. After the patient has moved up, the therapist relaxes her pressure into the foot to allow the pelvis to come back to the bed. If the patient is to move up again, the feet are repositioned closer to the hips and the process repeated. To move down in bed, the therapist uses the same hand placements. After the patient has lifted her pelvis, the therapist's hands exert a forward pressure on the knees as well as a downward message into the heels.

11
Rolling

CONCEPTS AND PRINCIPLES

The ability to roll in bed allows us to change position (side/side, front/back) while we are resting or sleeping and is a step in moving to sitting on the edge of the bed. Variations in the initiation of rolling patterns allow the body to respond to motivational demands—to get a glass of water on the bedside table, to move the legs off the bed, and to provide automatic adjustments for comfort. The movement task during rolling from supine to sidelying is to change the base of support from the dorsal aspect of the trunk and limbs to the lateral aspect of one side of the body. There are three initiation patterns for rolling: the upper body (upper trunk and arm) can initiate the movement; the lower body (lower trunk and leg) can initiate the movement; or the upper and lower body can move as a "unit" ("log rolling"). Each individual may display a preferred pattern of rolling, based on body type and muscle strength.

Therapists help patients with hemiplegia learn how to roll for a variety of reasons. The patients in the acute stage of recovery need to roll to change position in bed and to position themselves to sit up. Therapists also teach the movement components of rolling to activate and strengthen paralyzed or weak muscles. Patients in later recovery stages practice rolling patterns to address the secondary impairments of shortened muscles, especially the latissimus dorsi, quadratus lumborum, and pectoralis muscles, and to treat loss of range or muscle stiffness in the spine and rib cage. We reeducate movement control by teaching varied initiation patterns and by retraining the ability to sequence trunk and limb movement in functional combinations.

Rolling to the involved side helps the patient experience tactile and proprioceptive sensations on the hemiplegic side, teaches trunk and extremity patterns that can be practiced with minimal manual contact, strengthens the pelvic and hip muscle on the involved side, and begins to increase balance control in sidelying (Fig. 11-1). In patients with hemiplegia, the presence of shoulder pain interferes with rolling or resting on the involved side. This secondary impairment of pain needs to be assessed and eliminated as rolling to the involved side is practiced.

Rolling to the uninvolved side helps the patient develop the control necessary to begin moving the trunk and hemiplegic arm and leg in coordinated, assisted patterns (Fig. 11-2). As we train rolling in our patients, it is important to reeducate and sequence compatible arm and leg limb movements with the selected trunk pattern. Lying on either side is often difficult for the patient with severe weakness and loss of balance control.

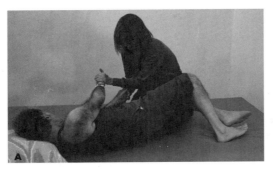

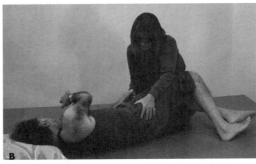

FIGURE 11-1 (*A & B*) Patient with left hemiplegic practicing rolling to the left. Therapist encourages him to roll using a symmetric initiation pattern as she uses her right hand to support and protect his left arm.

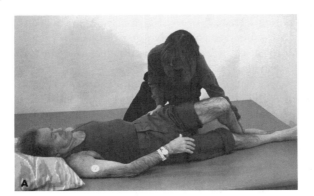

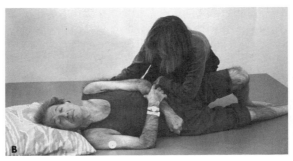

FIGURE 11-2 (*A & B*) Therapist teaches patient to initiate a lower body pattern with his left hemiplegic leg. She uses her right hand behind his left shoulder to assist the movement of the upper body as he comes to sidelying.

This chapter analyzes three trunk initiation patterns and identifies the common trunk and limb interrelationships during rolling movements. Of the three trunk initiation patterns, two are segmental patterns and one is nonsegmental. *Segmental rolling* patterns are ones in which the pattern of rolling is initiated by either the upper body or the lower body. Segmental rolling is done in several stages in which portions of the trunk move as separate units, upper trunk on lower trunk or lower trunk on upper trunk. In contrast to this, *nonsegmental rolling* occurs when the upper and lower trunk remain aligned over each other as the movement is initiated. Nonsegmental rolling is performed with the trunk moving together as one unit.

ROLLING MOVEMENT COMPONENTS

Rolling Initiated from the Upper Body

When rolling from supine to the right side is initiated from the upper body, the head and upper body move up off the bed on a diagonal toward the right. This movement of the upper trunk places the spine in flexion and is described as *flexion rotation right* (Fig. 11-3). In the initial phase of the movement, the head, left shoulder, and upper rib cage move away from the bed so they are anterior to the left pelvis. The left lower trunk and left leg remain on the surface. As rotation progresses down the spine, the left pelvis will rotate to the right and leave the support-

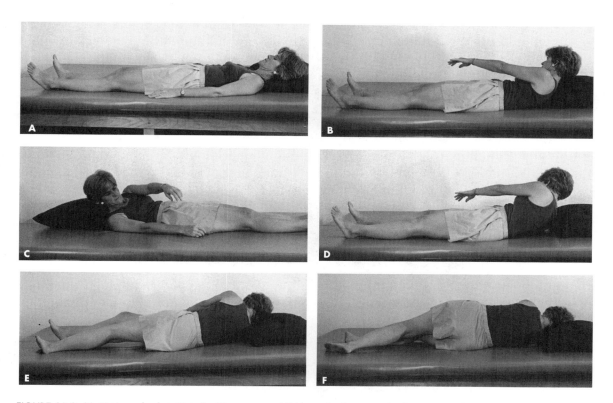

FIGURE 11-3 (*A–E*) Upper-body-initiated rolling pattern. (*C*) Upper-body-initiated rolling pattern/anterior view.

ing surface so that full body weight is shifted onto the right hip/pelvis and shoulder. In the final phase of rolling, the left leg leaves the bed and rests on the right leg or on the bed, and the lower body moves into the same plane as the upper body. When the pelvis and lower body are in the sidelying position, the spine will have moved out of flexion rotation to a neutral position.

The arm is often used to assist the flexion rotation pattern of the trunk. The arm on the non-weight bearing side can reach across midline to provide rotational assistance or can lift off the supporting surface and reach forward to provide flexion assistance.

Rolling Initiated from the Lower Body

When rolling from supine to the right is initiated from the lower body, the left side of the pelvis and lower trunk move away from the bed on a diagonal toward the right. This movement of the lower trunk is described as *extension rotation right* because the movement of the lower body places the spine in extension (Fig. 11-4). As the movement is initiated, the left pelvis moves anterior to the left shoulder. The head and upper body remain on the surface. As rotation moves up the spine, the left upper body will rotate right and leave the supporting surface so that full body weight is shifted onto the right pelvis/hip and shoulder. At the completion of the

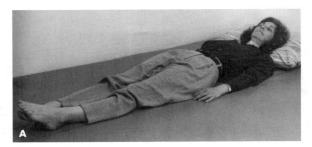
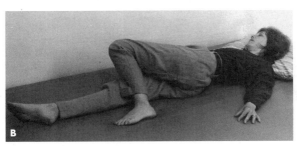
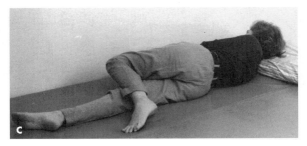

FIGURE 11-4 (A–C) Lower-body-initiated rolling pattern.

movement, the upper body rotates into the plane of the pelvis, and the sidelying position is attained.

The leg is used to assist the extension rotation pattern of the trunk. The amount of leg movement varies with the amount of trunk/pelvic extension rotation control: the foot can push into the surface with the knee flexed or with the knee extended to assist with lower trunk extension rotation, or the leg can lift off the surface and move across midline (with the knee extended or flexed) to assist with pelvic rotation. The arm is used to assist the upper body as it rotates to sidelying. It also helps as a balance assist to the trunk throughout the movement.

Nonsegmental Rolling

During nonsegmental rolling from supine to the right, the left shoulder and left pelvis remain aligned in the same plane, and the whole trunk moves together as one unit (Fig. 11-5). The upper and lower trunk are in neutral alignment as the movement is initiated so that head, shoulders, and pelvis leave the bed at approximately the same time. This movement is initiated by either the simultaneous activation of the trunk and extremities or by the activation of head, neck, and trunk rotation with minimal use of the extremities. During nonsegmental rolling to the right, body weight is shifted from the back onto the right shoulder and hip as the pelvis and shoulder leave the bed.

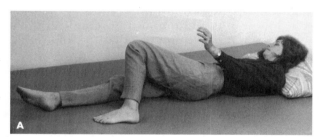

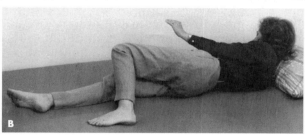

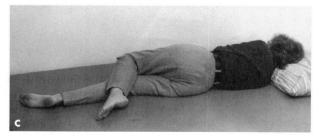

FIGURE 11-5 (A–C) Nonsegmental rolling pattern.

Movement Summary: Rolling

Starting position
  Supine
Initiation movement
  Upper trunk; flexion rotation
  Lower trunk; extension rotation
  Nonsegmental; neutral spine
Transition movement
  Upper trunk initiation; lower trunk rotates to meet upper trunk
  Lower trunk initiation; upper trunk rotates to meet lower trunk
  Nonsegmental initiation; upper and lower trunk move together
Extremity activity
  Upper trunk initiation; arm moves with trunk to assist
  Lower trunk initiation; leg assists trunk movement
  Nonsegmental initiation; trunk and limbs move together
Ending position
  Sidelying
Task
  Move the center of gravity from supine to sidelying

SIGNIFICANT IMPAIRMENTS THAT INTERFERE WITH PERFORMANCE

Extremity Hypertonicity

Hypertonicity in the arm and leg is not dominant in the acute stage of recovery, but attempts at rolling may result in inappropriate or unbalanced firing of the flexors of the elbow and wrist and the extensors of the knee and ankle to assist trunk movements. Flexor hypertonicity in the arm occurs in rolling either as a response to the patient trying to use the arm to assist the trunk pattern, as a result of tension in shortened or atypically aligned two-joint joint muscles as the upper or lower body initiates the roll, or as a balance response (Fig. 11-6).

Extensor hypertonicity in the leg occurs for similar reasons. The patient may use active knee extension to assist the lower-trunk-initiated extension pattern. If the patient cannot move the affected leg into a flexed position to assist the lower body

FIGURE 11-6 Flexor hypertonicity in the left arm as the patient initiates a lower body rolling pattern.

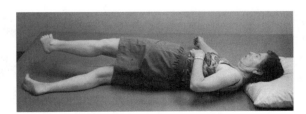

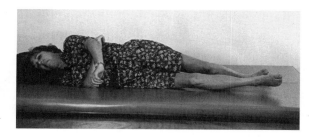

FIGURE 11-7 Patient with a right hemiplegia trying to initiate rolling with strong use of her left arm, can not coordinate the compatible trunk pattern.

initiate the roll, the leg often pushes down excessively into the bed with knee and ankle extension but does not assist the trunk pattern. Leg extensor hypertonicity may also occur as a balance response when rolling to the uninvolved side. When rolling toward the involved side, the leg becomes extended and stiff if the two-joint hip/knee muscles are stretched beyond their available range.

Over time, if abnormal alignment and atypical movement patterns in the arm and leg result in soft tissue tightness and persistent extremity posturing, compensatory rolling patterns will predominate, and reeducation of movement components will be more difficult. These atypical extremity patterns (arm flexion and leg extension) influence the starting position and subsequent recruitment patterns of muscle control available to the patient. Therefore, the therapist must identify the cause of the hypertonicity—muscle shortening, poor trunk control, abnormal muscle recruitment—and decrease it enough to allow reeducation and strengthening of needed movement components.

Loss of Trunk Control

Rolling can be initiated with flexion rotation patterns in the upper body, extension rotation patterns in the lower body, or with the upper and lower trunk working in a symmetric, nonsegmental pattern. The inability to select and vary trunk initiation patterns makes it difficult for patients with hemiplegia to roll to either side. In acute patients, weakness and loss of control of the trunk musculature makes rolling difficult, if not impossible. Often, the spinal pattern and the extremity pattern that patients try to combine are incompatible. They struggle to use these patterns, and the result is inefficient, laborious movement (Fig. 11-7). In treatment, therapists use rolling to reeducate and strengthen trunk musculature by retraining each of the initiation patterns. The trunk muscles continue to be strengthened as arm and leg patterns are added to the practice pattern.

Extremity Weakness

If the paretic arm and leg cannot assist the trunk by moving up off the bed, the patient will have to work harder with his trunk musculature or use compensatory movements with the uninvolved limbs. The lack of extremity participation will make rolling to either side difficult.

Upper Extremity Weakness

Upper-body-initiated rolling requires upper trunk flexion rotation and the participation of the arm with this trunk movement. The arm reaches forward and up across the body to assist the upper trunk pattern. In patients with hemiplegia, severe weakness in the arm limits the reaching pattern of the arm during rolling. Weakness causes

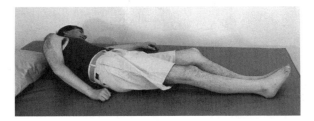

FIGURE 11-8 Patient's weak right arm is left behind his body as he initiates the roll with an upper trunk flexion rotation pattern.

the arm to either fall forward in front of the chest in shoulder flexion, internal rotation, and adduction or to get left behind the body in hyperextension as the trunk rolls forward (Fig. 11-8). Passive hyperextension of the shoulder during upper-body-initiated rolling makes it more difficult to move the trunk forward and complete the roll. Excessive passive hyperextension of the shoulder during lower-body-initiated rolling interferes during the transition phase, when the upper body must rotate forward into the plane of the pelvis. Excessive, passive adduction/flexion of the shoulder during upper-body-initiated rolling places the weight of the arm in front of the body and interferes with the grading and slowing down of the forward/rotational upper trunk movement to move into sidelying. The heavy weight of the arm may cause shoulder joint pain if the arm is not incorporated into the trunk initiation pattern.

Weakness in the Lower Extremity

Lower-body-initiated rolling requires the leg to assist the movement of the lower trunk. Weakness in the leg on the initiating side makes it more difficult for the lower trunk to initiate and rotate into the sidelying position. If the leg cannot assist the trunk, the patient often struggles to roll to his uninvolved side. This often causes the hemiplegic leg to become excessively extended or stiff (Fig. 11-9). Weakness of the leg may result in an inability to roll onto the involved side because of difficulty accepting and controlling body weight. When rolling onto the involved side, activity in the muscles of the lower trunk and leg provide stability. Without this stability, the patient is unable to balance comfortably and rest in the sidelying position. Many patients experience difficulty with rolling to the hemiplegic side because as they roll onto the weak side, they do not have enough extremity strength or control to

FIGURE 11-9 (A & B) Patient with right hemiplegia initiating a lower trunk rolling pattern without an appropriate assistive pattern in the right leg.

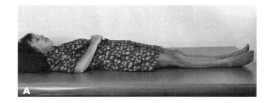

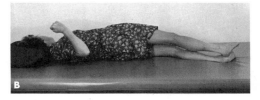

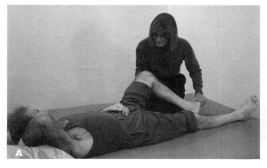
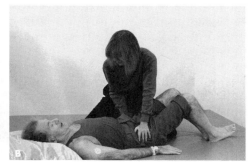
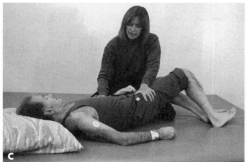
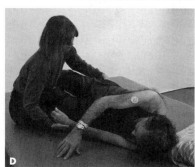

FIGURE 11-10 (A) Therapist teaches patient to move his weak leg into a position that will assist the trunk rolling pattern. (B) Therapist places her hands on patient's lower trunk. Her right hand will stabilize the left side and keep the pelvis from sliding as the patient rolls to the hemiplegic side. Her left hand will help the patient learn how to initiate with an extension rotation pattern. (C) As the patient initiates the roll, her left hand gives a diagonal message down towards the patient's left hip as weight is transferred onto it. (D) As the patient rolls into sidelying, the therapist supports his hemiplegic arm to help him avoid rolling onto it and causing pain.

balance on that side. If the patient cannot perceive tactile or proprioceptive messages from the hemiplegic side, they will have difficulty recruiting or sequencing appropriate muscle firing and will avoid moving onto that side.

In treatment, therapists must reeducate weak arm and leg musculature with compatible trunk patterns to allow patients to roll onto and balance on either side. To retrain rolling activities, when both the trunk and extremities are weak, the therapist must alternate her handling between assisting an extremity to focus on reeducating and strengthening the trunk and assisting the trunk to focus on reeducating and strengthening the extremities (Fig. 11-10).

Loss of Alignment Caused by Muscle Shortening

Loss of muscle length in the large multijoint muscles of the trunk and limbs (latissimus dorsi, quadratus lumborum, biceps, tensor fascia lata) will limit rotation of the spine and rotation between the upper and lower body. These patterns of muscle tightness change the alignment of the shoulder girdle on the upper trunk and of the pelvic girdle on the rib cage. This results in abnormal alignment of the body in supine and may lead to inappropriate muscle firing patterns or an inability to reeducate movement patterns during rolling. Prolonged muscle shortness may result in compensatory

FIGURE 11-11 (A) Therapist stabilizes the bottom of the rib cage with her right hand while she lengthens tight hip abductors and tensor fascia lata. (B) While maintaining the new length between her hands, she follows the initiation movement of the patient. (C) Therapist uses her right hand to correct and support the scapula while with her left hand she supports the glenohumeral joint. She uses both hands to maintain glenohumeral joint alignment while she lengthens shoulder girdle elevator muscles.

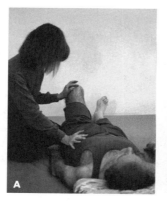 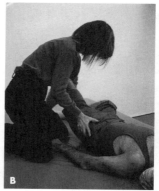 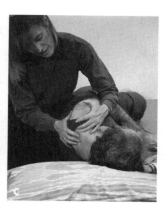

movements since, in the presence of abnormal alignment, the patient finds it harder to strengthen weak or missing muscle patterns. Loss of muscle length between the rib cage and shoulder girdle and humerus and between the ribs and the pelvis and femur will affect the ability of the limbs to appropriately assist the trunk during rolling. When muscle shortening is a problem, the therapist must lengthen the shortened muscles to prevent the tightness from interfering with activation or reeducation of specific movement components. She can lengthen tight muscles as a preparatory activity, or she can lengthen them specifically during a portion of the roll (Fig. 11-11).

Shoulder Pain

Shoulder pain will prevent the patient from attempting to roll to or rest on the hemiplegic side. Shoulder pain occurs during rolling if the arm is flexed greater than 45 to 60 degrees without corresponding scapular movement. As the patient approaches sidelying, the involved arm and shoulder joint must be positioned forward of the trunk, so that body weight does not rest directly on the joint. If the scapula does not move and the shoulder is trapped under the trunk as the patient moves to sidelying, joint pain from poor alignment and capsular pinching will be present. During upper-body-initiated rolling treatment, the therapist must be sure to maintain alignment of the shoulder joint and keep the shoulder joint forward as the body rolls toward the arm (Fig. 11-12A–C). If pain is present while these precautions are observed, the patient should not lie on the involved arm until the cause of pain is eliminated. When rolling to the uninvolved side, the therapist must teach the patient how to move the hemiplegic arm with the trunk movement to prevent pain (Fig. 11-12D & E).

ATYPICAL MOVEMENTS

Inappropriate Spinal Extension

If the patient initiates rolling from the lower body with an extension rotation pattern, he must be able to stop the extension rotation during transition and bring the upper body forward with trunk flexors. If this is not possible, the extension rotation pattern may continue and the patient gets "stuck" half-way onto his side and cannot move into the sidelying position. Excessive spinal extension may also result from strong extensor hypertonicity in the affected leg. The leg normally assists the movement of the pelvis and spine by moving forward with the trunk. If the foot and leg

FIGURE 11-12 (A) The base of the therapist's left palm is on the top of the shoulder to prevent shoulder elevation and her left fingers are on the back of the scapula. The web space of her right hand is under the axilla to support the joint, while the fingers of her right hand are controlling the rotation of the humerus. (B) This hand grip is maintained as the patient initiates an upper body rolling pattern. (C) As he rolls onto his hemiplegic arm, the therapist's hands work together to assist scapula and humeral movement to prevent pain. (D & E) Therapist supports the back of the shoulder joint as the patient initiates the rolls. When he can roll without pain with her assistance, she teaches him how to hold and protect his arm.

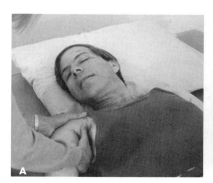

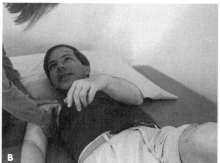

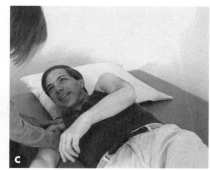

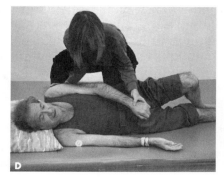

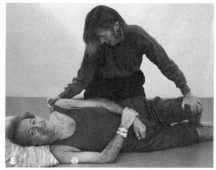

push forcefully into the bed, the pelvis lifts up but may not rotate forward. This strong extension pattern reinforces the spinal extension pattern not only in the lower trunk but causes overflow into the upper trunk as well, resulting in spinal extension but little rotation or rolling.

Inappropriate Spinal Flexion

Inappropriate spinal flexion occurs when the lower body initiates rolling, but strong flexion of the leg and trunk is activated instead of the pattern of spinal extension. Usually, both legs flex to roll to either side. Inappropriate spinal flexion also occurs when the patient initiates rolling from the upper body using flexion rotation, but he cannot vary or adjust muscle firing patterns to stop the flexion rotation pattern during transition. Since the patient cannot control the firing patterns, he rolls far forward "curled up into a ball."

UNDESIRABLE COMPENSATORY PATTERNS

Compensatory rolling patterns occur when the patient adopts a one-sided movement strategy resulting from severe weakness of the trunk, arm, and leg, or when there is an inability to control appropriate alignment of the upper and lower trunk because of loss of initiation or sequencing of muscle activation.

1. Grabbing and pulling with the unaffected arm. This compensation prevents developing control and strength in the trunk. While pulling on bedrails during the acute stage of illness is convenient, it does not teach the patient to use and strengthen available movement patterns that will be needed later in recovery (Fig. 11-13A & B).

2. Use of excessive hypertonicity in the arm and leg (Fig. 11-13C).

FIGURE 11-13 (*A & B*) Pulling to a sidelying position with the unaffected arm. (*C*) Patient attempts to roll to the good side by using strong flexor hypertonicity in the arm and extensor hypertonicity in the leg.

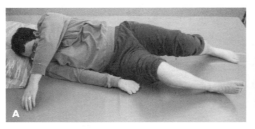
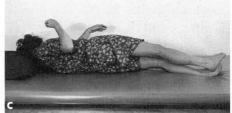
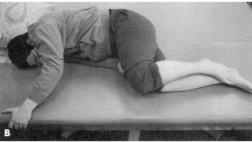

ASSESSMENT GUIDELINES

As the therapist begins an assessment, she may have the following thoughts as she answers the guideline questions. In supine, before rolling, is the patient's arm or leg posturing or stiff? Is the position of the head and trunk extremely asymmetric? Can she move the trunk and limbs into a more symmetric position and will they stay there? If not, are secondary problems of soft tissue, poor muscle tone, or joint stiffness present?

When the patient is asked to roll, how is the task performed? What normal components are present? Are there initiation patterns that the patient cannot perform? Can the hemiplegic limbs move appropriately with the trunk? Are the limbs active or do they assume an atypical posture? If the limbs posture during the roll, do the limbs stop posturing once the movement is complete?

I. Describe the preferred rolling initiation pattern; to the right and to the left.

II. Can the patient roll with each of the initiation patterns to the right? To the left?

III. What asymmetries or secondary problems do you observe during rolling?

IV. Can the patient roll to the hemiplegic side without shoulder pain? If pain is present, how is it relieved?

V. What improves when you put your hands on the trunk to correct asymmetries and to assist the trunk pattern?

VI. What improves when you put your hands on the arm or leg to correct asymmetries and allow the arm or leg to move with the trunk?

THERAPY GOALS

Functional Goals

Treatment to retrain the movements of rolling is necessary to help the patient meet the following functional goals:

1. Rolling to either side to allow bed mobility

2. Rolling to the sidelying position in preparation for sitting up on the side of the bed

3. Lying on the hemiplegic side safely without pain or fear

Treatment Goals and Techniques

Treatment goals appropriate for the task of rolling fall into three categories: reeducation of trunk movements and sequencing of trunk and limb movements, prevention of muscle shortening and joint alignment problems that may interfere with muscle reeducation or lead to asymmetric posturing, and establishment of balance control in sidelying.

Treatment Goal: To provide painfree arm movement during rolling. To provide a model of the movement components.

Treatment Technique: Establish sufficient muscle length between trunk and shoulder girdle to allow appropriate shoulder joint mechanics (Fig. 11-14). Additional treatment suggestions are included in Chapter 10.

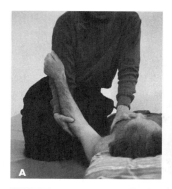
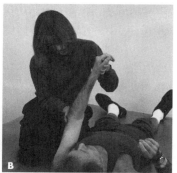
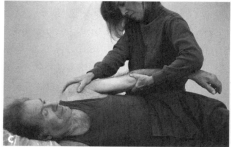
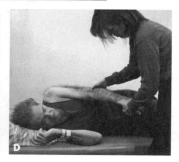
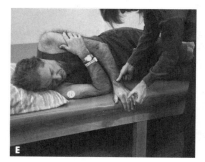

FIGURE 11-14 (*A*) Therapist's left hand stabilizes the lower rib cage as her right hand maintains humeral rotation and glenohumeral alignment while moving the humerus into 45 degrees flexion. (*B*) Therapist maintains glenohumeral joint integrity with her right hand while she moves her left hand to the patient's hand. With her left hand she controls forearm rotation and elbow position as she assists movement of the arm into more forward flexion in preparation for combining arm movement with the trunk rolling pattern. (*C*) In sidelying, the therapist holds glenohumeral joint alignment with her right hand, and her left hand holds the humerus in neutral rotation. In this position, she lengthens shortened shoulder elevators, pectorals, and biceps muscles. (*D & E*) Her right hand continues to support the shoulder joint, as her left hand helps the arm come across the body and make contact with the mat.

Treatment Goal: Reeducate nonsegmental rolling in patient with severe right hemiplegia and loss of trunk and arm control.

Treatment Technique: Early training of rolling: sensory preparation and guided movement (Fig. 11-15).

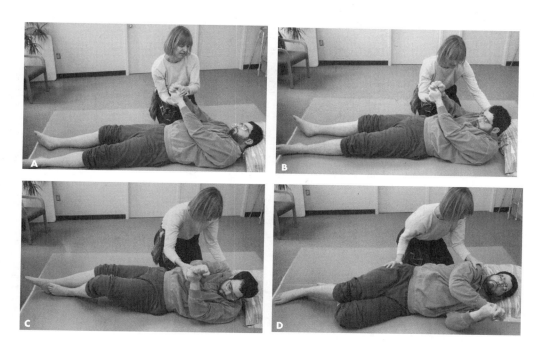

FIGURE 11-15 (*A*) Therapist asks patient to hold his right arm with his left arm to allow him to assist the upper trunk portion of the roll. (*B & C*) She asks him to activate a trunk flexor pattern by encouraging him to lift his head before he moves his trunk to the left. (*D*) With her right hand, the therapist assists the movement of the lower trunk as her left hand assists the movement of the upper trunk. Her left hand, on top of the shoulder girdle, prevents shoulder elevation, and her right hand, while rotating the pelvis to the left, delivers a downward message into the patient's left hip. Both hands stop the movement once the patient is in sidelying to help him learn to rest and balance on his hemiplegic side.

Treatment Goal: Reeducate lower-body-initiated rolling pattern.

Treatment Technique: Therapist teaches patient with a right hemiplegia to initiate rolling with a lower body extension rotation pattern (Fig. 11-16).

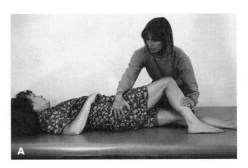

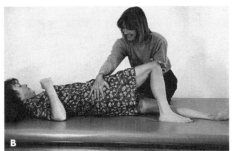

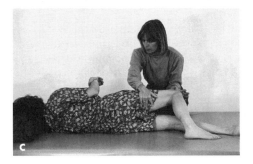

FIGURE 11-16 (*A*) The therapist's left hand directs a downward pressure into the foot to help stabilize the lower leg, while her right hand is over the back of the patient's hip joint. Her right hand and forearm assist pelvic rotation to the left. As the pelvis comes forward off the mat, the therapist's right hand delivers a downward message toward the left hip. (*B*) As the pelvis rotates further to the left, the therapist asks the patient to increase lower trunk extension rotation. The therapist helps reeducate leg strength and control by lessening her manual input on both the leg and trunk. (*C*) Therapist asks patient to rotate the upper body into sidelying as she assists the position of the leg.

Treatment Goal: Reeducate upper-body-initiated rolling pattern.

Treatment Technique: Hand placements to assist rolling (Fig. 11-17).

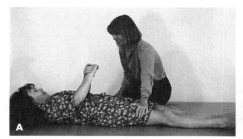
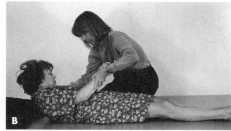
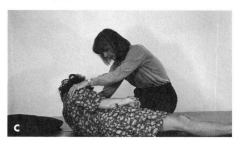

FIGURE 11-17 (*A*) Patient holds her affected right arm in preparation for practicing the trunk portion of upper-body-initiated rolling. (*B*) Therapist uses her left hand to guide the arms and assist the upper trunk as it moves up off the mat. Therapist's right hand is on the patient's left shoulder as a reminder to stay back behind the forward moving right shoulder. (*C*) The therapist moves her left hand to the patient's upper body to assist the rotation portion of the task. The patient tries to move her right arm with the trunk as it rotates.

Treatment Goal: Reestablish or maintain length in shoulder girdle and pelvic girdle musculature to prevent or eliminate the secondary problems of muscle shortening, poor joint alignment, or pain.

Treatment Technique: Shoulder mobilization followed by assisted movement (Fig. 11-18). Additional treatment suggestions are included in Chapter 10.

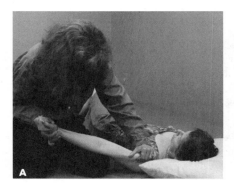
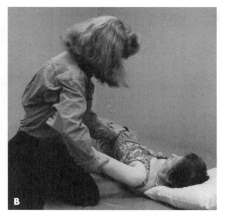

FIGURE 11-18 (*A*) Therapist's left hand is lengthening shortened pectoral and biceps muscles at the shoulder. As muscles at the shoulder lengthen, her right hand extends the elbow and/or externally rotates or abducts the arm. (*B*) Therapist supports the patient's forearm against her trunk while the right hand holds the patient's humerus. Therapist lengthens the latissimus and quadratus muscles. She stabilizes the upper body and arm with her right hand and uses her left hand to depress and rotate the pelvis.

Treatment Goal: Reeducate and strengthen leg and arm components.

Treatment Technique: Guiding and active assistive exercise (Fig. 11-19).

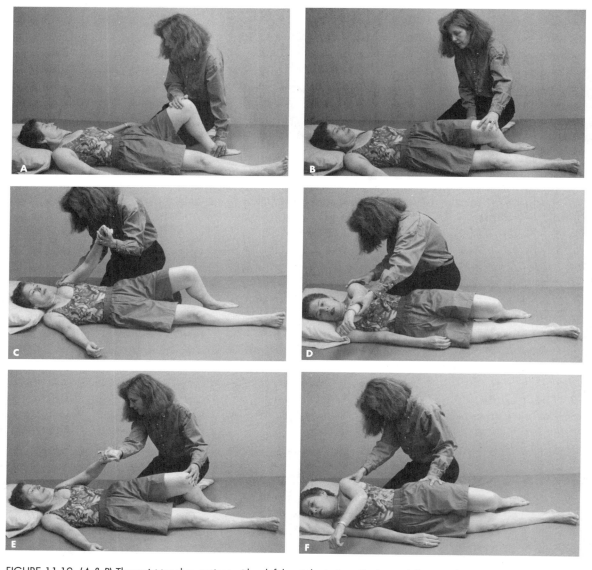

FIGURE 11-19 (*A & B*) Therapist teaches patient with a left hemiplegia to activate weak leg muscles to assist the rotation of the lower trunk. (*C & D*) Patient holds the leg position she has just practiced as the therapist helps her activate arm muscles that will allow her to move the arm across the body. Therapist's right hand corrects glenohumeral joint alignment, and her left hand teaches the patient's lower arm to initiate the movement. (*E & F*) As the patient activates shoulder and elbow muscles, the therapist moves both hands more distally. The patient initiates the trunk portion of the roll. The therapist is using minimal assistance to help the arm and leg as the patient initiates the activity and moves into sidelying.

Treatment Goal: Unassisted practice without using undesirable compensations.

Treatment Technique: Practice with verbal reminders (Fig. 11-20).

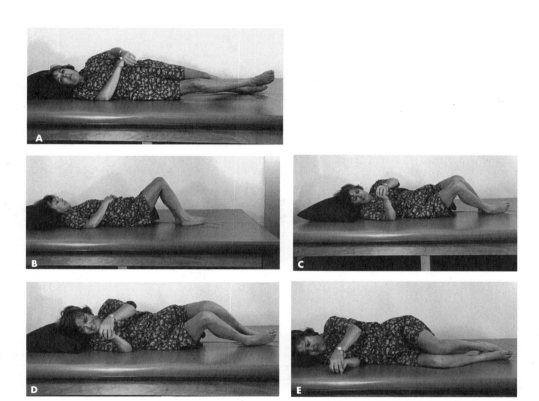

FIGURE 11-20 (*A*) Before treatment, patient with a right hemiplegia attempts to roll with incompatible trunk and extremity patterns. (*B–E*) Patient practicing rolling with verbal reminders, incorporating her hemiplegic side; she flexes both legs, supports her right arm to prevent it from getting caught underneath her, and uses a nonsegmental rolling pattern to roll onto her hemiplegic side.

Treatment Goal: Increase strength and control in trunk and limb muscles.

Treatment Technique: Independent practice (Fig. 11-21).

FIGURE 11-21 (*A & B*) Patient with a right hemiplegia is using the components of an upper-body-initiated rolling pattern to increase control of trunk flexion rotation patterns. She is increasing her ability to control her right arm as she rolls up and onto her forearm.

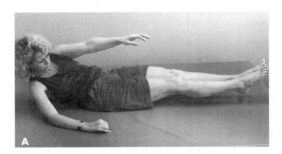

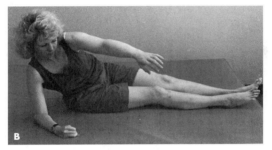

12

Sidelying to Sitting

CONCEPTS AND PRINCIPLES

The movements from sitting on the edge of a bed to moving into sidelying and the reverse, from lying on our side in bed to sitting up over the edge, are ones that we use several times each day. The available strategies from which we can choose can be identified and analyzed by the preferred trunk movement pattern. We may prefer one pattern over another because of our own body type, muscle strength, and our purpose or motivation for the movement. This is a movement in which the use of our extremities is critical. The arms are used to reinforce and assist the trunk patterns, and the legs need to be able to move on and off the bed with appropriate timing and strength. The timing of the movement of the legs on and off the bed is important to each of the strategies because the legs constitute a large percentage of total body weight, which influences the use of momentum, strength, and balance control throughout the task.

The movement of sidelying to sitting provides the transition from the supine or prone position to sitting. Transitional movements are difficult movements to relearn after a central nervous system insult because they require the coordination of control between the trunk and the extremities to maintain balance between two more stable positions—here, sitting and sidelying. In patients with hemiplegia, moving onto either side to get out of bed or back into bed is extremely difficult because of the need to combine movement patterns of the arm, leg, and trunk. Patients need to learn a strategy for moving between sitting and sidelying as part of regaining independence in daily life. Therapists use this position in treatment to increase trunk and extremity strength, to maintain muscle length and spinal mobility, and to train control between the trunk and extremities. This chapter analyzes the movement from sitting to sidelying to sitting with three trunk initiation patterns: upper trunk flexion rotation, lower trunk lateral flexion, and upper trunk lateral flexion.

MOVEMENT COMPONENTS
IN SITTING TO SIDELYING TO SITTING

Upper-Trunk-Initiated Flexion Rotation

Sitting to Sidelying

To lie down on the left side of the body using a flexion rotation pattern, we initiate the movement with the upper body (Fig. 12-1). The weight shift is on a forward diagonal over the left femur. The shoulders turn to the left, and both hands are

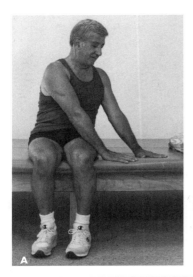
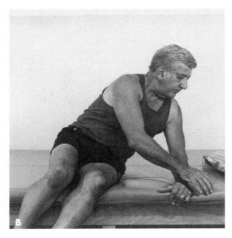
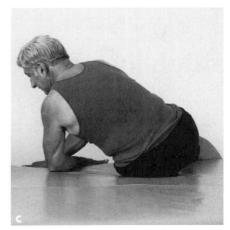
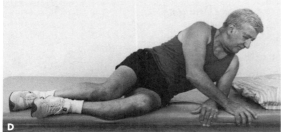
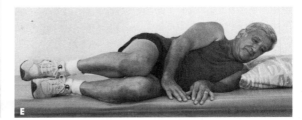

FIGURE 12-1 (*A–E*) Upper-trunk-initiated flexion rotation sitting to sidelying pattern.

placed down on the bed, lateral to the left thigh. This movement results in spinal flexion with vertebral rotation to the left. The right shoulder girdle and rib cage are rotated forward relative to the left shoulder. As weight shifts farther to the left, the left hip and thigh take more weight than the right, and the right arm supports more body weight than the left arm. As the trunk moves closer to the bed, the weight of the trunk is supported by the hands as a result of controlled elbow flexion (left greater than right). The elbows flex as the trunk moves down until the left elbow makes contact with the bed. The arms provide a balance assist for the trunk and leg movements. As both legs lift up onto the bed, the upper body rotates out of flexion rotation so that the right shoulder and rib cage are above the left shoulder and rib cage. As we complete the movement, the left shoulder moves back behind the left elbow as the trunk moves on a slight diagonal down to the bed. At the end of the movement, with the body in the sidelying position, the left arm is extended on the bed at an angle of 30 to 45 degrees to the body.

Sidelying to Sitting

To reverse this movement and move from sidelying to sitting with an upper-trunk-initiated flexion rotation pattern, the right hand and arm reach forward and up across the body to the side of the bed. The head and upper trunk follow the move-

---

Summary of Movement: Upper Trunk Flexion Rotation

Trunk
   Upper trunk flexion rotation to the left
Upper extremity
   Extended-arm weight bearing to forearm weight bearing; right arm more extended, left arm more flexed
Lower extremity
   Body weight taken on left hip and thigh

---

ment of the arm. This puts the spine in flexion with vertebral rotation to the left. As the upper trunk rotates, the left shoulder, elbow, and forearm gradually lift the trunk off the bed. At this transition point of the movement, the right shoulder girdle and rib cage are anterior to the left shoulder, and the left shoulder is above the left forearm. As weight shifts back onto the pelvis and thighs, both arms depress and push into the bed. The elbows and wrists extend. This active movement of the arms assists the movement and control of the trunk as it moves from flexion rotation into a sitting position. During this movement, the movement of the arms assists the weight transfer back from the left hip and thigh to the right hip and thigh until both legs are in contact with the bed. As the legs become the new base of support, the spine rotates from the left to neutral. At the end of the movement, the arms come off the bed as the upper body extends and balances over the lower body in the sitting position.

Lower Trunk Lateral Initiation/Extended Arm

Sitting to Sidelying

To lie down on the left side of the body using a lateral trunk movement pattern with extended arm, we initiate the movement with the lower trunk (Fig. 12-2). As weight shifts to the left, the left arm extends and moves to the bed, lateral to the left hip. The movement of the lower trunk results in lateral spinal flexion with the convexity of the spinal curve to the left. The right side of the pelvis elevates, and the left hip and thigh support more body weight. As the body continues to shift laterally, the demand for strength and control on the left pelvis and hip increases. The lateral movement of the trunk moves the left shoulder above the left hand. The left arm remains extended and reinforces the trunk pattern. At the transition point of the movement, strong coordinated muscle activity in the right lateral trunk and pelvic musculature provides stability so that both legs can lift up onto the bed. When the legs are supported on the bed, the trunk begins to move down. As the trunk moves out of lateral flexion, the left elbow flexes and assists the control of the body to the bed. The left forearm and left thigh accept more weight, and the right arm assists with balance control, if needed. At the completion of the movement, as the body moves back and down on a slight diagonal behind the left shoulder, the left elbow extends and rests on the bed.

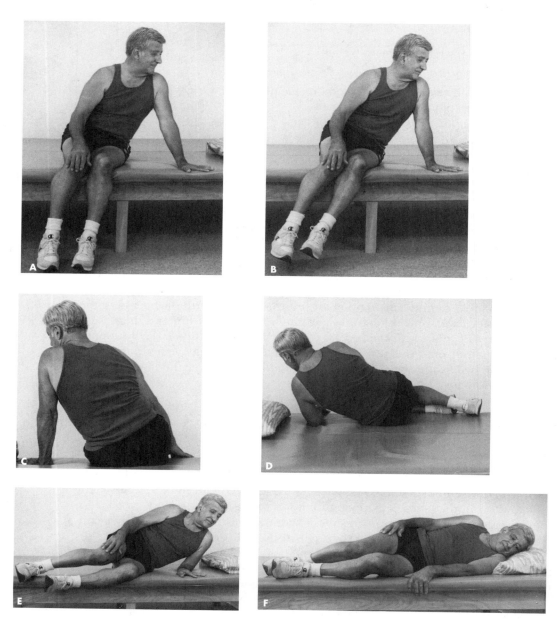

FIGURE 12-2 (A–F) Lower-trunk-initiated lateral flexion pattern to the left using support of the extended left arm.

Sidelying to Sitting

To reverse this movement and move from sidelying on the left to sitting using this pattern, the left forearm and shoulder push into the bed as the head and upper trunk lift up toward the right. This puts the spine in lateral flexion with the convexity to the left. At the initiation of this movement, the left arm is close to the body with the elbow slightly flexed. As the left arm assists the lift of the upper trunk off the bed, the shoulder moves over the elbow and the humerus becomes more abducted in relationship to the trunk. The left pelvis, hip, elbow, and forearm become the base of support. As both lower legs move off the side of the bed, the left arm extends and the trunk moves to 45 degrees of the vertical. The completion of the movement occurs as the right pelvis drops down and the hip and thigh come in contact with the bed. During this part of the movement, the spine moves from a position of lateral flexion to a neutral sitting position and weight shifts off the left hand.

Summary of Movement: Lower Trunk Lateral Initiation/Extended Arm

Trunk
   Lower trunk lateral flexion to the left/convexity on the left

Upper extremity
   Unilateral (left) extended-arm weight bearing to forearm weight bearing

Lower extremity
   Body weight taken on the left hip and thigh

Upper Trunk Lateral Initiation/Flexed Arm

Sitting to Sidelying

To lie down on the left side from sitting using an upper trunk lateral initiated pattern, the head, shoulder, and arm move down to the left, and the elbow flexes to accept weight (Fig. 12-3). The left shoulder is in abduction as the elbow and forearm are placed down on the bed near the left hip. This movement results in lateral flexion of the spine with the concavity of the curve on the left. The left forearm, hip, and thigh support the body weight. As the legs lift up onto the bed, the right side of the pelvis elevates and the left concavity of the spine changes to a neutral position. This allows the upper body to move down closer to the bed. While the legs lift up, the left shoulder also moves over the left elbow so that the position of the shoulder changes from abduction to adduction. At the completion of the movement, weight shifts from the left forearm onto the left shoulder and upper arm as the body balances in sidelying.

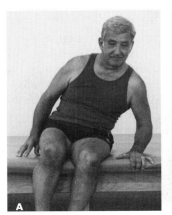
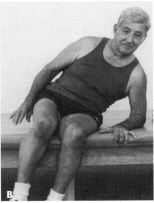
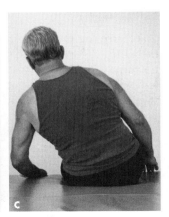

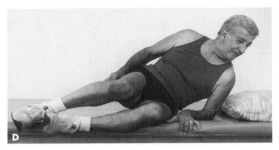

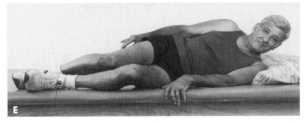

FIGURE 12-3 (A–E) Upper-trunk-initiated lateral sit to sidelying pattern using support of the flexed left arm.

Sidelying to Sitting

To return to a sitting position using this pattern, both lower legs move over the edge of the bed. The pelvis drops down on the right but does not make contact with the bed, and the left elbow and forearm push into the bed. This moves the spine into lateral flexion with the concavity on the left. As the left arm continues to push into the bed and extend, the concavity of the spinal curve increases. This shifts body weight to the right onto both hips and thighs. When the right side of the pelvis makes contact with the bed and the lower body is stable, the upper trunk moves up and laterally to the right until both shoulders are aligned over the lower body. This movement results in the spine moving from a position of lateral flexion to a neutral position in sitting.

Movement Summary: Upper Trunk Lateral Initiation/Flexed Arm

Trunk
  Upper trunk lateral flexion to the left/concavity on the left
Upper extremity
  Unilateral left forearm weight bearing;
Lower extremity
  Body weight taken on the left hip and thigh

SIGNIFICANT IMPAIRMENTS THAT INTERFERE WITH PERFORMANCE

Weakness in the Trunk and Extremities

Weakness and/or paralysis of the muscles of the trunk and extremities is a major cause of loss of ability to move from sitting to sidelying or sidelying to sitting. Severe weakness of the trunk muscles and loss of trunk movement patterns in sitting or supine results in an inability to recruit trunk patterns to initiate movement or to select the appropriate trunk pattern for a desired function. Weakness in the trunk makes it difficult for the patient to move onto and up over the affected side. And if the patient tries to sit up over the unaffected side, trunk weakness results in the affected side feeling heavy and unable to move forward and up. If trunk control is impaired, initiation of this movement in the three possible patterns is difficult or impossible to perform. Loss of trunk control results in the strong use of the uninvolved side to perform this task. The exclusive use of the uninvolved side may result in an inability to perform the task independently and, if allowed to persist, will make the reeducation of additional muscle strength more difficult. In early treatment, the therapist must help the patient learn to activate these weak trunk muscles in patterns that will allow him to perform the activity with more variety and less struggle. She must begin teaching the patient to incorporate the involved side by teaching him to use the appropriate trunk initiation pattern as he uses his uninvolved side to support body weight (Fig. 12-4). Reeducation of these trunk movement patterns can be begun in sitting or from sidelying. In sitting (see Ch. 5),

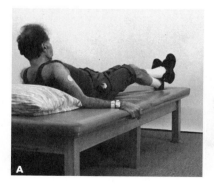 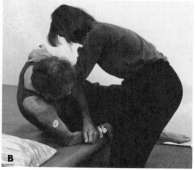

FIGURE 12-4 (*A*) Patient with left hemiplegia and severe loss of trunk control attempting to use uninvolved side to move to sitting. (*B*) Therapist assists patient by incorporating the hemiplegic left side into the movement pattern. Since the patient is using his right arm in a flexion pattern, the therapist is using her manual cuing to help the patient initiate with an upper-body lateral-initiated pattern (see Fig. 12-3).

trunk movement patterns can be strengthened with an emphasis on those that are needed for independence in any of the three possible sidelying/sit patterns.

The loss of trunk control influences the ability to use the extremities. In sitting to sidelying and vice versa, the arms and legs are used to assist and reinforce the trunk patterns. When the trunk is not active during arm or leg movements, or if the trunk and attempted extremity pattern are not compatible, the extremities cannot move freely and the patient will be required to use compensatory strategies. The loss of trunk control and resultant loss of balance may also result in arm or leg hypertonicity, as a balance response.

Weakness in the extremities results in an inability to use the arm to assist the trunk patterns and difficulty moving the legs on and off the bed. Weakness in the arm may decrease the ability of the trunk to perform the desired initiation pattern, either because of loss of assistance of the compatible components or because of poor alignment and increased heaviness of the arm. Weakness in the arm results in an inability to use the arm to follow and assist the trunk movements and to support body weight in either the forearm or extended-arm pattern. Since each of the patterns requires the use of one or both arms, the reeducation of extended and forearm upper extremity weight bearing movements, described in Chapter 7, must be trained in sitting and eventually combined with the accompanying trunk pattern throughout the movement of sidelying to sitting.

Weakness in the leg affects the ability of the hip and thigh to support body weight as the trunk shifts laterally or rotationally during these movements. In each movement pattern, one hip and thigh become the weight bearing point as the legs are moved on and off the bed. Strength in the flexors, extensors, abductors and adductors of the hip, knee, and ankle are needed in this weight acceptance and balance portion of the task. If leg strength is insufficient to support the trunk and balance, the patient may fall backwards and/or the leg may become stiff and spastic (Fig. 12-5). Strength in the entire leg, especially the lower leg, is also needed to lift the leg on and off the bed. When the foot and ankle muscles are weak or return is unbalanced, the foot may fall or push into plantarflexion. This heavy or stiff foot position often makes it harder to sequence the proximal muscles as the patient tries to lift his legs. In treatment, the therapist must address these distal problems along with any proximal leg problems before she helps the patient combine the trunk and extremity portion of the movement (Fig. 12-6).

When muscle weakness of the extremities is the cause of loss of functional ability, treatment can improve performance by reeducating and strengthening the needed extremity patterns. For this movement, reeducation and strengthening of weak extremity muscles should occur in both sitting and in sidelying and during the

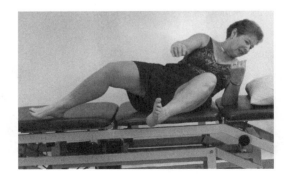

FIGURE 12-5 Patient with a left hemiplegia moving from sidelying to sitting over the affected side. Insufficient strength and control in the left hip contribute to her difficulty in moving forward.

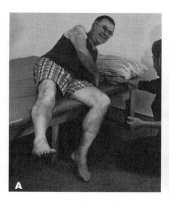
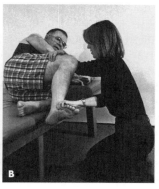

FIGURE 12-6 (*A*) Patient with a right leg weakness trying to lift his leg as he moves to sidelying. (*B*) Therapist assists patient as he attempts to activate weak leg muscles during the movement.

entire movement pattern to each side. In treatment, the therapist must assess both trunk and extremity strength and control to determine which pattern will be the easiest and most successful for the patient to perform. Then the specific weak or incomplete trunk patterns can be strengthened before sequencing of extremity and trunk control are practiced.

The trunk component of the upper body flexion rotation pattern can be taught, during early treatment, as the patient practices moving up over the unaffected side. The therapist assists the trunk pattern while the patient uses the uninvolved arm to lift the body up (Fig. 12-7A). As trunk control increases and the therapist begins to train weight bearing use of the hemiplegic arm and leg, the patient can practice rotating to the hemiplegic side. During treatment, the therapist should support the glenohumeral joint, prevent shoulder pain, and grade the amount of weight that the affected arm and leg control as the body moves up to sitting. The hemiplegic arm does not need to control full body weight since the stronger arm is in an advantageous position to assist during this initiation pattern (Fig. 12-7B).

FIGURE 12-7 (*A*) Therapist helps patient with a right hemiplegia learn an upper-body flexion-rotation–initiated pattern. The therapist's right hand is rotating the bottom of the right rib cage forward as her left hand introduces the flexion component of the movement. Both hands are directing a message down into the left hip as the patient moves up to sitting. (*B*) Therapist teaches patient to move up to sitting using an upper-body flexion-rotation–initiation pattern to the right. The therapist's right hand and forearm are supporting the upper trunk and glenohumeral joint to protect the joint and grade the amount of weight the patient can actively control with her right arm. The therapist's left hand is guiding the left shoulder forward in a flexion rotation pattern. Both hands are again directing a downward message into the patient's right hip as she moves up.

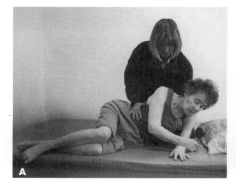
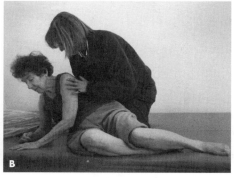

Therapists can reeducate the upper-trunk-initiated lateral pattern to the hemiplegic side in patients who have enough strength in their affected arm and leg to support and control body weight. This pattern is often performed with incorrect trunk and arm components. During an upper-body-initiated lateral weight shift, the elbow and forearm should move down towards the bed. The spinal pattern is lateral flexion with the concavity on the weight bearing side. When the trunk and arm pattern are incompatible, the arm postures, and the patient cannot balance and support body weight on the affected side (Fig. 12-8). The therapist assists the trunk and arm portion of the pattern during initiation, but during transition, when the legs must move up onto the bed, she moves one of her hands to assist the timing of the movement of the legs up onto the bed.

When patients use the lower-trunk-initiated lateral flexion pattern with an extended arm, they first choose to move onto their unaffected side and use the stronger arm to reinforce the trunk pattern. The difficult portion of the trunk movement for them will be to activate weak lateral trunk flexors concentrically on the hemiplegic side as the legs move up onto the bed. This requires strength and control of the lower trunk to stabilize the pelvis enough to allow the hemiplegic leg to initiate the lift of the legs onto the bed. The lower leg and foot must fire and sequence with the hip movement as the leg moves on or off the bed. This is a pattern that can be used in therapy to strengthen the trunk and hemiplegic leg in non-weight bearing movements.

If a goal of treatment is upper extremity movement control in extended-arm weight bearing, the therapist can chose the lower trunk lateral flexion/extended-arm pattern and have the patient move onto the hemiplegic side. She will assist the control of the supporting hemiplegic arm and hip to allow appropriate trunk and extremity patterns to be reeducated and decrease her handling as the patient's strength and control increase. This pattern requires strength and control on the

FIGURE 12-8 (A) Patient with right hemiplegia attempting to move down onto her hemiplegic arm with incompatible trunk/arm patterns; the concavity of the spinal curve should be on the right when the arm is flexed. (B) Therapist teaching patient to combine appropriate trunk and arm patterns. The therapist's right hand is on the patient's left shoulder, and her left hand is maintaining alignment of the humerus as both hands direct a message to the upper trunk to move down and to the right. (C) Therapist reeducating the shoulder, elbow, and forearm portion of the task. The therapist's left hand is under the axilla, and the back of her hand and forearm are resting against the upper trunk. This hand controls glenohumeral joint alignment and gives a message to the right rib cage to remain "tucked." Her right hand is pronating the forearm and stabilizing distally so that the patient may practice forearm weight bearing.

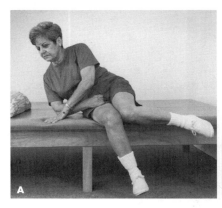
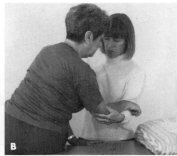
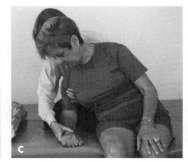

hemiplegic side and is a difficult pattern to relearn (see Fig. 12-11 wherein the patient attempts to perform lower-body-initiated pattern and loses the ability to control her right arm). Since this pattern is initiated from the lower body, if the patient is going to lie down onto the unaffected side, it is also used in treatment to increase pelvic and hip strength and control. If moving to the affected side, the hemiplegic hip and thigh must have enough stability to hold the position while the upper trunk and affected arm control the descent of the body.

In any of these patterns, if the patient's hemiplegic arm is weaker than his trunk, the therapist can support the glenohumeral joint, and the patient can independently practice the trunk movement. At the point in the movement when the legs must lift on or off, the therapist protects the shoulder joint with one hand and, with her other hand, assists the patient's practice of the leg movement.

Loss of Alignment of Trunk and Extremities

Loss of joint alignment in the trunk and extremities from prolonged weakness, loss of control, and shortened muscles significantly affects the ability to perform all three trunk initiation patterns and interferes with the ability to use the arm and leg.

In the trunk, loss of spinal alignment may result in neither symmetric nor asymmetric changes that affect the patient's ability to perform movement patterns. The symmetric problem, excessive flexion, is common in patients with severe weakness and loss of control. The asymmetric change, rotation or shearing of the spine and rib cage, makes it difficult to move completely into the sidelying position. It results in a pull-to-sit pattern and strong reliance on the uninvolved side (Fig. 12-9).

Any of these changes in alignment affect the initial starting position and the ability of the patient to strengthen weak muscles in any desired pattern. In treatment, when training any of these patterns, the therapist must try to manually correct the trunk asymmetries to increase the possibility of strengthening muscles. In the acute patient, correction of the trunk position may occur easily and result in activation of muscles. However, as time after injury increases, muscle shortening may restrict the mobility of the trunk, scapula, and pelvis. If this occurs, the muscle length problems will have to be treated before the reeducation process.

Upper extremity weight bearing in sitting (see Ch. 7) is frequently used to lengthen shortened muscle to correct trunk asymmetries and simultaneously activate and strengthen associated trunk patterns. Correction of the rotational asymmetries is performed with the therapist's hands on the ribs, using equal yet opposite manual pressure. To correct the lateral spinal asymmetries, the therapist uses one

FIGURE 12-9 Patient with left hemiplegia and severe weakness. Strong flexion across the lumbar spine and rotation backwards of the left rib cage makes it difficult for him to move into the sidelying position or move to sitting independently.

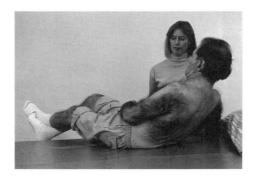

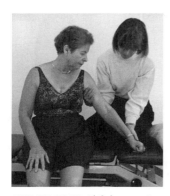

FIGURE 12-10 The therapist's right hand corrects humeral position, while her left hand pronates the forearm and assists with active elbow extension as the patient places her hand on the bed.

hand on the lateral aspect of the flared rib cage to tuck it in and the other hand under the opposite axilla to lengthen that side. When specific tightness is identified, the therapist lengthens the shortened muscle during the movement pattern.

Loss of alignment in the shoulder girdle and arm results in an inability to reach the arm down to the bed to assist the trunk. Correction of scapular position and glenohumeral subluxation must precede any attempts at training upper extremity weight bearing. As the joint is repositioned, the therapist assists the reeducation of either extended-arm or forearm weight bearing. The therapist corrects alignment and immediately asks for active arm or arm and trunk movement into or out of sitting to use the new muscle length and to strengthen weakness (Fig. 12-10).

Alignment problems of the lower trunk and leg can be assessed as the body moves over one hip. As body weight shifts to one side, tight pelvic or hip muscles cause the leg to slide into adduction or the pelvis to spin forwards or backwards (Fig. 12-11). To lengthen these muscles during the activity, the therapist stabilizes the thigh and pelvis or trunk and pelvis as she asks the patient to perform portions of the movement that will specifically and slowly stretch tightness. If multiple muscles are shortened, the therapist may have to use supine or sitting to lengthen each muscle systematically in preparation for movement reeducation. It is important to remember that the large multijoint muscles of the lower trunk and thigh (latissimus, quadratus, tensor fascia lata, hamstrings) shorten quickly if the patient does not regain the ability stand and walk or if he remains in a wheelchair for more than a few weeks.

Inability to Accept Weight on Extremities

The inability to accept weight on the arm or the leg results from a combination of weakness, loss of control, and poor joint alignment.

All three sitting to sidelying patterns can be used in treatment to introduce weight transfer onto the hemiplegic hip when the patient has enough strength and balance control in the trunk, pelvis, and hip to maintain appropriate alignment during the activity. It is common to see the trunk pattern initiated or assisted appropriately, but at the point in the movement when weight is taken on the hemiplegic hip, the patient's pelvis spins or the trunk shears to the stronger side.

FIGURE 12-11 Patient with right hemiplegia moving from sidelying to sitting. Her right leg slides into adduction as weight is placed on her right hip and the accompanying stretch exceeds the limit of tight pelvic and hip muscles.

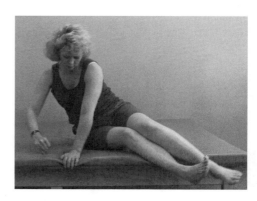

The upper body flexion rotation pattern and the upper body lateral flexion patterns are good to use when initially teaching the patient to lie down toward the hemiplegic side. With the flexion rotation patterns, the more extended outside arm (the stronger arm) assists the trunk with the body movement so the therapist can assist with the leg demands. The patient can grade the amount of weight placed on the hemiplegic arm, and if necessary only place minimal demands on it (see Fig. 12-16D). The upper body lateral flexion pattern gradually lowers the upper trunk over the affected side and allows the patient to practice supporting weight with a flexed arm. This pattern allows the patient and therapist to grade the trunk movement according to the patient's ability to use and balance over the affected arm and leg (see Fig. 12-17B).

Hypertonicity of the Extremities

Hypertonicity in the affected arm and leg interferes with the performance of all of the sit-sidelying-sit patterns because each initiation pattern requires the use of the arm and leg in combination with the trunk. Both flexor and extensor hypertonicity in the arm are common impairments during sitting to sidelying movements. Flexor and extensor hypertonicity prevent the arm from actively and appropriately supporting body weight in either forearm or extended-arm weight bearing. When the arm is stiff, either in flexion or extension, the arm cannot move to assist trunk movements. If the patient tries to force weight on the flexed elbow and forearm or if a tight muscle is additionally stretched, the arm may internally rotate and extend, resulting in a loss of balance control. In some patients in whom the arm hypertonicity is due to a severe loss of alignment and loss of control at the shoulder girdle, the arm extends and internally rotates, resulting in an inability to use the arm for support (Fig. 12-12).

Flexor posturing of the arm is often observed as the patient initiates the movement into or out of sitting. This hypertonicity in the arm may be a result of weakness and poor trunk control. The flexor muscles are recruited to assist the attempted trunk movement. If this is the case, the hypertonicity in the arm will be immediately decreased if the therapist stabilizes the lower trunk and strengthens or assists the active recruitment of trunk muscles (Fig. 12-13). If the posturing occurs during the transition point of the movement, it may be occurring as a balance reaction.

Hypertonicity in the leg manifests itself as body weight is shifted to the hemiplegic leg. This hypertonicity may be due to tight hip muscles. If asymmetries in the hemiplegic hip exist as a result of tight or shifted thigh muscles, as weight is trans-

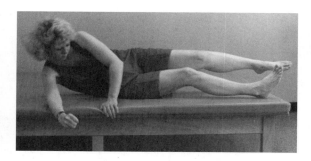

FIGURE 12-12 Patient attempts to use her right arm for support. As her hand slips out from under her shoulder, she is unable to use it to assist the trunk movement and loses her balance.

FIGURE 12-13 (A) Patient attempts to move up off the bed. Her left arm has flexor hypertonicity as she recruits muscles to assist the trunk pattern. (B) Therapist helps patient use her left leg to stabilize her lower trunk and assists the patient to activate trunk flexors. Note the decrease in arm flexor hypertonicity.

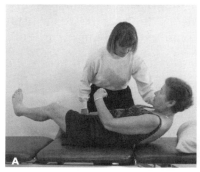
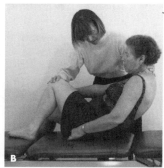

ferred to the hip and the limit of the tight muscles is reached, the leg will posture in extension, or if trunk control is poor, the leg will posture in an extensor pattern as it tries to assist the trunk movement (see Fig. 12-13A). Hypertonicity in the leg is also found when the body is in transition between sidelying and sitting and the legs move up on or off the bed. As the patient attempts to move the leg, abnormal patterns of muscle activation or incomplete muscle recruitment results in either extension or flexor hypertonicity (see Fig. 12-18A).

Treatment of these patterns of hypertonicity is selected according to the presumed cause. If hypertonicity is a result of poor alignment, the therapist corrects the alignment and asks for the pattern of movement again; if the hypertonicity results from a loss of balance as a result of poor trunk control, the therapist's hands move to the trunk to provide assistance to the trunk movements, and she spends a portion of the treatment time reeducating trunk control (Fig. 12-14). If the increase in tension is related to excessive or abnormal patterns of muscle activity, the hypertonicity is lessened by active assistive and active movements to change patterns of muscle firing or by reeducation of weak or missing muscle patterns. When the therapist treats the correct cause of the posturing, the hypertonicity decreases immediately in treatment.

UNDESIRABLE COMPENSATORY PATTERNS

The most common abnormal pattern in patients with hemiplegia is the tendency to sit straight up and to use the unaffected arm to pull the body up out of bed. During this movement, the legs tend to fly up off the bed. As the legs lift up, body weight shifts back onto the pelvis and makes the trunk movement more difficult. The arm

FIGURE 12-14 (A) Patient with poor trunk control struggles to sit up. As she tries to pull herself up with her left arm, her right arm and leg posture. (B) Therapist helps patient use her trunk appropriately. Note the decreased hypertonicity in the right arm and leg.

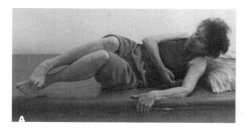
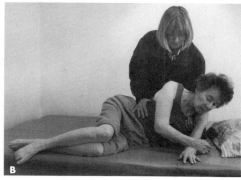

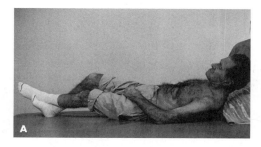

FIGURE 12-15 (A) Patient with severe left hemiplegia starting to move to sitting by tucking his right leg under the left leg. (B) Patient pulls on the edge of the bed with his right arm and uses a strong total flexor pattern to lift his upper body and bring his legs over the edge of the bed. (C) Patient is unable to bring himself to sitting. Note the inability to recruit sufficient spinal extension and to move his hemiplegic side forward.

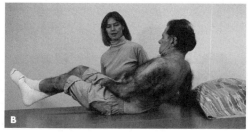

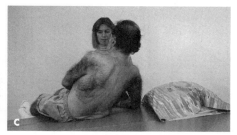

may posture in flexion as a result of loss of balance and excessive recruitment. When half way through the sit, the patient pivots over the unaffected leg and arm as he passively lifts the affected leg off the bed (Fig. 12-15).

ASSESSMENT GUIDELINES

Assessment of sitting to sidelying to sitting should be started by asking the patient to lie down to either side. As he attempts the movement, the therapist should note the following to gather appropriate information.

I. Describe the trunk pattern used as the patient lies down to the right/to the left.

II. Describe the ability to use the hemiplegic upper extremity. Is the upper extremity pattern compatible with the trunk pattern?

III. Describe the ability to lift the legs onto the bed. Can he lift the hemiplegic leg independently? What pattern/muscles are used?

IV. Does the hemiplegic arm or leg posture during the movement? If so, when? Does it posture because of poor alignment, poor trunk control, or active recruitment to assist the movement?

V. If you assist the trunk pattern, can the patient use the affected arm more appropriately? If you assist the trunk pattern, does the hypertonicity, if present, decrease?

VI. Are there asymmetries in the hemiplegic arm and/or leg? If you correct the alignment problems, does the strength or control of the arm or leg movement improve? How?

THERAPY GOALS

Functional Goals

The functional goal for the task of moving from sitting to sidelying and the reverse, sidelying to sitting, is to perform the movement independently with as much use of the affected side as possible. The movement is trained toward the affected side to help the patient gain the strength and control to accept weight and support movement of the body with the hemiplegic arm and leg. While patients learn to move to the unaffected side without as much training, they need to learn how to use their hemiplegic side as much as possible during the activity to maximize their potential for strength and control and to minimize the development of secondary impairments.

1. To move from sitting to sidelying to sitting to either side independently
2. To use the involved arm and leg to assist the movement to either side

Treatment Goals and Techniques

Treatment Goal: Reeducate and strengthen the trunk component of the activity

Treatment Technique: Upper-trunk-initiated flexion rotation sitting to sidelying pattern (Fig. 12-16A–E).

Treatment Technique: Decrease manual assistance to allow independent practice (Fig. 12-16F–H).

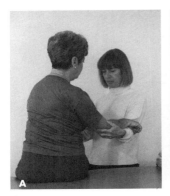 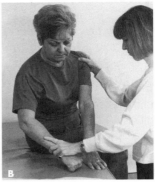

FIGURE 12-16 (*A*) Therapist uses a bilateral symmetric arm grip to teach the patient upper trunk rotation movement components. Her left hand supports the hemiplegic arm giving a message to the right upper quadrant to move back while her right hand on the patient's humerus is giving a message to the left upper quadrant to move forward. The therapist is careful not to shift the upper trunk forward but tries to teach the patient to rotate the upper trunk over the stable lower body. (*B*) Therapist's right hand helps the patient keep the upper trunk rotation while she moves her left hand down to the bed. This movement of the arms down to the mat introduces trunk flexion. The therapist's left hand assists this trunk flexion component as she helps the patient's right hand make contact. Note: During the upper body flexion rotation pattern, the front arm assists the trunk pattern even if the back arm cannot participate equally in the movement. *(Figure continues)*

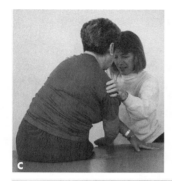
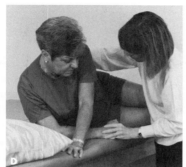
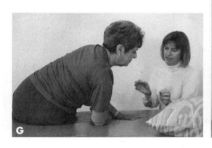
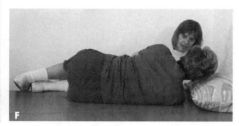
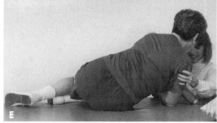
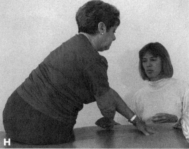

FIGURE 12-16 (*Continued*) (*C*) The therapist's hands continue to assist the rotation of the upper body while the patient practices combining the arm components with the trunk pattern. (*D*) Patient practices moving her trunk out of the flexion rotation pattern to a neutral sidelying position. The therapist's right hand is on the back of the upper trunk guiding the body into a neutral spinal position as the patient moves her legs up to the bed. (*E*) Patient continues to move her body down into sidelying. The therapist's left hand is controlling the right humerus to prevent atypical joint mechanics as the patient lies down onto her hemiplegic side. The therapist's right hand on the patient's left shoulder directs a diagonal message into the patient's right hip to assist the movement of the pelvis and lower trunk as the patient lies down. (*F–H*) Therapist uses verbal reminders to help the patient practice initiating sidelying to sitting with upper trunk flexion rotation. The patient uses her left arm to stabilize the trunk pattern and uses her hemiplegic right arm in forearm weight bearing during the first stage of the movement sequence.

Treatment Goal: Combine reeducation of active use of arm and trunk components during sitting to sidelying.

Treatment Technique: Reduce subluxation, protect glenohumeral joint, and teach weight bearing use of hemiplegic arm while training active trunk patterns in patient with right hemiplegia and weakness of trunk, arm, and leg (Fig. 12-17A–C).

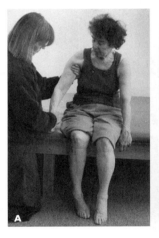
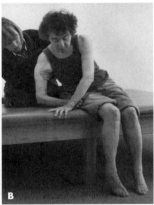
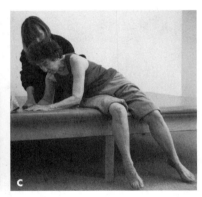

FIGURE 12-17 (*A*) Therapist uses her left hand to maintain alignment and support the glenohumeral joint while her right hand helps pronate the forearm and slowly extend the elbow as the patient's hand moves to the mat. (*B*) Therapist's left hand continues to protect and support the glenohumeral joint as her right hand on the patient's right lower rib cage assists lateral flexion of the trunk as the patient initiates an upper body lateral movement pattern. As the right side of the patient's trunk shortens, the therapist's right hand directs a message down into the right hip as her left hand moves the patient's upper body laterally and down over the flexing elbow. (*C*) Patient moves her left shoulder forward and down as the therapist's left hand supports the glenohumeral joint and grades an appropriate amount of weight onto the hemiplegic arm as she assists the rotation backward of the right upper trunk. The therapist's left forearm is against the patient's right rib cage. Her forearm can guide the movement of the upper body over the right hip and pelvis as increased weight is accepted on the right hip and thigh. (*Figure continues.*)

Treatment Technique: Therapist supports the glenohumeral joint as she reeducates active use of the hemiplegic right arm with a lower-trunk-initiated extension rotation trunk pattern (Fig. 12-17D & E).

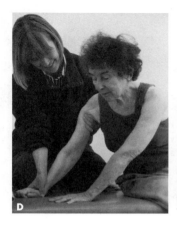
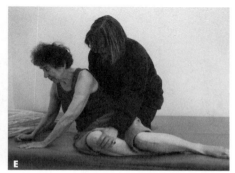

FIGURE 12-17 (*Continued*) (*D*) The therapist's righthand thumb and index finger stabilize the distal portion of the radius as the patient weight bears on a fisted hand. The hand is fisted to preserve the palmar arches since she does not have sufficient length of the long finger muscles across the wrist to allow open-handed weight bearing without severe compensation. As the patient moves from forearm weight bearing to extended-arm weight bearing, she moves her trunk from flexion rotation to more extension rotation. The therapist's right hand assists pronation of the forearm as her left hand moves the shoulder up and back. The patient depresses into the bed with her right arm and extends her elbow as she moves her body up and back into more extension. (*E*) As the patient learns how to control the arm movements, the therapist moves her hands so that her right hand now assists the upper trunk rotation and protects the glenohumeral joint, and her left hand directs a message back through the femur toward the hip joint to help the patient move over her right hip.

Treatment Goal: Reeducate and strengthen leg components

Treatment Technique: Train distal initiation, combine distal and proximal leg movement sequences, teach timing of leg movements with trunk movement pattern (Fig. 12-18).

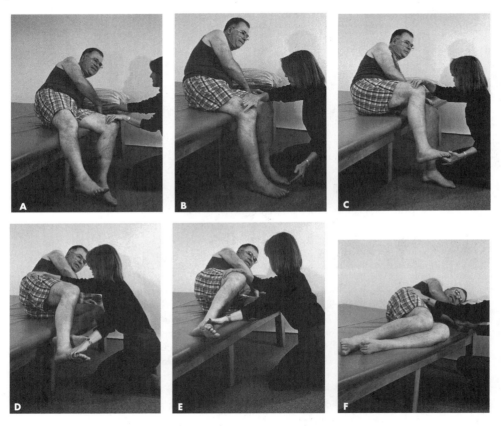

FIGURE 12-18 (A) Patient with a right hemiplegia using active knee extension to try to lift his right leg up onto the mat as he moves to sidelying. He initiated the pattern with an upper trunk lateral movement, but as he tries to lift his leg, his leg abducts and his right trunk rotates back. (B & C) Therapist helps him keep his thigh from abducting and encourages him to lift his foot and knee up off the surface. Note how his trunk is more active and his right arm postures less. (D–F) Therapist's right hand is over the right hip assisting the lateral movement of the pelvis and preventing the pelvis from rotating back as the patient controls his thigh and lower leg. The patient lifts his legs onto the bed as the therapist prevents the leg from abducting.

Treatment Goal: Reeducate trunk and arm components to allow independent practice.

Treatment Technique: Teach patient to practice trunk components, arm and leg movements, and to combine trunk and limb movements (Fig. 12-19).

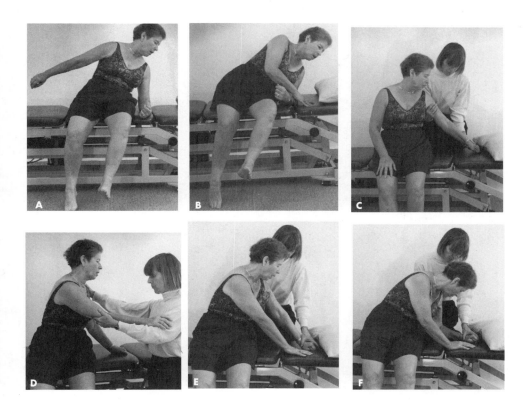

FIGURE 12-19 (*A & B*) Patient with a left hemiplegia moving to sidelying. As she moves onto her right side, the trunk and limb components are not compatible; her right arm and leg posture. (*C*) Therapist lengthens shortened forearm and elbow tissues as patient practices extended-arm lateral weight bearing. (*D*) Therapist practices upper trunk flexion rotation movements with patient. The patient maintains left extended-arm weight bearing as the body rotates over the left arm. (*E & F*) Patient practices moving her trunk with the arms as her arms move from extended-arm weight bearing to forearm weight bearing. Therapist assists the arm portion of the movement because it is the more difficult component for the patient to control.   (*Figure continues*)

FIGURE 12-19 (*Continued*)
(*G & H*) Therapist decreases her
manual guidance as the patient
practices placing her hemiplegic
hand on the support and initiates
compatible trunk movement. The
therapist chooses which component needs a "reminder" as
patient moves to independent
practice. (*I–K*) Patient practices
the movement sequence independently.

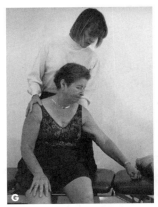
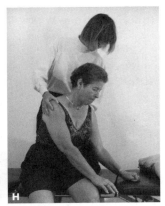
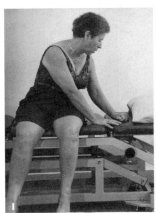
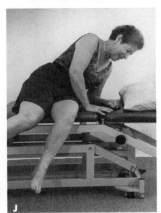
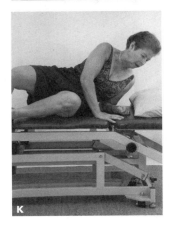

13
Sit to Stand

CONCEPTS AND PRINCIPLES

To stand up from a sitting position, we must have trunk control, lower extremity strength, and dynamic balance. Critical components of this task include the ability to control the upper trunk over the lower trunk during anterior/posterior weight shifts, to maintain both feet in contact with the floor, and to produce extension power in the legs. The ability to stand up from a sitting position—sit to stand—marks the beginning of movement in an erect posture. From standing we can transfer to chairs or other seats, we can begin to walk and eventually run, and we can "reach higher" into our environment.

In patients with central nervous system (CNS) dysfunction, moving from sitting on the edge of the hospital bed into a chair is usually their first attempt to stand. The loss of trunk and extremity control makes it difficult for them to move from sitting into standing. They may not have enough strength in the hemiplegic leg, their leg or arm may stiffen or posture, and they may lose their balance and be afraid of falling.

Weakness, posturing, and poor alignment of the upper extremity on the upper trunk significantly influence the ability to control the upper trunk over the lower trunk during sit to stand and create an abnormal starting position for the movement. Treatment of the upper extremity as a preparation for this movement must be included in goal setting and sit-to-stand training, when upper extremity problems interfere with normal movement components.

The task of retraining the movement of sit to stand in patients with hemiplegia requires the reestablishment of trunk movement components, sufficient control to combine trunk movements with extremity movements, and an ability to minimize common secondary impairments that interfere with the development of trunk and extremity control. The practice of sit to stand in patients who can stand up but rely heavily on the use of the uninvolved side is used to decrease undesirable compensations, to improve movement deficits, and to prevent further secondary impairments.

Kinesiology

The movement goal of sit to stand is to change the center of gravity from an area defined by our hips, thighs, and feet to an area defined only by our feet.

During sit to stand, *initiation* is defined as the movement that occurs from the sitting position to the point where the hips leave the support. Initiation is the movement of the trunk forward over the legs and feet. During initiation, our center of gravity is over a large base of support and is relatively close to that base.

Transition is defined as the period when the hips leave the support and the body moves up over the feet. At this point in the movement sequence, the trunk moves up and back as the pelvis continues to move forward over the feet. The difficulties in transition result from the fact that lower extremity strength and power are required to lift the body from the support, and balance control is needed to move the center of gravity from behind the new base of support to a position over the new base.

Completion of sit to stand is defined as the final movement of the trunk back over the feet and the final movement of the pelvis that occurs to establish midline and maintain balance in the standing position. At completion, the base of support (the feet) is small and the center of gravity is high above the base.

In normal sit to stand, there are three different trunk movement strategies for accomplishing the task. These strategies result in three sit to stand initiation patterns: lower trunk initiation (upper trunk aligned over lower trunk); lower trunk/pelvic initiation (trunk extension); upper trunk initiation (trunk flexion). These strategies exist because of differences in length of body segments, differences in strength, and differences in muscle length and joint range. Efficiency of movement and body structure dictate the trunk pattern we choose. Additionally, individual variations can occur in foot placement, starting position of the trunk, arms and feet, performance speed, and the amount of force produced or the amount of momentum used, but all individuals initiate the task with one of the three strategies.

SIT TO STAND MOVEMENT COMPONENTS

Lower Trunk Initiation

During lower trunk initiation (Fig. 13-1), the upper trunk remains aligned over the lower trunk with the spine in a neutral position. The upper trunk, lower trunk, and pelvis incline forward so that the hips flex and the shoulders move in front of the hips. The hips are the fulcrum of the trunk movement, and weight is evenly distributed over both femurs and feet. The balance demands are minimal since the center of gravity is still within the base of support.

FIGURE 13-1 *(A–D)* Lower trunk initiated sit to stand pattern.

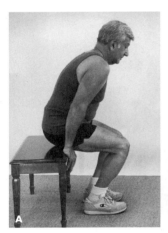 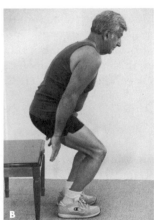 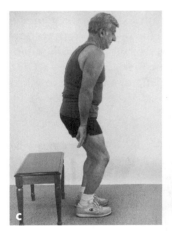 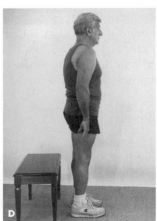

During early transition, the trunk and pelvis move forward and up on a diagonal, the hips begin to extend, and the thighs leave the supporting surface. The ankles continue to dorsiflex as the knees and lower leg move forward. The head remains in neutral during transition, and the eyes are oriented horizontally to the environment. The shoulder and upper trunk are anterior to the hips and the spine is in a neutral position as the hips begin to leave the surface. This is a difficult phase of the movement because the center of gravity is behind the feet, and both lower extremities need to produce extension power to allow the body to move symmetrically forward and up over the feet. Some individuals use the arms or momentum of the trunk to assist in the initiation and transition phases of this pattern.

In late transition, the hips, knees, and ankles continue to extend to allow erect standing, but the arc of trunk movement changes from one of a forward diagonal to a posterior diagonal as the upper body moves back up and over the feet. The upper trunk moves up and back over the feet at the same time as the hips and knees extend and move anteriorly. This counterbalancing of the trunk and the lower extremities allows the body to come to the full standing position. At the completion of the movement, the body "sways" or shifts to balance over the new base of support.

Lower Trunk/Pelvic Initiation

In contrast to the above pattern in which the spine is in neutral, this strategy, a variation of lower trunk initiation, places the lumbar spine in more extension. During a lower trunk pelvic-initiated sit to stand (Fig. 13-2), the lumbar spine extends, the trunk inclines forward so that the hips flex, and the shoulders and upper trunk are anterior to the hips. Strong extension in the lumbar spine is accompanied by an anterior pelvic tilt, resulting in less upper body forward inclination than in the first pattern.

During transition, the arc of forward trunk movement is smaller than in lower trunk initiation. The arc of upper trunk movement posteriorly is also less. Since the

FIGURE 13-2 (A–D) Pelvis-initiated sit to stand pattern.

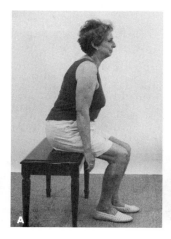
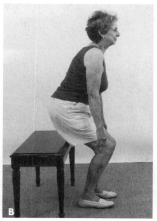
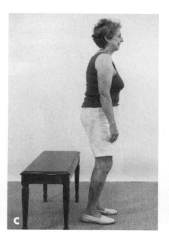
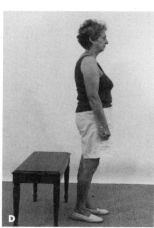

arc of trunk movement is decreased, the demand on the hips and legs to produce extension power to stand is greater than in the lower trunk strategy. At completion, body sway is present to balance the body in midline.

The major difference in this strategy is the lower spine extension, the corresponding decrease in forward inclination of the trunk, and the increased need for strength in the lower extremities.

Upper Trunk Initiation

The upper trunk initiation strategy (Fig. 13-3) differs from the other two strategies because the thoracic spine is in flexion during initiation and transition phases. During the initiation phase of the upper body strategy, the upper trunk flexes forward and down over the thighs and the hips flex. This movement places the head and shoulders over the knees so that the eyes are oriented down to the ground and places the center of mass of the body lower and closer to the feet. With this pattern, the arms are frequently used to push (into the thighs or onto chair arms) to assist the trunk and the extension movements of the legs.

In early transition, the hips extend and rise up from the surface and the thoracic spine remains in flexion with the shoulders anterior to the knees. This strategy uses the forward position of the upper body as a counterbalance to the pelvis, the location of the center of gravity. As the upper body moves forward and down, the hips lift up. During late transition, more strength and power are required to extend the hips, knees, and ankles because the upper body weight is forward of the feet. Additional trunk extension control is needed to move the upper trunk from its flexed forward position back up over the extending hips and knees.

At the completion of the movement, anterior/posterior body sway may be greater than in lower-trunk-initiated patterns to counterbalance the range of upper body movement forward at initiation. The major difference in the upper trunk strategy is the pattern of spinal flexion during initiation and early transition and the subsequent trunk extension control required to move the spine from flexion to an erect, neutral position for standing.

FIGURE 13-3 (A–C) Upper body initiation strategy.

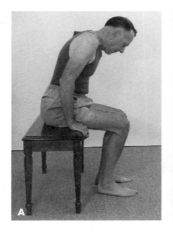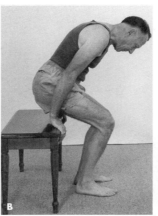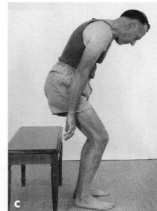

Movement Summary: Sit to Stand

Task

Move from sitting with a wide base of support and low center of gravity to standing with a small base of support and high center of gravity.

Beginning position

Sitting, upper trunk controlled over lower trunk, hips, knees in flexion, ankles in slight dorsiflexion.

Initiation

Trunk forward inclination with hip flexion.

Transition (early)

Hips leave supporting surface, ankles dorsiflex maximally, trunk continues to incline and move forward.

Transition (late)

Hips, knees, ankles extend, trunk moves posteriorly to return to an erect position.

Completion

Body balances in standing position.

SIGNIFICANT IMPAIRMENTS THAT INTERFERE WITH PERFORMANCE

Loss of Trunk Control and Alignment

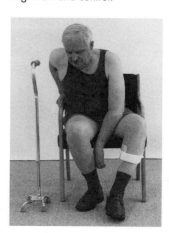

FIGURE 13-4 Arm weakness contributes to loss of upper trunk alignment and control.

Trunk asymmetry during sit to stand may come from any of the causes noted in Chapter 5: loss of alignment of the upper trunk over the lower trunk, pelvic and hip joint asymmetry, and the weight of a weak arm (Fig. 13-4). Patients who have trunk weakness and minimal balanced motor return have difficulty maintaining alignment of the upper trunk over the lower trunk in sitting. Their bodies quickly become poorly aligned because of this lack of postural control and weakness. In the sitting position, there can be excessive flexion of the thoracic spine, and/or rib cage rotation, lateral spinal curvatures with the concavity of the curve on the weaker side, or the convexity of the curve on the weaker side. When the upper extremity is weak, the dependent position of the arm reinforces upper trunk flexion and rotation. Poor control of the upper trunk makes it difficult for the lower trunk and extremities to initiate and control the weight shift and to produce the power and control in the legs that are necessary to stand.

During treatment of sit to stand, upper body asymmetry should be corrected and maintained, manually if necessary, to allow lower trunk and lower extremity initia-

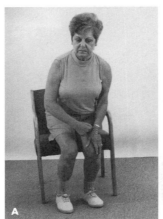
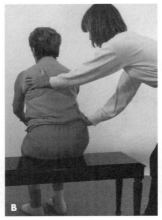
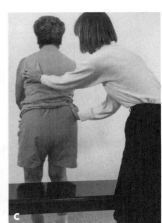

FIGURE 13-5 (A) Upper body shearing to the left with rib cage rotation. (B & C) Therapist corrects upper body shearing by using her left hand to move the upper body to midline while her right hand is used as counterpressure and stabilizes the lower rib cage and pelvis while the patient moves from sit to stand.

FIGURE 13-6 Excessive use of the right arm and leg to rise to standing results in inappropriate lateral trunk weight shift, trunk rotation, and decreased use of the left leg.

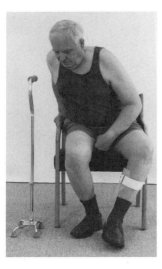

tion and transition patterns to be actively reeducated and to prevent further compensations (Fig. 13-5). Upper trunk reeducation should focus on increasing control of thoracic extension and correcting the rotational asymmetries necessary to increase upper body stability in both sitting and standing.

The inability of the body to control the weight of the weak, dependent upper extremity results in abnormal scapula positioning (scapular downward rotation and abduction) and poor rib cage alignment in sitting. These asymmetries result in an atypical trunk position throughout the movement and an uneven distribution of weight on the lower extremities. Therefore, the weight of the arm must be supported to correct the scapular and upper trunk alignment and allow proper lower extremity activity.

If the loss of trunk control and strength results in the rib cage on the involved/weaker side moving backwards, asymmetries between the rib cage and pelvis will result in difficulty using the hemiplegic leg during sit to stand. During the stand, this rotation will influence the upper extremity on the affected side. Often, the upper arm moves into internal rotation and hyperextension, and the elbow flexes with forearm supination. If the patient uses his uninvolved arm to assist the sit to stand, the initial weight shift is often lateral (to the uninvolved side) instead of anterior, resulting in decreased use of the involved leg. Trunk rotation is exaggerated by the exclusive use of one side of the body (Fig. 13-6).

At the completion phase, standing balance is difficult to control because the rotational asymmetry keeps the body's weight balanced over just one leg. Rotational disturbances in the spine, rib cage, and pelvis on the involved side eventually influence foot alignment and control, making it even more difficult to balance in standing (Fig. 13-7).

FIGURE 13-7 Loss of trunk alignment and poor control of the hemiplegic leg results in difficulty balancing as the patient moves to standing. The patient has kept all her weight on her uninvolved leg as she initiated the movement.

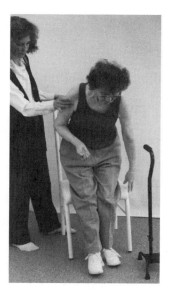

Inefficient Trunk Initiation Patterns

Lower trunk initiation patterns are difficult for patients with hemiplegia to perform because they require that the upper trunk remain aligned over the lower trunk as the body moves forward over the feet. Patients with weak trunk and lower extremity muscles do not have enough upper body control to maintain the alignment of the upper trunk over the lower trunk and initiate movement from the lower trunk.

Lower-trunk-initiated movements require shoulder girdle stability to maintain the position of the upper extremity on the rib cage (upper trunk) throughout the activity. The weight of the weak arm is significant, and because the arm easily moves in front of the body during sit to stand, it reinforces the tendency of the upper trunk to rotate forward and laterally. An important goal of therapy is to reeducate control of the upper extremity on the upper trunk and the control of the upper trunk over the lower trunk to allow the patient to use lower-trunk-initiated strategies for sit to stand movements (Fig. 13-8).

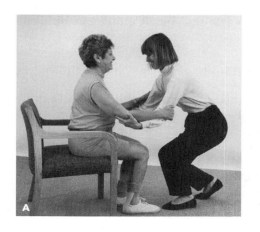

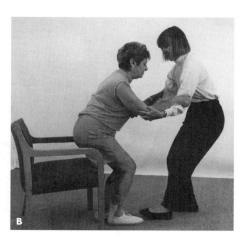

FIGURE 13-8 (A & B) Therapist uses bilateral lower arm grip to control alignment of upper body over lower trunk as patient practices lower-trunk-initiated pattern.

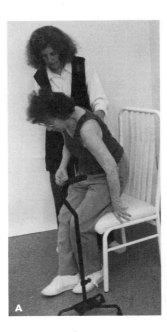

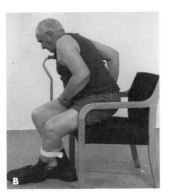

FIGURE 13-9 (*A*) Weakness in the right leg results in difficulty keeping the leg on the floor during sit to stand. (*B*) Weakness in the left leg results in patterns of asymmetry in leg and lower trunk.

Weakness and Asymmetry in the Lower Extremities

The patient with weakness in the leg will have difficulty activating the muscles of the affected lower extremity to lift the hips off the support (Fig. 13-9A). This weakness results in reliance on the unaffected leg, which produces an asymmetric weight bearing pattern. It also contributes to patterns of asymmetry in the involved leg. As the patient attempts to stand, his involved leg does not contract with enough strength to produce the normal components. Instead, the pelvis rotates and lists downwards, the knee flexes, and the heel comes off the floor (Fig. 13-9B). If trunk symmetry is not maintained, the patient's weight shifts off the affected leg and he learns to stand using his uninvolved arm and leg.

During the initiation and transition phases of sit to stand, it is critical to teach the patient to maintain the hemiplegic foot on the floor, to extend the leg appropriately for the task, and to sustain muscle firing throughout the completion of the activity. It is also important that sit to stand be practiced with the trunk in a symmetric position with weight on both feet, so that asymmetric movement and compensations do not develop. Activities to practice these components are described in the treatment section.

In some patients, the involved leg comes off the floor as they try to stand. This excessive hip and knee flexion during transition and the completion phases is a sign of poor trunk control and weak, disorganized lower extremity muscles (Fig. 13-10). During the acute phase of recovery, patients with excessive hip and knee flexion learn to weight shift to the uninvolved side and use the uninvolved arm and leg to lift the body. This weight shift to one side causes further trunk asymmetries and compensatory upper extremity movement patterns. As the patient begins to learn to stand relying solely on the uninvolved extremities, he will have extremely poor balance and will not be able to come to a stand without the use of a hemiwalker or a quad cane.

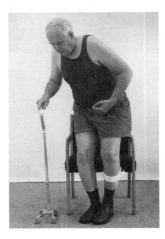

FIGURE 13-10 Excessive hip and knee flexion as a result of poor trunk and leg control.

Loss of Knee Extension Control

Two common knee extension patterns exist: One pattern is early knee extension, and the other is excessive knee extension.

Early Knee Extension

The most common reason for early knee extension is lack of ankle joint dorsiflexion range and control (Fig. 13-11). During early transition, the ankle should continue to dorsiflex as the hips leave the support. If the ankle joint moves into plantarflexion or cannot dorsiflex past neutral, the proximal portion of the tibia will move posteriorly and the knee will move into early extension during transition, when it should still be in flexion.

Excessive Knee Extension

If one side of the pelvis rotates forward excessively and the leg is not in full weight bearing, the femur on that side internally rotates with the pelvic movement. As weight is placed on the leg in standing, the line of gravity becomes anterior and medial to the internally rotated knee, and the knee begins to move into hyperextension.

If weight is placed on the leg and the pelvis rotates forward during the extension moment of the activity, the femur will internally rotate with the pelvis, but the tibia may not rotate with the femur. This results in an internally rotated femur and a relatively externally rotated tibia. This incompatible rotation between the segments contributes to excessive knee extension.

When one side of the pelvis rotates backward during sit to stand and there is less weight on that hip and thigh, the femur abducts and externally rotates with the pelvic movement. The lower leg follows the backward movement of the pelvis and femur. This results in ankle joint plantar flexion and excessive knee extension.

Loss of Ankle Joint Range

Loss of ankle joint dorsiflexion range due to muscle tightness in the gastrocnemius and hamstring muscles and edema in the foot and ankle is one the most common secondary impairments during the movement of sit to stand. Normally, the ankle requires 10 to 20 degrees of range during sit to stand. If the ankle cannot move into dorsiflexion during the transition phase of sit to stand, the patient will have difficulty moving up and over his feet, and the heel will not stay on the floor.

Muscle tightness in the hamstrings and gastrocnemius/soleus muscles across the knee results from prolonged sitting, and tightness in the gastrocnemius/soleus muscles across the ankle results from the inability to stand on the foot. Edema, which can restrict ankle joint range, commonly begins on the plantar surface of the foot and will perfuse the tissues of the entire foot until the swelling becomes obvious on the dorsum of the foot and around the ankle joint (Fig. 13-12).

In treatment, the loss of ankle joint range should be addressed immediately to maximize the patient's ability to perform sit to stand as efficiently as possible. This may be done through techniques to lengthen the muscles in standing (see Ch. 9) or during sit to stand.

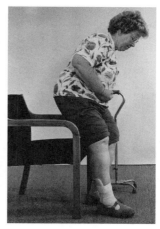

FIGURE 13-11 Early knee extension during sit to stand.

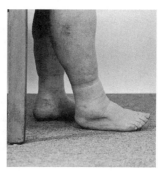

FIGURE 13-12 Edema of the foot and ankle resulting in limited ankle joint range.

Muscle and Soft Tissue Tightness

Loss of muscle length in large multijoint lower extremity muscles, specifically the hamstrings, gastrocnemius, soleus, and tensor fascia lata, in combination with the loss of stability of their proximal attachments contributes to poor alignment of the lower extremity and interferes with muscles reeducation in the hemiplegic leg. Tightness of these muscles either individually or in combination produces rotational asymmetries in the femur and tibia, which interfere with muscle reeducation and function during sit to stand.

Lower Extremity Extension Hypertonicity

Extensor hypertonicity in the lower extremity during sit to stand occurs for three reasons. First, it can be a response to *insufficient trunk control* for the task. If trunk control is poor and the trunk overshifts to the uninvolved side, leg extensor hypertonicity may occur as a part of a balance response to the atypical trunk movement (Fig. 13–13).

Extensor hypertonicity also occurs as a result of *poor alignment* in the leg, either hip joint malalignment or incompatible alignment between the thigh and the lower leg. Over time, poor joint alignment results in muscle shortening. Shifts in proximal alignment on the hemiplegic side place a stretch on these already shortened two-joint leg muscles. As the patient stands up and the leg begins to straighten, these tight, shortened muscles pull the knee into hyperextension either because the muscle has reached the limit of its length at the hip or because its line of pull has shifted. During sit to stand, incompatible alignment of the hemiplegic thigh and lower leg also contributes to knee hyperextension. Incompatible alignment occurs when the thigh internally rotates from loss of trunk/pelvic control while the tibia externally rotates as a component of strong foot inversion posturing. These opposite rotational forces make it difficult for the patient to control the hemiplegic knee and strong knee hyperextension results.

Extensor hypertonicity in the lower extremity during sit to stand may also occur as a result of the body attempting to produce the extension power to stand but with inadequate or *unbalanced muscle activation*. The quadriceps is an appropriate muscle to use to stand, but many other significant and necessary leg muscles must also be active. When these other muscles do not contract synergistically with the quadriceps, the knee extends too strongly or at the wrong time in the movement sequence.

Extensor hypertonicity in standing makes it difficult to balance because body weight is shifted laterally off the leg and patients must balance over a very narrow base—one foot. Therefore, the extensor pattern must be stopped through treatment intervention so that both legs actively participate in the sit to stand movement.

Upper Extremity Hypertonicity

Upper extremity hypertonicity affects the performance of sit to stand through its influence on the trunk. The upper extremity may posture in flexion as a balance response to poor alignment and control of the trunk or in response to poor hip stability and lower extremity control as the body moves from sitting to standing (Fig. 13-13). This hypertonicity interferes with the ability to align and control the upper trunk over the lower trunk, thus interfering with the patterns of trunk

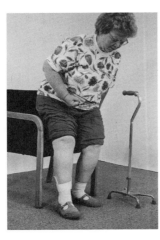

FIGURE 13-13 Extensor hypertonicity in the leg and flexor hypertonicity in the arm during sit to stand.

control. When hypertonicity maintains the upper extremity in an abnormally flexed position, the therapist may have difficulty correcting the patient's trunk and pelvis. In these patients, the shortened or spastic muscles that influence the arm and trunk must be lengthened as a prerequisite for reeducating sit to stand patterns. Techniques for treating flexor spasticity in the arm are described in Chapters 6, 7 and 10.

UNDESIRABLE COMPENSATORY PATTERNS

Compensatory movements of the trunk and extremities develop during sit to stand because of trunk asymmetries, limited ability to use the involved leg because of weakness and muscle shortening, inefficient patterns of movement initiation (lateral instead of anterior), and incorrect patterns of muscle activation. Common examples of compensations include the exclusive use of the uninvolved side to push up, pulling to standing with one arm, and mechanical locking of the involved knee joint to provide stability.

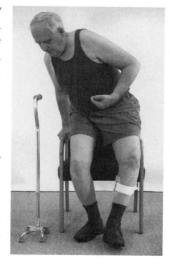

FIGURE 13-14 Undesirable compensatory pattern: exclusive use of uninvolved side.

1. Exclusive use of uninvolved side to push up. Shearing of the upper trunk and extremity posturing (Fig. 13-14).

2. Pulling to stand. Use of one arm to pull on a stable object and use of the uninvolved leg to push backwards.

ASSESSMENT GUIDELINES

Assessment questions for sit to stand require a review of the questions used for the assessment of trunk movements in sitting. The choice of a sit to stand initiation pattern often depends on the trunk control patterns available to the patient. The other critical area of exploration is the leg, both for strength and control and available range of motion.

I. Describe the position of the trunk as the patient performs sit to stand.

II. Identify the position of the arm and leg in sitting and during the sit to stand. Does the arm or leg posture?

III. Describe the change in the control of the trunk and leg during the sit to stand when you symmetrically support the arms.

IV. Describe the change in the trunk and/or arm during the sit to stand when you correct and support the hemiplegic leg. Describe the amount of ankle joint range in sitting with the knee bent and during standing when the knee is extended.

V. Can the patient stand and balance on both legs? If not, what effect does correcting trunk position have on balance and leg control?

VI. What hand placements/grips improve the movement pattern during sit to stand?

VII. What problems do not change immediately with handling and will require further treatment to improve the ability to move from sitting to

THERAPY GOALS

Functional Goals

Treatment for the task of sit to stand is performed to achieve the following functional goals:

1. Independent, safe sit to stand with equal weight on both legs
2. Independent transfers to left and to right from chair to chair, chair to bed, bed to chair, wheelchair to toilet/to chair

Treatment Goals and Techniques

Treatment Goal: Train components of task. Reestablish trunk control needed to maintain upper trunk alignment over lower trunk during anterior/posterior weight shifts in sitting and during lower-trunk-initiated sit to stand.

Treatment Technique: Upper trunk/lower trunk grips (Fig. 13-15).

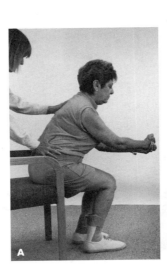 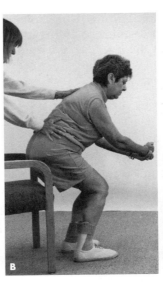 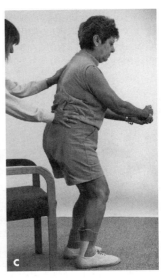

FIGURE 13-15 (*A*) Upper trunk/pelvic grip to maintain upper body alignment over lower body while patient practices lower-trunk-initiated weight shift. Patient is clasping her hemiplegic arm to help maintain upper trunk symmetry. (*B*) Therapist's left hand assists upper trunk while therapist's right hand stops pelvic asymmetries as patient practices controlling extension in her right leg. (*C*) Therapist's hands assist upper body alignment over legs and lower trunk as patient tries to balance in standing.

Treatment Goal: Correct glenohumeral joint subluxation and maintain alignment of the arm on the trunk during sit to stand to allow reeducation and strengthening of trunk initiation pattern.

Treatment Technique: Unilateral/bilateral arm grip (Fig. 13-16).

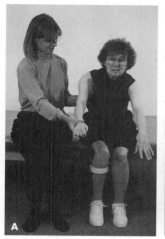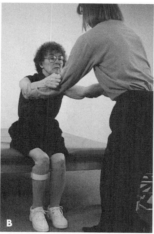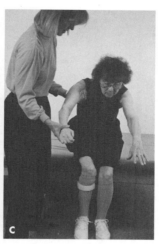

FIGURE 13-16 (*A*) Therapist uses her left hand with an axillary grip to correct scapular position, to support the glenohumeral joint, and to prevent humeral internal rotation. Her right hand maintains the wrist and forearm in neutral positions. With these grips, she maintains alignment of the upper body as the patient begins to practice sit to stand. (*B*) The therapist can move her hands to the distal humerus and forearm to assist upper trunk symmetry while the patient practices lower trunk initiated anterior weight shifts. (*C*) Patient practices with less assistance; patient helps keep her upper trunk over both hips while the therapist supports shoulder joint.

Treatment Goal: Decrease significant secondary impairments. Restore/maintain ankle joint dorsiflexion range to allow reeducation of lower leg and foot musculature during sit to stand.

Treatment Technique: Heel cord lengthening in non-weight bearing in preparation for sit to stand (Fig. 13-17).

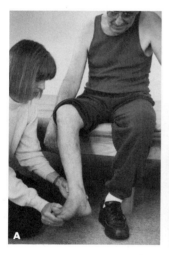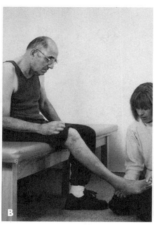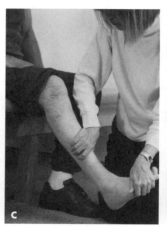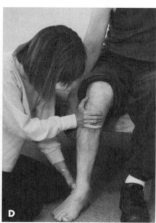

FIGURE 13-17 (*A*) Therapist supports forefoot and identifies calcaneal position and gastrocnemius/ soleus length with knee in flexion. (*B*) Therapist uses her right hand to assess length of gastrocnemius muscle and its effect on the rearfoot as the knee extends. (*C*) Therapist uses her hands to lengthen tight soft tissue structures in the lower leg and foot in preparation for maintaining heel and foot contact when the foot is placed on the floor. (*D*) Therapist continues to lengthen tight soft tissues with the foot firmly on the floor. Her right hand is directing pressure down through the tibia into the foot as her left hand maintains correction of calcaneus. This grip can be maintained to assure appropriate ankle joint movement as the patient practices the initiation phase of sit to stand.

Treatment Technique: Heel cord lengthening during function (Fig. 13-18).

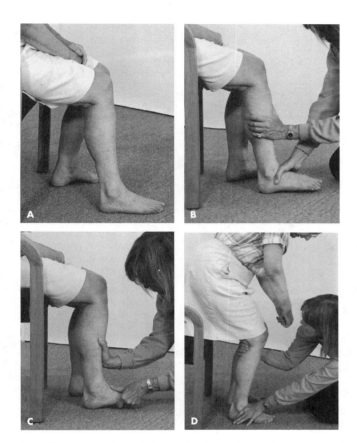

FIGURE 13-18 (*A*) Patient's foot and ankle position before treatment. The ankle is in plantarflexion and tight muscles limit dorsiflexion range. (*B*) Therapist uses her left hand to stabilize the foot and direct pressure back into the heel while her right hand gently glides the distal tibia posteriorly to lengthen the gastrocnemius tendon as it crosses the ankle joint. (*C*) Alternate hand positions for maintaining heel contact and lengthening posterior calf muscles to increase ankle joint dorsiflexion range. (*D*) Therapist maintains heel contact while assisting ankle joint dorsiflexion while patient moves from sit to stand. Therapist's left hand is over the talus, directing pressure on a diagonal back into the heel while her right hand is encouraging forward movement of the proximal tibia.

Treatment Goal: Maintain symmetric weight bearing through the legs to allow appropriate sequencing and strengthening of weak leg muscles

Treatment Technique: Bilateral leg grips (Fig. 13-19).

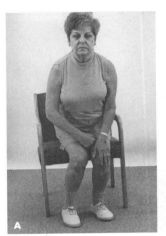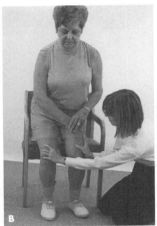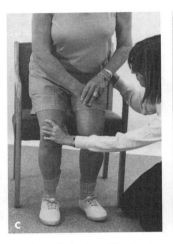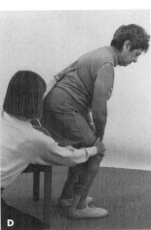

FIGURE 13-19 (*A*) Patient is unable to maintain symmetric weight bearing through the legs. The hemiplegic right hip adducts as the patient shifts to the left leg. The following figures provide alternate grips to align the leg so the patient can learn to activate leg muscles during sit to stand. (*B*) Therapist corrects leg position during initiation to allow patient to strengthen pelvic and lower trunk pattern. Therapist's left hand is preventing the femur from adducting while aligning the tibia over the foot. Her left hand is also directing a message to help the leg depress into the floor. (*C*) Therapist's left hand is providing the message as described in Figure B while her right hand is correcting the pelvic position. (*D*) Therapist's right hand is helping the patient maintain alignment of the thigh and lower leg over the foot. The therapist's left hand is helping the patient remember to keep the upper trunk over the lower body during the movement.

Treatment Progression: Use of varying hand placements to correct upper body and lower body asymmetries (Fig. 13-18).

FIGURE 13-20 (*A*) Initial sit to stand pattern. Excessive use of left arm, forward flexion, and rotation of upper body, minimal use of right leg, flexor posturing right arm. (*B*) Initial trunk position. (*C & D*) Therapist uses her left hand in an axillary grip to support and correct glenohumeral joint and to provide a message to the trunk to extend and move forward over the hips and thighs. Her correction prevents the right side of the trunk from rotating forward and stops the flexor posturing in the right arm.(*E*) Therapist continues to assist the upper body as the patient initiates the sit to stand. (*F–I*) Therapist maintains foot contact with the floor and assists lower leg movement so the patient can activate and strengthen leg musculature. Therapist's left hand provides a downward message to help maintain heel contact and encourages forward movement of the tibia over the foot during initiation. The left hand also prevents excessive knee extension during transition and in the full stand. (*J & K*) Therapist provides verbal cues as patient practices by himself. Note improved symmetry of trunk and improved weight bearing on right leg.

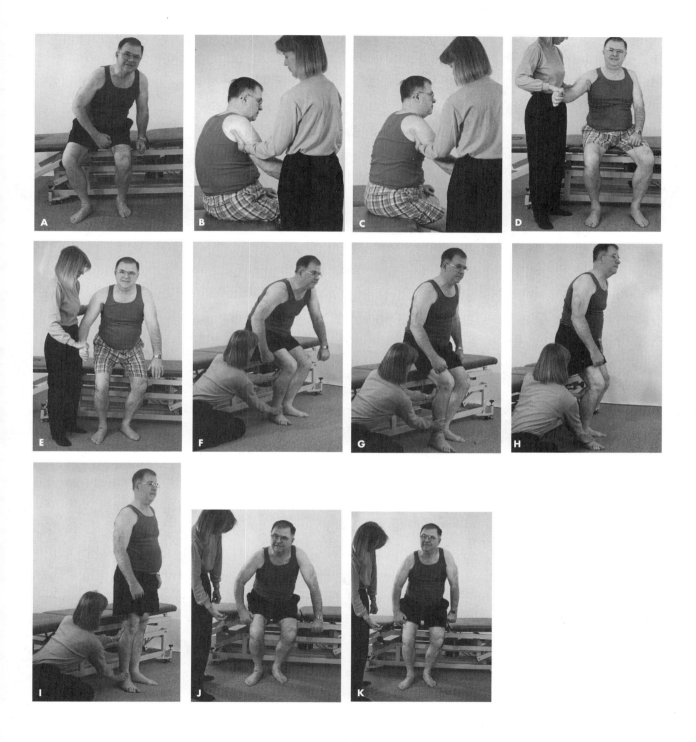

14
Transfers

CONCEPTS AND PRINCIPLES

During daily activities we *transfer*, i.e., move from one sitting surface to another sitting surface, when the surfaces are abutting or close enough to move from one to the other without walking. We transfer to an adjacent chair around a dining table or from seat to seat in a movie theater. Transfers from bed to wheelchair to bed are among the first transitional movements attempted by patients after a stroke. While transfers are initially performed with assistance to change position safely, they are later performed independently, often before the patient walks alone. Independent transfers are an important part of independence at a wheelchair level, but they are an interim phase of movement in rehabilitation. As movement control improves, the patient will no longer need to "transfer" as often from one surface to another but will walk from place to place.

The movement goal of a transfer is to change the center of gravity of the body from sitting on one surface to sitting on another surface. The control demands on the trunk and lower extremity during transfer activities will be similar to those in the movement of sit to stand: the upper and lower trunk need to remain aligned over one another, the body moves away from one surface as the legs produce extension power, and the legs control the descent to a second surface.

In patients with central nervous system dysfunction, the movement control goals for transfer training are similar to those of sit to stand (see Ch. 13). The upper trunk remains aligned over the lower trunk as the body inclines forward, the legs produce appropriate extension control, and the body balances over the feet. In addition to these sit to stand components, transfers require the body to pivot over the feet before the legs control the descent of the body back down into a chair or bed (Fig. 14-1). The teaching of transfers is used to establish postural control in the trunk and strengthen movement patterns in the lower extremities as well as to accomplish the functional goal. The therapist maintains proper alignment of the upper body over the lower trunk to minimize compensatory movements and to allow firing of appropriate muscles. Transfer training is used to build progressions that are based on the patient's needs and strengths. The therapist slowly increases the demands of the task according to the patient's level of movement control and recovery.

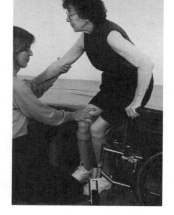

FIGURE 14-1 The body pivots over the feet during a transfer.

MOVEMENT COMPONENTS OF TRANSFERS

Transfers can be initiated by either the upper or lower trunk and can be performed in either of two ways: a *partial stand transfer* or a *full stand transfer.*

Partial Stand Transfer

A partial stand transfer is one in which we complete the transfer without standing erect. This transfer is performed in a partial stand as the pelvis and hips rotate toward the new surface. Partial stand transfers can be initiated with either the lower trunk or the upper trunk. While lower-trunk-initiated transfers are the more common patterns, the upper-trunk-initiated partial stand transfer is analyzed in this section because therapists use it during treatment of severely impaired patients.

Lower-Trunk-Initiated Pattern

In a lower-trunk-initiated partial stand transfer (Fig. 14-2A–C), the upper trunk must remain controlled over the lower trunk as the lower trunk initiates a forward weight shift and the hips flex. The legs actively extend into a half-stand during transition. The upper trunk remains aligned and stable over the forwardly inclined lower trunk as the pelvis and legs rotate over the feet. The feet remain in contact with the floor.

During treatment, the therapist allows the trunk and upper extremities to follow the movement of the lower body, since this is not a trunk counterrotational activity but a rotational movement of the pelvis and hips on the lower legs and feet. The completion of the task requires that the trunk remain stable as the leg muscles eccentrically contract and slowly lower the trunk and pelvis down to the new supporting surface. The therapist may choose to have the patient control the trunk position while she assists with the lift, or the therapist may assist the trunk while the patient focuses on using his legs to control extension and rotate the body into the chair or bed. This pattern is the preferred pattern to reeducate when the patient is expected to progress to independent transfers and ambulation because it uses trunk movements that are closest to those needed in sit to stand and in walking (Fig. 14-3). With acute, low-level patients, therapists may start treatment with upper-trunk-initiated transfers and progress to this pattern when the patient develops more trunk and lower extremity control.

FIGURE 14-2 (A–C) Lower-trunk-initiated partial stand transfer pattern.

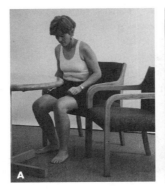 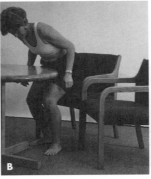 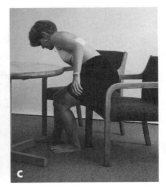

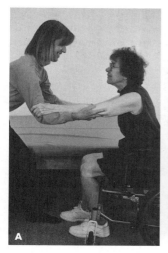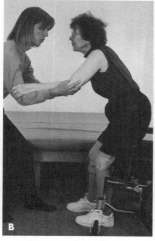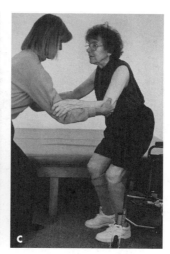

FIGURE 14-3 (A–C) Teaching a lower-trunk-initiated partial-stand assisted transfer.

Upper-Trunk-Initiated Pattern

Upper-trunk-initiated partial stand transfers require minimal trunk and leg control and are often taught to nursing staffs as a safe, maximal-assist transfer technique for low-functioning or severely involved patients. In an upper-trunk-initiated transfer, the therapist teaches the patient's upper body to move forward and down toward the floor as the spine and hips flex. As body weight shifts forward, the pelvis comes off the sitting surface as a result of the forward momentum of the trunk. To complete the transfer, the patient remains in upper trunk flexion while the therapist assists the rotation of the trunk and pelvis over the feet and assists the weight shift back down to the sitting surface (Fig. 14-4).

This transfer allows the center of gravity to be moved easily over the feet by the use of momentum and mechanical advantage, with less need for trunk control against gravity or power production in the legs. If the patient cannot activate trunk or leg muscles or if that is not a goal of treatment, this transfer can be safely performed by nursing or assistive staff.

Full Stand Transfer

The full stand transfer is more complex than the partial stand transfer because it requires more strength and movement control. It requires strength and control in the trunk and legs to move from sit to a full stand, additional strength and balance to unweight each leg and coordinate stepping movements of the lower leg, plus additional control in the legs to lower the body down to the sitting position. While full stand transfers can be performed with an upper-trunk-initiated pattern (see Ch. 13), we will analyze only the lower-trunk-initiated pattern. Full stand transfers are appropriate in treatment when the patient has some ability to control the trunk against gravity and to use the legs to support body weight. When these components are missing or require maximal assistance from the therapist, partial stand transfers are safer and more appropriate.

Movement Summary: Partial Stand Transfer

Lower trunk initiation
Initiation
  Spine neutral
Transition
  Legs control extension
Completion
  Legs control flexion

Upper trunk initiation
Initiation
  Spine flexion
Transition
  Legs less active
Completion
  Legs less active

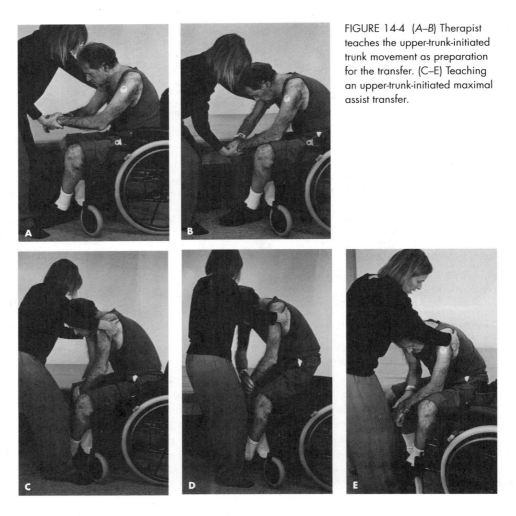

FIGURE 14-4 (*A–B*) Therapist teaches the upper-trunk-initiated trunk movement as preparation for the transfer. (*C–E*) Teaching an upper-trunk-initiated maximal assist transfer.

Lower-Trunk-Initiated Pattern

In the lower-trunk-initiated full stand transfer (Fig. 14-5), the sit to stand is performed with the spine in neutral extension. The lower trunk initiates a forward weight shift so that the trunk moves forward and the hips flex. The spine remains in extension as the hips and knees extend and the pelvis moves up off the surface. As the legs extend more completely, the trunk moves back up over the hips to a full standing position. To step or pivot the feet, the body must shift laterally to place the center of gravity over one leg and maintain this unilateral stance as the opposite leg is lifted off the floor and moved. Small diagonal steps are taken with each foot. The trunk must remain upright over the lower extremities until the body is parallel to the new supporting surface. Then the hips flex, the trunk inclines forward, while the legs control the downward movement of the body.

Nonambulatory patients who use a full stand transfer pattern rely on a quad cane or hemiwalker as their "second leg" because they do not have enough trunk control nor strength in the hemiplegic leg to balance and support body weight while they step the other leg around. They also have great difficulty stepping with the hemiplegic leg and, instead, pivot around the sturdy cane and the uninvolved leg (Fig. 14-6).

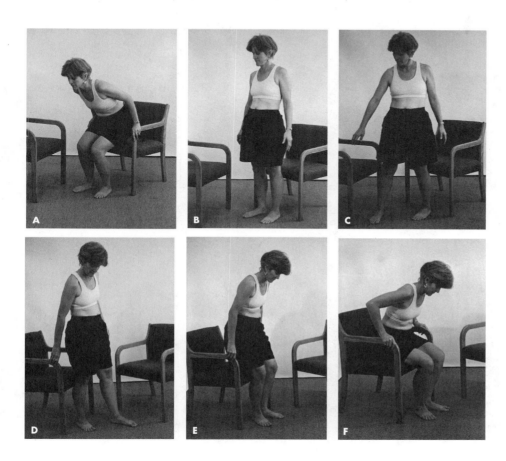

FIGURE 14-5 (*A–F*) Lower-trunk-initiated full stand transfer.

FIGURE 14-6 (*A–F*) Patient attempting full stand transfer pattern. He has difficulty standing and balancing on the left leg and relies heavily on the quad cane.

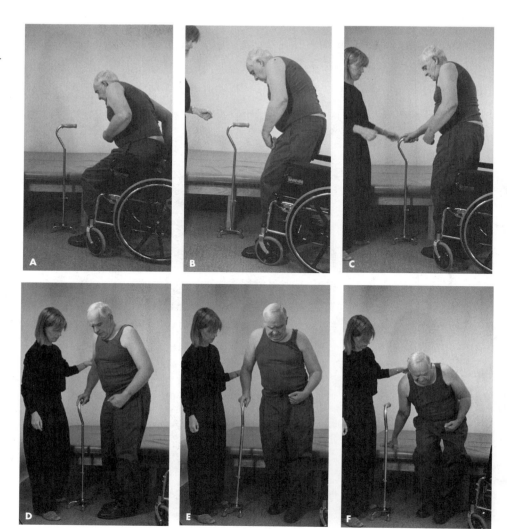

Movement Summary: Full Stand Transfer

Initiation
  Spine erect, trunk inclines forward, hips flex

Transition
  Full stand, feet step around

Completion
  Legs eccentrically control descent to chair

SIGNIFICANT IMPAIRMENTS THAT INTERFERE WITH PERFORMANCE

Lack of Ankle/Foot Joint Range

During the transition and completion phase of transferring, ankle joint range and control are significant prerequisites. Not only is ankle joint dorsiflexion range necessary (as with sit to stand), but since the lower extremities are rotating over the foot, the foot must have mobility and control in eversion and inversion and in supination and pronation (Fig. 14-7). When this range is not available, the leg will not be able to rotate appropriately and compensations will occur in the leg and lower trunk. The therapist should lengthen tight ankle and foot muscles before teaching the transfer or use her hands to reeducate movements of the ankle and foot as the patient learns the transfer.

Extensor Hypertonicity in the Leg

Extensor hypertonicity of the leg during a partial stand transfer occurs in the transition phase as the hips extend and rotate towards the new surface (Fig. 14-8). As the body rotates, the leg may posture in extension, either as an attempt to "help" the body move to the new surface or as an atypical response to maintaining contact with the floor.

During a full stand transfer, extensor hypertonicity may be observed as the patient attempts to step the hemiplegic foot around. Extensor hypertonicity in the leg causes extension of the knee, plantarflexion of the ankle, and supination of the foot. With severe hypertonicity, in addition to this knee and ankle pattern, the hip may internally rotate and adduct. Hypertonicity makes it difficult both to step with the leg and to keep the foot flat on the floor. Extensor spasticity develops in patients who have alignment problems in the leg as a result of hip muscle tightness, have improper initiation patterns for stepping, or have difficulty organizing firing patterns in the leg.

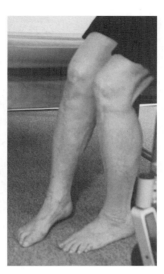

FIGURE 14-7 Loss of right ankle and foot range prevent the right leg from rotating over the foot during a transfer to the right.

FIGURE 14-8 Extensor hypertonicity in the left leg during a transfer to the left.

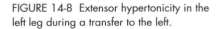

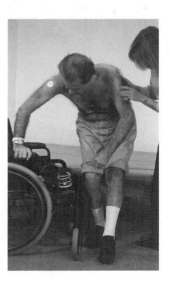

Inability to Step Affected Leg in Standing

During the full stand transfer, the patient must come to standing, balance in the standing position, and take small steps with each foot. Small diagonal steps are taken as the body shifts weight over each leg, while the trunk remains controlled over the lower extremities until the body is parallel to the new sitting surface. For the patient to step with his involved leg during the transfer, he must be able to control the trunk symmetrically as the weight is shifted onto the unaffected leg and control the pelvis on the affected side as the affected foot is lifted off the floor. To step the foot around, the foot and ankle initiate the movement, the knee and hip flex a small amount, and the entire leg rotates to position the foot (Fig. 14-9). Because it is almost impossible to teach the leg to move during the transfer (since patients who need to transfer have difficulty standing and usually cannot walk), this portion of the task must either be present or the patient must practice it before the transfer is attempted. If the patient can only move the affected leg by hiking the pelvis or excessively abducting the hip, compensatory patterns will be introduced in

FIGURE 14-9 (A–E) As patient's son attempts to help her with a maximal assist full stand transfer, her left leg does not have the strength to step around and he pivots her over the uninvolved leg.

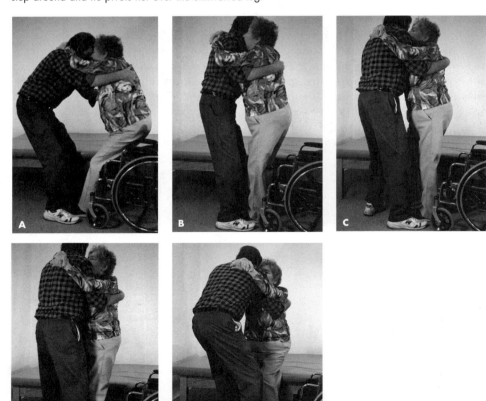

the leg that may carry over into walking. If the patient is unable to step with his affected leg, the therapist can show the patient how to shift body weight onto the hemiplegic side and how to keep the upper and lower trunk positioned symmetrically as the unaffected leg steps around.

UNDESIRABLE COMPENSATORY PATTERNS

The most common compensatory movement during a transfer is the use of only the unaffected side to move and support the body. If the trunk position is severely asymmetric during this movement, the affected leg will not be used and may actually come up off the floor; the affected arm will posture with flexor hypertonicity. This common compensatory movement is also present when the hemiplegic leg lacks the control or strength to support the body. If these patients are confronted with a transfer to their affected side, they will stand and pivot almost completely around to avoid using or placing weight on the hemiplegic leg.

Exclusive use of unaffected side:

1. Partial stand transfer avoiding use of left side (Fig. 14-10).
2. Full circle transfer (Fig. 14-11).

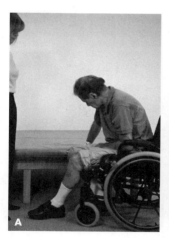
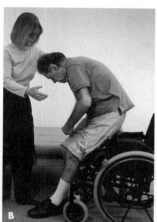
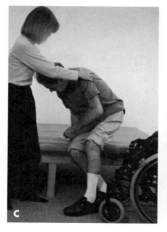
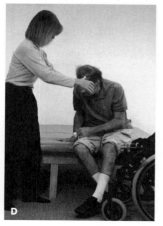

FIGURE 14-10 (*A–D*) Undesirable compensatory pattern: exclusive use of unaffected side during partial stand transfer.

FIGURE 14-11 (A–F) Undesirable compensatory pattern: full stand "circle" transfer relying on a quad cane to avoid placing weight on affected right leg.

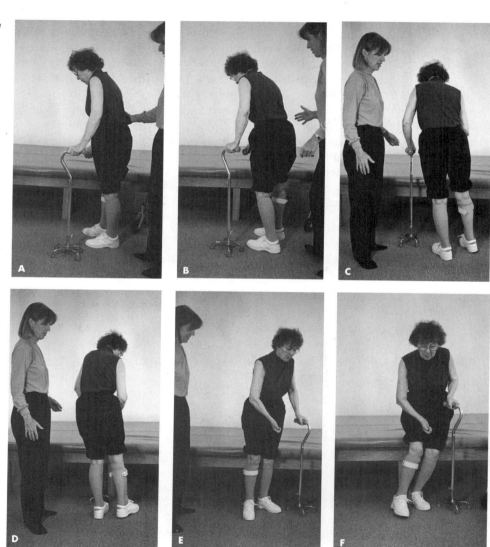

ASSESSMENT GUIDELINES

Assessment of the ability to perform transfers is the same as the assessment of sit to stand with the following questions added to gather information about the patient's ability to control the legs and trunk while performing a partial stand transfer and a full stand pivot transfer to either side. The full stand pivot transfer assessment requires information about the ability to move each leg while in the standing position.

I. Describe the position of the trunk, arms, and legs as the patient performs a partial stand transfer to the left, to the right.

II. Describe the changes in the legs that occur if you correct the trunk alignment and/or the alignment of the upper extremity on the upper trunk during the partial stand transfer.

III. Describe the change in ability to perform the transfer if you correct the affected lower leg and foot position during the partial stand transfer.

IV. Can the patient stand and balance on both legs? If not, what is the trunk position during attempts at standing? Can the patient use the affected leg to help the body rise to standing and balance?

V. In standing, can the patient move each leg enough to step around?

VI. Describe the position of the trunk, arms, and legs as the patient performs a full stand pivot transfer to the right, to the left.

VII. What asymmetries or impairments occur repeatedly as the patient performs the transfers?

What improves when you put your hands on the patient to either correct asymmetries or to facilitate or assist the transfers?

What problems do not change immediately with handling and will require further treatment to improve the ability to perform the transfers independently?

THERAPY GOALS

Functional Goals

The ultimate goal of transfer training is for our patients to safely and automatically transfer from one surface to another. However, treatment must focus on selected goals during the activity: trunk symmetry, muscle activity in the lower extremities during the weight bearing or loading phase, the ability to turn or rotate the body over the feet, and balance control to achieve patterns of movement that relate to standing and walking.

Transfers should be taught to both sides and should be practiced without and with the assistance of the upper extremities. While early transfer training is often practiced from a treatment plinth, functional training requires it be practiced in real life environments such as from a wheelchair to bed, to the toilet, and eventually to a car.

The training of transfers is necessary to help the patient meet the following functional goal: Ability to perform safe, independent transfers to either side in all relevant situations (transfers to toilet and tub, to a variety of types of chairs, and to the car) (Fig. 14-12).

FIGURE 14-12 (*A & B*) Teaching a partial stand transfer to and from the toilet.

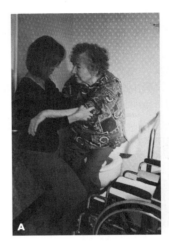
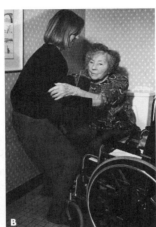

Treatment Goals and Techniques

Treatment Goal: Provide a model of movement during transfers to the left and right.

Treatment Technique: Partial stand transfer with arms supported—maximal assist (Fig. 14-13).

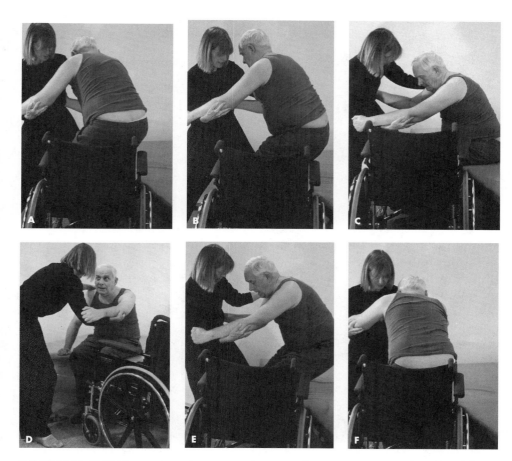

FIGURE 14-13 (*A&B*) Therapist provides upper trunk symmetry by supporting patient's hemiplegic left arm and by asking the patient to place his right arm against her waist. Therapist helps patient initiate a lower trunk anterior weight shift. He performs a partial stand transfer, working to keep the spine in neutral extension, maintaining weight on both feet as the therapist assists the pivot to the right. (*C*) Patient slowly lowers his hips to the mat while the therapist uses her hands to maintain symmetry of the upper trunk over the lower trunk and assist the movement. (*D*) Therapist's hands help the patient organize his trunk around midline. Her right hand supports the hemiplegic arm and provides an extension assist to the upper body; her left arm prevents the upper trunk from shearing to the right. Her right hand is delivering a diagonal message from the patient's upper body to his left hip, which corrects the upper body shearing and equalizes the weight distribution to both hips. (*E–F*) Therapist uses the same grip to maintain upper trunk alignment and helps the patient initiate a partial stand transfer to his left back into the wheelchair.

Treatment Goal: Align upper trunk over lower trunk to allow reeducation of lower trunk and leg components during the transfer.

Treatment Technique: Bilateral symmetric arm grip (Fig. 14-14).

Treatment Technique: Unilateral arm/trunk grip (Fig. 14-15).

Treatment Technique: Practice with less assistance: clasped hands (Fig. 14-16).

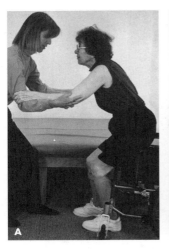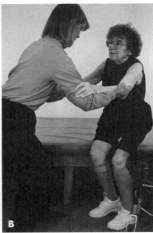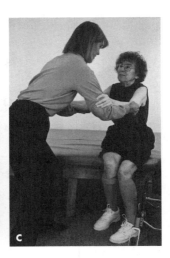

FIGURE 14-14 (*A & B*) Therapist uses bilateral symmetric arm grip to control upper body during the partial stand transfer to the patient's hemiplegic side. The therapist's hands support the patient's humerus, forearm, and hand. Her hands support the humerus in a neutral rotatory position, and by resting the patient's hand on her upper arm, she controls the position of the forearm. In this position, the therapist delivers an upward message through the humerus to assist spinal extension. The therapist does not pull on either arm but uses the arms to maintain alignment of the upper trunk over the lower trunk as the patient is asked to keep her back straight and move her body forward over the feet. As the patient initiates the partial stand, the therapist's right hand provides a lateral message to the upper trunk while her left hand encourages the patient to keep the upper trunk over the right leg. The patient pivots over her feet toward the mat without assistance from the therapist. (*C*) As the patient sits down, the therapist's hand are helping the upper trunk remain aligned over the lower trunk.

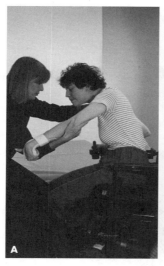
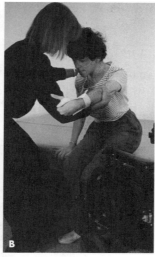
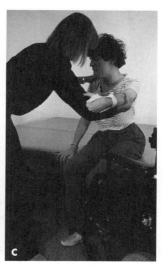

FIGURE 14-15 (A) This patient, with a left hemiplegia and athetosis, cannot transfer independently. The therapist's right arm supports the patient's left arm in the same manner as described above, but because of extensor spasticity in the arm, cannot maintain the humerus in a neutral rotatory position. The therapist's left arm is placed on the back of the patient's right shoulder and delivers a diagonal message through the trunk down toward the patient's left hip. These two hand placements and messages help assist trunk alignment. (B & C) The patient initiates the lower body weight shift to the best of her ability. Note that as the patient moves forward, the therapist moves her body backward. As the patient performs a partial stand, the therapist's hands continue to assist the alignment of the upper trunk over the lower trunk. The therapist pivots her body as the patient's body pivots. She does not have to block the patient's left knee because her left hand is continuing to deliver a downward diagonal message into the patient's left hip. This assists the alignment of the trunk over the legs. This grip is maintained as the patient organizes her body around midline at the end of the transfer.

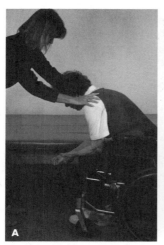
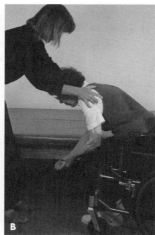
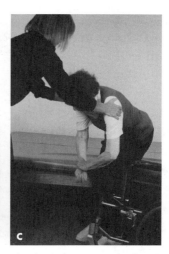

FIGURE 14-16 (A) As the patient gains more trunk control, she supports her hemiplegic arm. The therapist lightens her handling as she places her hands on the top and back of the patient's shoulders and corrects the shearing or lateral asymmetry of the patient's upper trunk with her left hand while her right hand stabilizes the upper body. Both hands assist the forward movement of the trunk over the hips. (B&C) The therapist's hands continue to give the same alignment message as described above, but now assist the upward lift of the trunk and legs. Note the therapist's arms follow the upward diagonal of the patient's trunk as she initiates the partial stand and pivots to the mat.

Treatment Goal: Reeducate the movement components in the leg. The legs provide the power that allows the body to move up out of the chair. The leg movement components must be reeducated as soon as the patient can control the correct trunk pattern with minimal assistance.

Treatment Technique: Reestablish normal alignment in the hemiplegic leg and foot (Fig. 14-17).

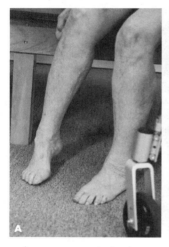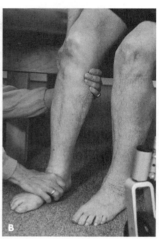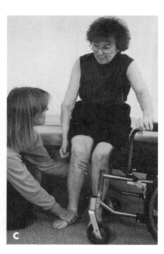

FIGURE 14-17 (*A*) Atypical alignment in the right lower leg and foot. Patient's right heel cord is shortened, the heel is off the floor, the foot is supinated, and the lower leg is externally rotating with the foot posturing. (*B*) Before beginning the transfer, the therapist must realign the leg and foot to allow the foot to come in contact with the floor and to allow muscles to be activated and reeducated. Her left hand is behind the top of the lower leg. She uses her left hand and wrist to control tibial rotation and simultaneously exerts a downward pressure to assist heel contact. The web space of her right hand is over the talus and places pressure back into the heel. The palm of her hand is over the midfoot to stop supination, if necessary. (*C*) This hand placement is maintained as the patient begins the transfer. Since the therapist is assisting with alignment and reeducation of the leg and foot, the trunk portion of the transfer must have been previously practiced. The therapist gives verbal reminders to help the patient sequence trunk and leg movements.

Treatment Technique: Teach active control of leg during the transfer (Fig. 14-18).

FIGURE 14-18 (*A & B*) Using the leg grip described above, the therapist uses her right hand to keep the heel in contact with the ground as the patient initiates the partial stand. Her left hand guides tibial rotation, maintains a downward pressure into the heel, and assists ankle dorsiflexion as the hips begin to extend. The therapist's left hand is in a position to prevent excessive or early knee extension, by keeping the tibia forward.

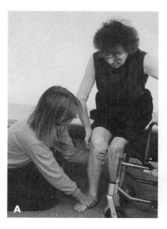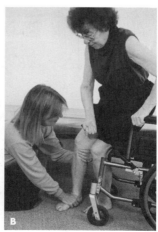

Treatment Technique: Combine reeducation of trunk and leg movement components (Fig. 14-19).

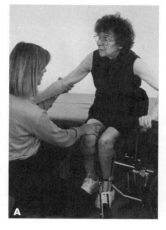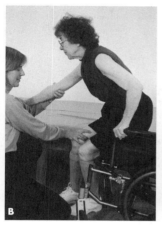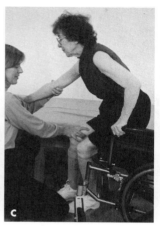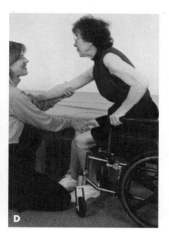

FIGURE 14-19 (*A*) Patient uses her left arm for support as the therapist teaches her how to use her hemiplegic leg. The therapist places her right hand on the top of the patient's right lower thigh. Her hand gives a downward pressure to assist heel contact and maintains alignment of the leg over the foot to minimize foot supination posturing. The therapist's left hand externally rotates the patient's arm to neutral and gives an upward message through the humerus to the upper trunk to extend and remain symmetric over the lower trunk as the patient's left arm holds the armrest of the wheelchair towards which she is moving. (*B*) The patient initiates the transfer, and the therapist uses her manual contact to assist the alignment of the leg and upper trunk. (*C & D*) As the patient pivots toward the chair, the therapist's right hand allows the lower leg to follow the movement of the pelvis and lower trunk and her left hand maintains upper trunk extension by giving a message up through the right humerus as she supports the patient's arm.

Treatment Goal: Increase independence in the task.

Treatment Technique: Decrease manual assistance and use verbal reminders during practice (Fig. 14-20).

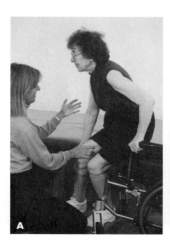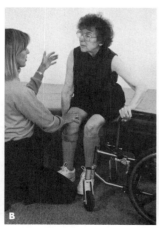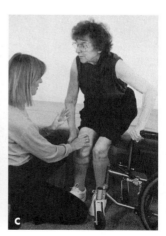

FIGURE 14-20 (*A*) Therapist uses her right hand to assist the lower leg and foot components of the task but decreases the manual cues. She gives verbal reminders to the trunk during the initiation phase. (*B & C*) During the transition and completion phase, the therapist alternates between manual assist and verbal reminders.

15
Walking

CONCEPTS AND PRINCIPLES

Walking is described as "... the manner of moving the body from one place to another by alternately and repetitively changing the location of the feet, with the condition that at least one foot is in contact with the walking surface."[1] Normal walking moves the body forward in space with a smooth, rhythmical progression. While there are movements of the center of gravity side to side and up and down, the overall result is a large, continuous forward movement of the body.

Although each individual's walking has its own distinctive differences, we all walk with the same general pattern. Even in stroke patients with hemiplegia, the gait pattern is not lost; what appears is a predictable alteration of the stance and swing phases. Hemiplegic gait is characterized by its slow speed and cycle time, uneven step length, (shorter step with the hemiplegic leg), shorter stance and longer swing times on the affected side, and the patient's impaired balance and excessive use of adaptive equipment. Normal walking has been studied, measured, and documented more than any other functional movement, and our intent is not to duplicate that but to highlight and emphasize those characteristics of normal walking that are relevant to therapists who treat stroke patients.

In the patient with neurologic damage, independent, functional walking is difficult because it requires a refined degree of trunk and extremity control. The trunk must remain balanced and controlled over the legs as the legs change position. The legs support the weight of the trunk, initiate weight shifts between each other, and move in space. As the patient walks faster, the requirements for strength and muscle timing in the trunk and legs are more complex. A goal of therapy is to help stroke patients learn to walk as safely and as functionally as they can. Therapists try to help patients achieve this with as few compensations as possible, to maximize muscle return and to minimize the number and amount of secondary complications that will develop in the future. The first portion of this chapter analyzes normal walking in functional segments as a model for understanding impairments and setting treatment goals. The second portion of the chapter relates impairments of the trunk, lower extremity, and upper extremity to these functional gait segments. Higher-level walking activities are presented after the treatment section of the chapter.

Definitions and Kinematics

During an analysis of walking, measurements and components are described within one *walking cycle*. A walking cycle (Fig. 15-1) starts when one foot contacts the floor and continues until that same foot makes contact again. Each cycle is divided into stance and swing phases (Fig. 15-2). The *stance phase* is the period when one foot is in contact with the ground. This is the part of walking when the leg is in weight bearing. Stance phase begins as the foot makes contact with the ground and ends when that

FIGURE 15-1 (*A*) Distance and (*B*) time dimensions of walking cycle. (From Inman et al.,[2] with permission.)

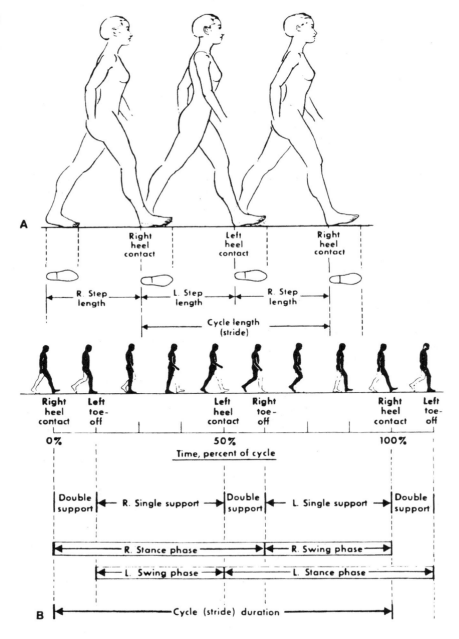

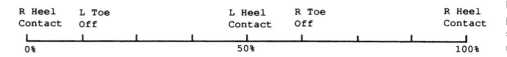

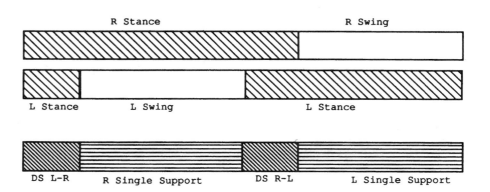

FIGURE 15-2 Stance and swing phases of walking. DS, double support. (From Smidt,[3] with permission.)

same foot leaves the ground. It is divided into three periods: heel contact, midstance, and heel off. Stance phase is 60% of the gait cycle. *Swing phase* is the period when the foot is in the air. It begins as the foot leaves the ground and ends when that foot makes contact with the ground again. Swing phase is divided into two periods: early swing and late swing. Early swing is the period from the moment when the foot comes off the ground and the leg is behind the body to the point where the foot is directly underneath the body. Late swing starts as the leg moves in front of the body and ends as the foot makes contact with the ground. Swing, the non-weight bearing phase of gait, is 40% of the gait cycle.

During each walking cycle there are two periods of *double limb support* when both feet are on the ground and one period of *single limb support* when each leg is on the ground alone. The period of single limb support composes the majority of the stance time and is the only time in the gait cycle when the center of gravity lies outside the base of support. Because of this, the single limb support period is a critical time for strength and balance control. The periods of double limb support occur at the transition from stance to swing and swing to stance. During the double support periods, both feet are in contact with the ground as weight shifts forward between the two legs.

Time and distance factors are used to measure the walking cycle. Time measures, which quantify the speed of walking, include cycle time, stance time, and swing time. *Cycle time*, the amount of time of one gait cycle, is usually measured in seconds. *Stance time* of one gait cycle is the amount of time that one foot is in contact with the surface, and *swing time* of one gait cycle is the amount of time that one foot is not in contact with the surface. As walking speed increases, the double stance time decreases. During jogging and running, both feet are off the ground for a brief period. Distance measures include stride length, step length, and step width and are usually measured in centimeters or inches (Fig. 15-3). *Stride length* is the length of one walking cycle. *Step length* is the distance between two consecutive steps, left-right or right-left, and *step width* is the perpendicular distance between two consecutive midheel placements.

FIGURE 15-3 Distance factors in walking. (From Smidt,[3] with permission)

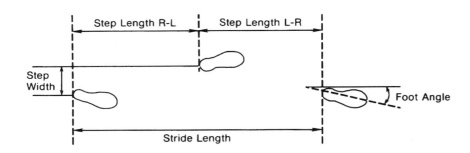

MOVEMENT COMPONENTS—
FUNCTIONAL SEGMENTS OF GAIT

The starting body position for walking is upright standing, in which the upper trunk is aligned and stable over the lower trunk. The base of support is defined by the two feet and the area between them. In this book, the lower extremity starting position for analysis will be the step/stance position (see Ch. 9). To begin to walk, the lower extremities initiate the movement forward and the upper and lower trunk respond and adjust to the lower extremity movements to keep the body balanced as it moves in space (Fig. 15-4). To help organize the assessment and treatment planning processes, walking can be broken down into three functional segments: *forward progression* (foot contact through midstance), *single/double limb support* (midstance to heel off), and *swing* (early and late).[2]

FIGURE 15-4 (*A & B*) The trunk remains upright and adjusts to leg movements as the body progresses forward.

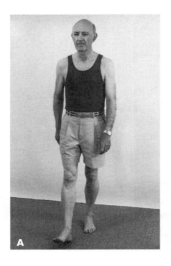

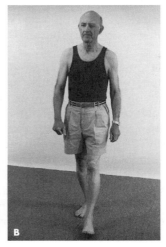

Forward Progression

This first functional section describes the demands on the body at the beginning of stance phase. At right foot contact, the right leg is ahead of the body and the upper trunk is aligned and controlled over the lower trunk. As the body moves forward, the hip extends toward neutral from its previously flexed position. The ankle moves from dorsiflexion at heel contact into plantar flexion as the entire foot moves onto the floor. As the body moves to the mid-stance position, the ankle joint moves from plantar flexion to dorsiflexion (Fig. 15-5A–C). Hip extension control is a critical component of this phase. The two related components necessary for the development of hip extension control are range and control of the ankle joint and alignment and control of the trunk and arms.

Three major demands on the body during forward progression are important considerations for treatment planning. First, the *foot makes contact with the ground with the leg in front of the body.* As the body moves forward, the ankle must have available joint range into dorsiflexion. When the right foot makes contact (right step/stance), the upper body is upright and perpendicular to the plane of progression and the lower trunk and pelvis are slightly rotated to the left. The right hip is in flexion, with knee extension and ankle dorsiflexion. The left leg is behind the body in hip and knee extension. In normal walking, the heel makes initial contact with the ground. For years this has been called heel-strike, but recently Winter[5] described this moment as "gentle heel landing," which implies more of a need for control in the trunk and leg (Figure 15-2D). To allow strength and control at the ankle and foot during this phase of walking, the body must also have sufficient muscle length, especially in the hamstrings and gastrocnemius, to allow hip flexion and knee extension with ankle joint dorsiflexion.

The second demand during forward progression is *sufficient trunk control to respond to the forward motion of the body.* While the legs are in a step stance position, the upper trunk follows the forward movement of the lower body so that the trunk position remains erect and symmetric. Both the upper and lower trunk must remain responsive to the initiation movement of the legs (see Ch. 9).

The third demand requires that *muscle activity in the lower extremity provide stability to the leg in weight bearing as it moves the body forward* over the foot. Stability and adjustments of the femur and lower leg maintain an appropriate amount of knee extension while allowing the entire body to move forward. This leg activity keeps the femur aligned with the lower leg and makes the ankle the fulcrum of the movement (Fig. 15-5E–F).

Summary of Critical Demands—Forward Progression

1. Muscle length at pelvis, hip, knee, and lower leg to place leg in front of the body (step/stance position)
2. Strength in the legs to control forward momentum
3. Coordinated trunk and leg control to allow the body to move over foot
4. Ankle joint range and control from plantarflexion into dorsiflexion as the body moves forward

FIGURE 15-5 (*A*) Forward progression, right heel contact. (*B*) Forward progression, right foot contact. (*C*) Forward progression, right midstance. (*D & E*) Forward progression of the leg. Note the forward movement of the leg and the muscular activity in ankle and toes.

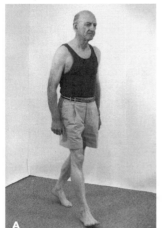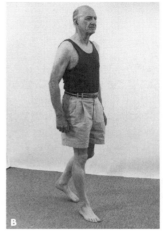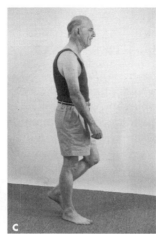

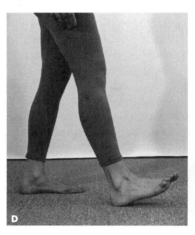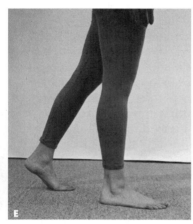

Single/Double Limb Support

Single limb support is the phase from midstance to the start of heel off. During single limb support on the right leg, the left leg is swinging forward. As we stand on the right leg, the right body moves forward and laterally over the supporting foot. At the end of single limb support, the knee extends and the ankle joint continues to dorsiflex (Fig. 15-6A).

Single limb support phase presents a difficult balance control task and a difficult lower extremity control task. The upper trunk must remain aligned over the lower trunk as the right leg continues to initiate the forward movement of the body. Trunk control must be refined enough to allow the pelvis to stay relatively level yet rotate as the swinging left leg lifts and moves forward. Ankle joint dorsiflexion range and control must be present to allow the right leg to move forward over the foot. Unilateral right knee control is also essential at this critical point (see Ch. 9). The knee responds to the changes at the hip and ankle and remains appropriately extended as the body balances and moves over the foot.

At the end of this phase, as the right heel lifts up and the left heel makes contact, a *double support* period occurs (Fig. 15-3B). At right heel off, the body is ahead of the leg. The right pelvis rotates backward, and the hip extends. The right knee is in a small amount of flexion, and the forefoot remains on the ground. As the heel lifts up, weight is transferred to the left leg, which has stepped forward. The hip extends with ankle plantarflexion to maintain enough limb length to keep the front of the foot on the floor as the body continues to move ahead of the leg.

To balance on both legs in this left step/stance position, as the body is progressing forward, weight shifts to the toes of the right leg; the leg "depressors" control and grade the movement onto the forefoot as a balance assist (Fig. 15-6C). This weight shift places the toes in relative dorsiflexion and prepares the body for swing phase. From the beginning of single limb support to the end of double limb support, weight shifts from the lateral border of the right heel to the medial aspect of the forefoot (Fig. 15-6D–E).

Summary of Critical Demands— Single/Double Limb Support

Balance control in unilateral stance

- Line of gravity moves outside single limb base of support
- Trunk must remain aligned over one leg and adapt as weight is shifted forward

Knee extension control

Hip extension control with ankle dorsiflexion

Body moving ahead of foot; foot must remain in contact with ground

Transfer of weight through foot

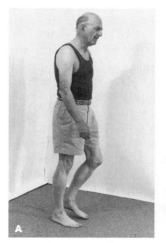
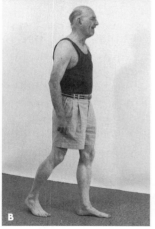
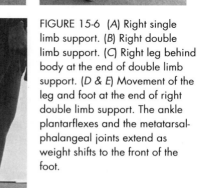
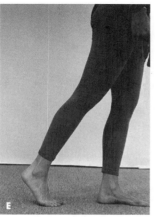

FIGURE 15-6 (*A*) Right single limb support. (*B*) Right double limb support. (*C*) Right leg behind body at the end of double limb support. (*D & E*) Movement of the leg and foot at the end of right double limb support. The ankle plantarflexes and the metatarsal-phalangeal joints extend as weight shifts to the front of the foot.

Swing

In swing phase of walking, the *leg moves from behind the body to in front of the body while the body continues to move forward.* At *early swing* on the right, the right hip is in extension, and the pelvis is rotated to the right. The upper trunk is in a rotation pattern opposite the pelvis, so the body remains balanced. To initiate swing, the foot and toes lift off the floor to allow clearance as the leg swings forward. The shift from ankle and foot plantarflexion control at the end of stance to dorsiflexion control at early swing is critical to the initiation of swing. Activity in the long toe extensors reinforces ankle dorsiflexion activity and provides additional lateral stability to the foot during swing (Fig. 15-7A & B). The pelvis rotates forward with the swinging leg. The upper trunk rotates opposite the pelvis to keep the body in the line of forward progression.

Late swing phase begins as the right leg begins to move in front of the body. As the leg reaches forward, the pelvis continues to rotate forward and the knee extends to within a few degrees of neutral. The ankle remains dorsiflexed to neutral and the toes are dorsiflexed as the right leg reaches forward and down toward the ground (Fig. 15-7C).

Swing phase is accomplished by a combination of three factors: active non-weight bearing control of the leg and foot, the "pendulum-like" movement of the leg as a result of trunk and pelvic position, and the continuing movement forward of the body and stance leg. The forward movement of the leg occurs as muscular activity in the foot and ankle clear the toes from the ground. At toe off, the pelvis is rotated back in its most posterior position of the gait cycle and the hip extended. As body weight shifts forward off the leg, the leg swings forward. During swing, the stance limb is in single limb support and is moving forward with the body.

Swing phase also presents challenging demands for the trunk. While the trunk remains aligned over the pelvis and the pelvis remains relatively horizontal over the supporting limb, the trunk must adjust to the rotational movements of the pelvis and the movement of the swinging leg from behind the body to in front of the body. This trunk adjustment occurs as the entire body is continuing to progress forward.

FIGURE 15-7 (*A & B*) Early swing phase. (*C*) Late swing phase.

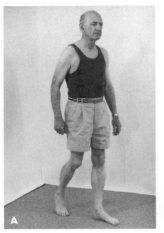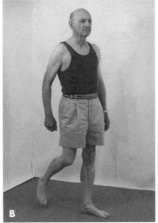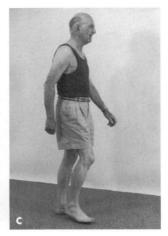

SIGNIFICANT IMPAIRMENTS THAT INTERFERE WITH PERFORMANCE

Therapists, treating patients with a hemiplegia, face an immense set of impairments as gait training begins.[6,7] Common movement impairments lead to similarities in compensatory gait patterns. These compensations are predictable and are a result of the primary neurologic impairment, the secondary impairments, resultant atypical movement patterns, and the type of therapy the patient receives. The impairments that were described in standing (Ch. 9) are applicable in walking. Problems of loss of trunk control and alignment, weakness and loss of alignment in the lower extremities, inappropriate initiation patterns, and abnormal tone are present during standing and walking. During walking these impairments become more noticeable because of the additional demands of forward movement and balance control.

This second portion of the chapter discusses impairments of the trunk, lower extremity and upper extremity in stance (forward progression, single/double limb support), and swing. Problems in stance phase differ from the problems in swing phase, yet they are interrelated. We realize that it is difficult to separate these problems into categories, but to simplify analysis, we will consider each body segment separately. The key to producing significant, lasting carryover is to plan a treatment program that combines trunk and extremity movement patterns during reeducation, functional sequencing, and performance.

TRUNK IMPAIRMENTS

Stance

Loss of Control of Upper Trunk over Lower Trunk

In *forward progression*, the upper trunk must remain balanced over the lower trunk and pelvis with the shoulders perpendicular to the line of progression. This alignment is maintained as the body moves forward to midstance. The lower trunk and pelvis begin to rotate backward as the body moves over the foot. Patients with hemiplegia have difficulty maintaining control of the upper trunk over the lower trunk as the body moves forward over the leg. Loss of upper trunk control results in *improper initiation patterns* of stance on the hemiplegic leg. Patients compensate by initiating with the upper trunk instead of the lower extremity or by moving in an inappropriate direction. Common atypical patterns include upper body forward flexion and rotation with hip flexion, upper trunk rotation forward with lower trunk rotation backward, and lateral trunk flexion with the concavity on the hemiplegic side. In patients who do not walk independently, with severe trunk and leg weakness, we often see the upper body forward-flexed position. During walking, if the forward initiation pattern comes from the upper body, the direction of the leg movement is backward, instead of forward. This results in ankle plantarflexion, knee hyperextension, and hip flexion (Fig. 15-8A). Loss of trunk control and early reliance on a quad cane or hemiwalker can result in the pattern of upper trunk rotation forward and lower trunk rotation backward. The upper trunk in these patients shears laterally toward their uninvolved side, and the pelvis elevates. Extensor hypertonicity in the leg is commonly present as a result of the trunk asymmetry (Fig. 15-5B). Other patients with loss of trunk control and

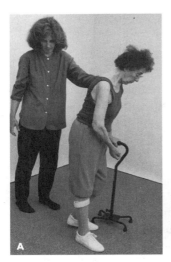 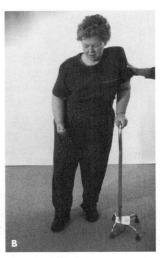 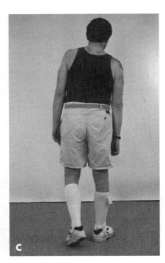

FIGURE 15-8 (*A*) Patient with a right hemiplegia with loss of control of the upper trunk over the lower trunk in forward progression. (*B*) Patient with a right hemiplegia with upper trunk rotation forward and lower trunk rotation backward. Her upper trunk shears laterally as she shifts to the left to rely on the quad cane for balance. (*C*) Patient with a right hemiplegia. His upper trunk is laterally flexed and shortened during forward progression.

FIGURE 15-9 Treatment in forward progression with a patient with a right hemiplegia. The therapist's right hand corrects upper trunk forward flexion and rotation, and her left hand provides counterpressure for the right hand. She helps the patient practice initiating the forward movement from the legs.

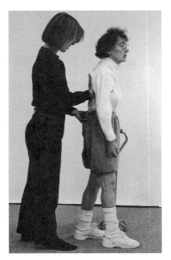

arm weakness or paralysis have a trunk pattern of lateral flexion with the concavity to the affected side (Fig. 15-8C).

During treatment of the forward progression period of walking, therapists must include *two trunk treatment goals.* One is to reestablish trunk and lower extremity alignment to allow reeducation of lower extremity patterns; the other is to train trunk control during lower-extremity-initiated weight shift with the feet in step/stance (Fig. 15-9). Treatment of upper trunk control over the lower trunk during walking must include assessment and treatment of the hemiplegic arm (see Chs. 5 to 7).

In *single limb support,* the upper and lower trunk must move forward with and remain balanced over the pelvis. The trunk provides much of the control that keeps the pelvis appropriately positioned. If the trunk becomes asymmetric, control of the pelvis is lost (Fig. 15-10A). This period of gait requires precise trunk and balance control because it is the time in the gait cycle when the center of gravity moves outside the base of support for a brief moment. Precise control of the upper and lower trunk is needed to keep the pelvis level and the body from falling. This is the most difficult phase for patients to control and therapists to treat.

At heel off, the end of *double limb support,* the requirement for upper trunk control is to remain balanced over and adapt to the movements and position of the lower trunk and pelvis. The upper trunk remains relatively perpendicular to the line of progression, and the lower trunk and pelvis rotate backward as the body moves forward of the stance leg. When loss of trunk control results in upper trunk asymmetries, the lower trunk and pelvic movements are difficult to retrain (Fig. 15-10B). The alignment and control of the trunk in this period is also difficult for patients because of the loss of upper trunk extension control and weakness in the

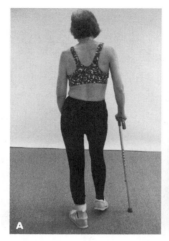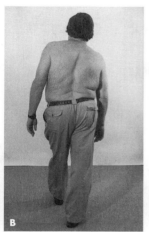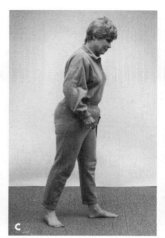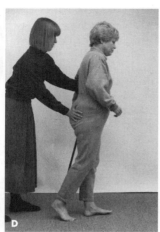

FIGURE 15-10 (A) Left single limb support phase of walking in patient with left hemi-plegia. Her trunk cannot remain aligned over the pelvis as she stands on her left leg. (B) Patient with a right hemiplegia. His trunk is laterally flexed with the concavity on the right, and his pelvis is elevated. (C) Patient with a right hemiplegia at the end of right double limb support. Her lower trunk is rotated backward and her pelvis is ele-vated. Her lower leg and foot spin into external rotation as she unweights her leg. (D) In treatment, the therapist uses her left hand on the anterior lower aspect of the left rib cage and her right hand on the right pelvis to assist with trunk alignment and control as the patient practices forward/backward movements. The therapist corrects the rota-tion with her left hand (she does not push the right side forward); she rotates the left side backward and uses her right hand to assist the weight shift over the left leg.

arm. Retraining upper and lower trunk control as the body moves ahead of the leg is an important trunk treatment goal for this phase of gait (Fig. 15-10C & D).

Swing

Loss of Trunk Control and Alignment

In swing phase, the upper and lower trunk remain aligned, rotate on each other a small amount, and continue to move forward. The difficulty of the trunk task increases because during swing, only one leg is supporting the trunk. With one leg swinging forward, the lower trunk and pelvis must stay oriented horizontally, pro-vide stability for the swinging leg, and continue to maintain the forward movement of walking.

In preparation for trunk reeducation during swing, the therapist must make sure there is enough muscle length (abdominals, latissimus, quadratus lumborum) to allow the upper trunk to remain aligned over and respond to the moving lower trunk and leg. Treatment can be divided into *three parts*. In the first part of treat-ment, the therapist supports the upper body while the lower trunk movements are practiced in patterns that lengthen areas of tightness. The therapist then corrects leg asymmetries and retrains upper body responses to assisted movements of the lower trunk and leg. Thirdly, the therapist retrains trunk control with forward momentum; she assists the trunk control as the affected leg swings forward and the body continues to move over the stance leg.

FIGURE 15-11 (*A*) Patient with left hemiplegia, in forward progression with left pelvic rotation forward and left hip internal rotation. (*B*) Patient with right hemiplegia in forward progression with right pelvic rotation backward and elevation with right hip flexion. (*C*) Patient with left hemiplegia in forward progression with left pelvic elevation and right hip flexion and adduction.

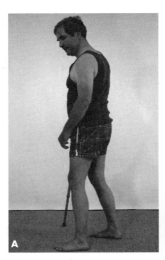 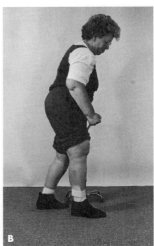 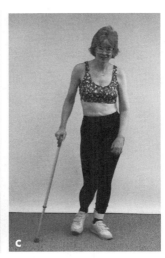

LOWER EXTREMITY IMPAIRMENTS

Stance-Forward Progression

Loss of Lower-Extremity-Initiated Forward Weight Shift

During forward progression, the movement is initiated from the lower extremity in a forward direction. Atypical leg movements occur either because the upper body initiates the weight shift or because the direction of the movement is incorrect. If the upper trunk is flexed or rotated forward, hip extension movements are blocked. If the hip does not extend, the leg cannot initiate the forward weight shift. With loss of hip extension, the ankle remains plantarflexed and the knee either hyperextends or flexes excessively. Common atypical leg patterns during forward progression include

Pelvic rotation forward with hip flexion and internal rotation (Fig. 15-11A)
Pelvic rotation backward and elevation with hip flexion (Fig. 15-11B)
Pelvic elevation with hip flexion/adduction (excessive lateral weight shift—hanging on hip) (Fig. 15-11C)

Hip weakness, especially hip extensors/abductors, results in difficulty initiating lower extremity movements during forward progression. This is more obvious in patients with poor trunk control who sit more than walk. Hip extension strength and control is a requirement of safe, functional walking because it is a critical component of the entire stance phase. Winter[8] remarks that the single most important correlation with improvement of hip extension control is alignment and control of the head, arms, and trunk. In treatment, we have found that increasing upper body extension control leads to improved strength and control of the hip in standing and walking. In patients with excessive hip flexion caused by hip extensor weakness, the line of gravity of the hip falls anterior to the knee joint. This results in knee hyperextension and ankle joint plantarflexion. Prolonged plantarflexion results in loss of joint range, shortened muscle tissue, and limited or absent heel contact.

Leg treatment must establish compatible proximal and distal movement control. The proximal goals should focus on increasing hip extension in conjunction with increasing trunk extension control to maintain alignment over the pelvis. Distal treatment goals should include ankle dorsiflexion range and control and alignment and control of lower leg over foot. Distal treatment goals are then sequenced and combined with proximal goals during movement through stance.

Loss of Ankle Joint Range and Control

For the heel to contact the ground at the beginning of forward progression, the ankle and foot must dorsiflex as the leg reaches down to the floor. If ankle dorsiflexion range is limited because of tightness or if the muscles are too weak to lift the foot, the leg pattern for the rest of stance phase is affected. When ankle dorsiflexion is not available as the leg reaches to the floor, the forefoot makes contact with the floor. If the forefoot contacts the ground, the patient shifts his weight backward to place the entire foot on the ground. The ankle plantarflexes and the hip flexes with this posterior leg movement. To move the body forward from this position, the patient compensates with his trunk, either by inclining forward or rotating the uninvolved side forward (Fig. 15-12A)

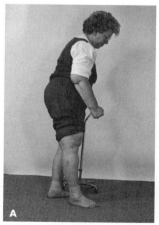
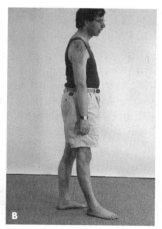
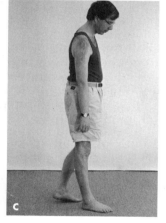
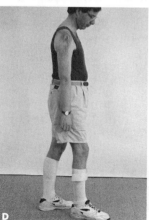
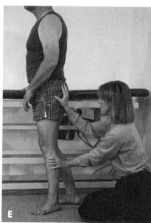

FIGURE 15-12 (A) Loss of ankle joint dorsiflexion range in a patient with a right hemiplegia. Her hip stays flexed as she moves forward. (B) Patient with loss of ankle joint dorsiflexion range and control on the right. (C) As he shifts forward, his ankle remains plantarflexed, his knee hyperextends, and his hip flexes. (D) With a semisolid ankle foot brace, his leg begins to move forward, and the knee hyperextension is corrected. (E) Patient with a left hemiplegia in left step/stance. Therapist helps the patient learn the timing necessary to move his thigh and lower leg forward over a dorsiflexing ankle.

Loss of ankle joint dorsiflexion range in forward progression and single/double limb support is one of the causes of knee recurvatum. When patients cannot activate ankle dorsiflexion muscles, an ankle-foot brace must be provided to allow the heel to make initial contact (Fig. 15-12B–D). Initial heel contact is an important component of initial stance, for it sets the foundation of the forward body movement during walking. If weakness is present in the leg, a brace provides distal stability, thus making it easier to reeducate proximal patterns. Ankle foot braces should be flexible enough to allow some ankle joint movement, or they should be trimmed to allow forward movement as trunk and leg control increase.

During treatment the therapist should set goals to maintain correct trunk and pelvic position, initiate the weight shift from the legs in a forward direction, and reestablish ankle joint range and control (Fig. 15-12E).

Single Limb Support

Instability of the Hip

In hemiplegia, the hip is often unstable in the lateral direction. When the lateral muscles of the hip are weak, the patient moves further laterally than forward during forward progression. This excessive lateral shift occurs because there is little muscular activity controlling the movement of the pelvis and femur. The patient shifts laterally to the point where ligamentous tension provides lateral stability. Therapists refer to this as "hanging on the hip" (see Fig. 15-10A). The pelvis is usually elevated and rotated and the femur adducted and internally rotated. In some patients who use this atypical pattern, there is a large bulging area over the lateral aspect of the upper thigh. This prominence is the superior aspect of the greater trochanter that has shifted to a more lateral position. As the femur adducts and internally rotates, the line of gravity moves anterior to the knee, and the knee hyperextends.

In treatment, the therapist must help the patient learn to move forward instead of laterally by assisting with trunk/leg alignment and reeducating hip muscles in standing (Fig. 15-13A and B).

FIGURE 15-13 (*A*) Patient with a right hemiplegia hanging on her right hip in single limb support. The therapist is providing a balance assist to the trunk but is not correcting the atypical leg pattern. (*B*) Therapist corrects trunk alignment and supports the lateral aspect of the hip joint with her left hand while the patient practices stepping with her left leg.

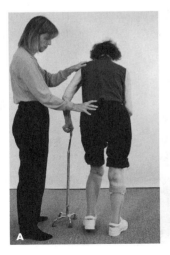
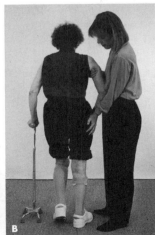

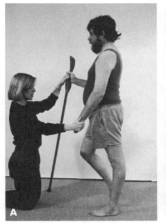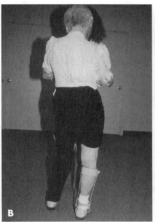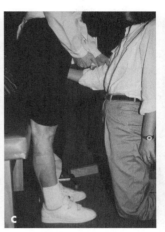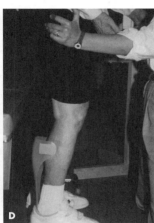

FIGURE 15-14 (*A*) Knee hyperextension in single limb support phase of walking. (*B*) Patient with a right hemiplegia who is not independently ambulatory. She moves excessively laterally during single limb support, and her knee hyperextends. Although she wears a Klenzak brace with a T-strap, the brace does not control the recurvatum. When the cause of the recurvatum is a hip problem, a brace will never be able to control the knee. However, a treatment program aimed at improving hip control and the assistance of a well chosen brace will begin to correct the knee position. (*C*) Patient standing with severe knee recurvatum and ankle joint plantarflexion. She wears a polypropylene ankle/foot brace that can hold her ankle at 90 degrees, but the recurvatum pushes it into plantarflexion. (*D*) Therapist corrects lateral hip position and helps the patient shift forward. Ankle range is available and the knee moves out of recurvatum.

Loss of Knee Control

In single limb support, the most common lower extremity problem is loss of knee control. During normal stance, the knee maintains a relatively constant position of extension while the position of the hip and ankle change as the body moves over the foot. The two knee problems in single limb support—hyperextension and excessive flexion—are directly attributable to alignment and control problems at the hip and ankle.

Knee Hyperextension

Knee hyperextension results from hip instability, loss of ankle joint dorsiflexion range and control, shortened and shifted two-joint muscles (hamstrings and tensor fascia lata), or from a combination of these causes. Activation of the rectus femoris muscle often causes knee hyperextension, but in other patients, the knee hyperextension is a passive result of control and alignment impairments of the hip or ankle, or both (Fig. 15-14A). The causes of knee hyperextension are also described in Chapter 9. During walking, the need to control forward momentum and the need for balance during unilateral stance exaggerate the knee problems.

Loss of lateral hip control and excessive lateral weight shift in single limb support place the femur in a relatively adducted position. As the patient "hangs on his hip" and the femur adducts and internally rotates, the line of gravity shifts in front of the knee. Since this "hanging" is not accompanied by active trunk or leg control, the knee is pushed or locked mechanically into a hyperextended position (Fig. 15-14B–D).

FIGURE 15-15 (A) Patient with a right hemiplegia in forward progression with knee recurvatum. (B & C) As he moves through right single limb support, he pushes his right knee into flexion to avoid recurvatum.

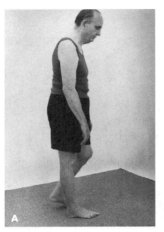 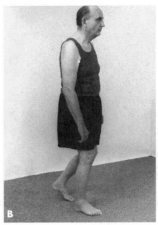 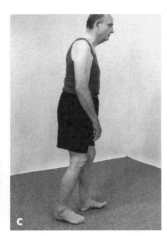

The second reason for knee recurvatum, *loss of ankle joint dorsiflexion* range or control, is described above in the forward progression section and in Chapter 9. If the ankle joint does not dorsiflex to allow the leg to move over the foot, the knee hyperextends as the body moves forward. Muscle shortening of the gastrocnemius, lack of proximal (hip and trunk) alignment and control, a sensory "need" to find the ground, or ankle and foot edema are possible contributing reasons for loss of ankle joint dorsiflexion. Treatment must prevent the development of foot and ankle edema and must maintain length in both the posterior calf muscles across the knee and ankle and in the large multijoint muscles of the hip and knee to keep adequate ankle range.

In hemiplegic patients, *muscle shortening* may occur in the long two-joint muscles that attach to the pelvis and femur and tibia and in the small, deep rotator muscles of the hip. As the patient stands, if the trunk, pelvis, and femur become asymmetric, the length and line of pull of these muscles change. As the knee continues to extend, these shortened and shifted muscle tendons affect knee position. With the pelvis elevated and the femur flexed and internally rotated, tight lateral hamstring or tensor fascia lata muscles pull the knee into hyperextension.

Excessive Knee Flexion

Knee flexion is the other common knee problem that occurs during stance. Excessive knee flexion during single limb support is often adopted as a strategy to prevent the knee from hyperextending. Excessive knee flexion allows tibial movement forward over the foot without recurvatum, but results in atypical movements at the hip and foot. When the knee is pushed into flexion and held there, the pelvis rotates forward, the hip flexes, internally rotates, and adducts. The ankle may remain in plantarflexion, while the midfoot is pushed into a pronated position with severe midfoot collapse and resultant forefoot abduction and toe clawing (Fig. 15-15A–C). The flexed or "crouch" knee position may prevent overstretching of the posterior knee capsule, but it results in inappropriate hip positioning and a destructive collapse of the midfoot. Therapists should plan a treatment program to improve the hip and ankle impairments that are causing the recurvatum to develop active control of the knee before training a strategy that may produce new, unwanted problems.

Toe Curling and Clawing

Toes curl or claw during stance phase, and especially during single limb support, for two reasons: as part of a balance or *equilibrium response* and as a result of *abnormal alignment* of the lower leg, ankle, and foot. During walking, when trunk and extremity control is insufficient to maintain balance, the toes "grab" the floor as part of the body's response to prevent falling. In single limb support, as the line of gravity falls outside the stance foot, balance demands are at their greatest and toe curling or clawing increases (Fig. 15-16). Loss of foot alignment is the second reason for toe curling or clawing. Loss of alignment is due to weakness in the trunk and leg or shortened muscles in the ankle and foot. With loss of ankle joint dorsiflexion range, the calcaneus moves into a position of equinus and inversion. Patients compensate for this limitation with various atypical midfoot and forefoot patterns. Some patients move through stance with their foot inverted and internally rotate their leg to get the foot in contact with the floor. Others, with less structural integrity of foot tissues, push or collapse the midfoot into the floor. In both cases, the arches of the foot become altered, tissues tighten, and long toe muscles shorten.

Toes that curl are in phalangeal joint flexion, and the toe nails dig into the floor. The midfoot of this foot is more inverted and long toe flexor tendons are shortened (Fig. 15-17).

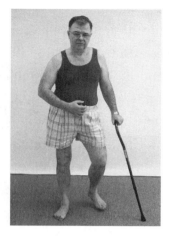

FIGURE 15-16 Toe curling in single limb support in patient with a right hemiplegia.

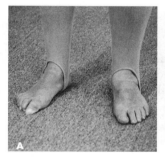
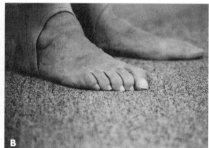

FIGURE 15-17 (*A & B*) Right toe curling. (*C*) Therapist lifts leg and foot off the floor to correct ankle and foot position to stop curling. Her left hand corrects tibial rotation as her right hand holds the foot and slowly dorsiflexes the ankle to stretch the posterior compartment muscles. (*D*) Her left hand moves distally to align the rearfoot on the midfoot. Note the forefoot plantarflexion. She lengthens tight foot tissues and corrects the midfoot position. (*E*) She continues to hold the rearfoot as she places the foot back down on the floor.

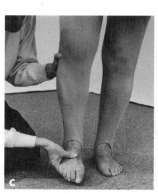
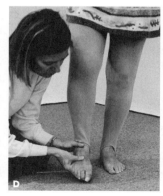
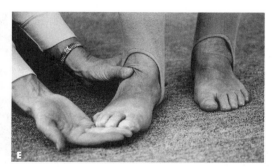

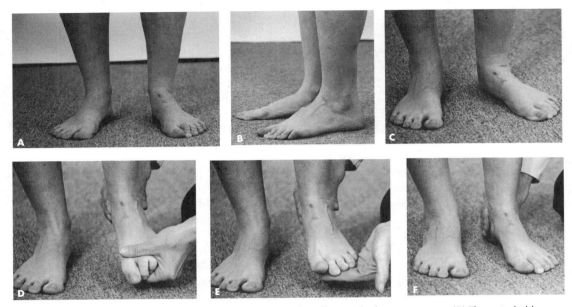

FIGURE 15-18 (*A & B*) Left toe clawing. (*C*) Left midfoot pushed into pronation. (*D*) Therapist holds rearfoot and forefoot as she lifts foot off the floor to correct the cause of the toe clawing. While her hands are in a position similar to that in Fig. 15-17D, they are applying different messages. Her right hand holds and moves the calcaneus out of equinus while her left hand lengthens tight toe extensor tendons. Her left fingers are lengthening tight plantar tissues to reestablish a longitudinal arch. (*E*) As the tissues release and alignment is reestablished, the toes straighten. (*F*) As she places the foot on the floor, she continues to align the rearfoot. Note the arch of the foot in comparison to C.

Clawed toes are in metatarsophalangeal joint extension, proximal phalangeal joint flexion, and distal phalangeal joint extension. In stance, the midfoot collapses or pushes into pronation. Muscle tightness exists in both the long toe flexor and extensor tendons (Fig. 15-18).

Double Limb Support—Heel Off

Inability to Keep Foot on Floor

At the end of double limb support, the hip is extended, the heel rises off the floor, and the weight of the body is on the ball of the foot and the dorsiflexed toes. The body is moving in front of the leg, but the foot–leg remains in contact with the ground. This position is maintained by appropriate alignment and control of the trunk and leg. The body grades the muscular control to adjust the amount of pressure on the ball of the foot as a balance assist to keep the foot on the floor as long as possible. This is a difficult position for patients to assume and control. Tightness of pelvic and hip muscles makes it hard for them to place their legs in the step/stance position: to keep the upper trunk forward, the pelvis rotated back, and the leg behind the body (Fig. 15-19A). They have difficulty grading ankle and foot movements to keep the foot in contact with the ground while the leg is extended behind the body.

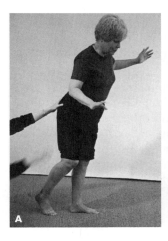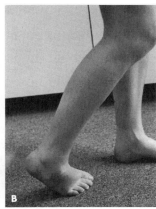

FIGURE 15-19 (*A*) Patient trying to keep the leg and trunk aligned in double limb support. (*B*) The right foot postures in inversion as weight is shifted off the right leg onto the left.

Treatment of this portion of gait requires lengthening shortened muscles to position the leg in step/stance with appropriate trunk alignment. Treatment must reeducate control of the foot on the floor: depression of the leg behind the body, as the hip extends and the body moves forward. As weight shifts onto the ball of the foot and the heel lifts off the ground, the patient's foot tends to posture in inversion (Fig. 15-19B).

Swing

Atypical Muscle Firing

In swing, atypical muscle firing, inappropriate initiation patterns and the inability to sustain appropriate firing are more noticeable. Patients have difficulty moving the swing leg with appropriate speed and smoothness, and changing the firing pattern from one of hip extension and knee flexion with the leg behind the body, to hip flexion with knee extension with the leg in front of the body. Patients typically stop the forward progression as they attempt to lift and swing the involved leg forward. They stop to "get their balance" when trunk and leg control is inadequate. Forward momentum is lost. Without forward movement, the gait pattern is halting and swing phase is performed atypically. They initiate with pelvic elevation or rotation backward, a posterior pelvic tilt, or by using the uninvolved side and a stable cane. When they initiate with pelvic rotation backward or elevation, the hip flexes slightly and internally rotates. The patient may then use rectus femoris firing to increase hip flexion and extend the knee. Since the ankle is usually plantar flexed, the patient overshifts to the unaffected side or circumducts to clear the foot from the floor (Fig. 15-20).

Patients with strong backward rotation of the pelvis and lower trunk at late stance initiate swing by rotating the entire trunk forward. Other patients posteriorly tilt the pelvis to initiate swing. In this pattern, the hip externally rotates and abducts with knee flexion. This flexion pattern of the leg is usually accompanied by strong foot inversion.

In treatment, these problems of muscle timing and firing in the leg are trained with stance leg forward movement to replicate the demands of the swing cycle. Carryover into walking will not occur if these problems are treated only in a stationary position.

FIGURE 15-20 Patient with a right hemiplegia uses pelvic elevation to initiate swing. Her knee is strongly extended and her foot postures in supination.

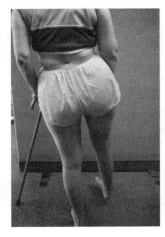

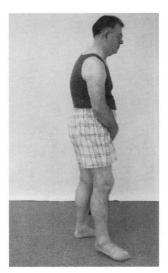

FIGURE 15-21 Patient with a right hemiplegia with insufficient ankle joint dorsiflexion in swing.

Insufficient Ankle Dorsiflexion

If the foot and ankle muscles are not active to help clear the floor, atypical movements are used in the trunk and pelvis to clear the toes. Common atypical patterns such as pelvic rotation backward, pelvic elevation, excessive lateral shift to the cane to unweight the foot, vaulting on the unaffected side, or combinations of these are used to initiate movement in space. When the foot and ankle muscles are weak and cannot clear the foot from the floor, bracing can be used to prevent these atypical patterns from occurring. Proximal compensations become strong habits and, once established, are difficult to change. The therapist must take care to reassess active foot and ankle movement continually, and when it improves, reduce the amount of bracing control to allow the ankle and foot muscles to become stronger (Fig. 15-21).

Foot Posturing

When the foot inverts in swing, the inversion is a result of either firing of the anterior and posterior tibialis muscles, while the ankle remains plantarflexed, or from the influence of a shortened gastrocnemius muscle on the calcaneus as the knee extends, or a combination of these factors. Strong foot inversion with slight knee flexion eventually produces *excessive tibial external rotation*. This pattern of foot and lower leg rotation occurs frequently in patients with muscle return that has a quality of cocontraction. Inversion of the foot during swing sets up an atypical foot contact pattern at initial stance. The inverted foot contacts the ground on the lateral aspect of the forefoot (Fig. 15-22). The body then shifts weight posteriorly and medially to place the entire foot on the ground. This results in knee recurvatum with pelvic and hip internal rotation at the start of forward progression.

To avoid the pattern of inversion in swing and the atypical foot contact position, the foot must initially be aligned in a brace during walking. Bracing that controls the ankle position may not control foot position. Foot control in a brace requires specific rearfoot and midfoot control, long medial and/or lateral borders to control forefoot asymmetries, and a toe plate, if necessary, to stop forefoot plantarflexion. The therapist must also work to strengthen and reeducate firing patterns in the foot and ankle from the end of stance through heel contact, so that bracing control can be decreased and minimized.

UPPER EXTREMITY IMPAIRMENTS

Stance and Swing

Weakness

Upper extremity problems during walking are the result of muscle weakness, trunk asymmetry, and poor balance control. Weakness in the arm creates an abnormal force on the upper trunk. The heaviness of the weak arm pulls on the upper trunk and results in upper trunk asymmetries. A weak arm that is unsupported causes the upper trunk to flex forward or laterally (Fig. 15-23). If the arm contributes to upper trunk asymmetries, the process of reeducation of leg musculature required for walking is harder because alignment and control of the upper trunk and arm are prerequisites for reeducation of hip control. Treatment of weak arm muscles

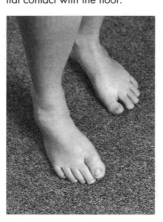

FIGURE 15-22 Strong foot inversion in swing. The lateral aspect of the forefoot makes initial contact with the floor.

includes reestablishing alignment of the scapula on the trunk, reduction of subluxation followed by active strengthening of shoulder girdle muscles, and reeducation of compatible trunk and arm patterns in standing.

Hypertonicity

Poor balance control in single limb support and in swing results in flexor hypertonicity of the arm. Abnormal, nonpurposeful arm posturing occurs during walking because of a lack of trunk or hip control during unilateral stance. The flexor posturing is, in part, a component of a balance response to keep the trunk balanced over one foot. During swing, if the patient uses an atypical initiation pattern, the center of gravity may be displaced closer to or outside the edge of the base of support. Because of weakness and loss of trunk and extremity control, patients need to recruit equilibrium responses earlier in the weight shift. For example, if a normal individual laterally overshifts during single limb support, he uses additional available leg or trunk muscle strength to keep from falling, or an equilibrium response in the foot. In patients with leg weakness, the same overshift during single limb support may result in an early equilibrium response, (i.e., arm posturing). We often see this as soon as the patient begins to walk. In standing, the arm may rest in extension by his side, but as soon as he begins to walk, the arm begins to posture (Fig. 15-24A & B). The hypertonicity of the arm may be a nonvolitional use of available muscles to assist the trunk to stay upright. As trunk or trunk and hip control improves, the arm hypertonicity will decrease. In this instance, the hypertonicity is not a primary arm problem but reflects the status of trunk or trunk and lower extremity control.

To decrease flexor hypertonicity in the arm in walking, treatment must focus on the trunk and hip control problems to improve strength, control, and balance. In chronic cases, or in cases in which trunk and lower extremity control never become sufficient to balance the body in sitting, standing, or walking, the arm may posture constantly and eventually have muscle shortening or joint contractures. When this happens, the arm postures because of the primary lack of trunk or lower extremity control and a secondary problem of tissue tightness or joint contracture as a result of prolonged abnormal alignment.

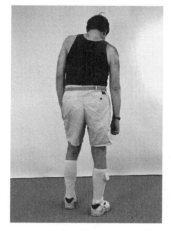

FIGURE 15-23 A weak right arm contributes to the lateral trunk asymmetry in stance.

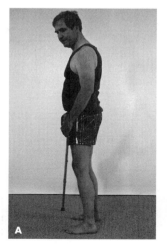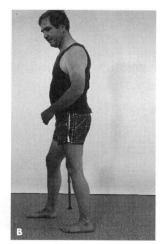

FIGURE 15-24 (A) Patient with a left hemiplegia in standing. His left arm is by his side. (B) As he begins to walk, his left arm begins to flex more.

Summary of Significant Functional Impairments

Forward Progression—Heel Strike to Midstance

Poor trunk control
  Loss of alignment of the upper trunk over lower trunk
  Loss of control of upper trunk as leg initiates weight shift forward
Lack of proper initiation pattern and direction
  Excessive forward trunk flexion
  Excessive lateral weight shift
Insufficient ankle joint dorsiflexion range
  Muscle tightness
  Loss of control
  Edema
Inappropriate foot contact
  Weakness of foot and ankle muscles
  Muscle tightness
  Foot posturing

Single/Double Limb Support

Insufficient trunk control to maintain position over one leg
  Asymmetries during unilateral stance
  Loss of control of upper trunk over lower trunk
Poor lower extremity control
  Hip instability
  Loss of knee control in unilateral stance
  Loss of ankle joint dorsiflexion range
  Toe clawing or curling
Loss of ability to transfer weight through foot
Inability to maintain leg on floor behind body
  Muscle tightness
  Weakness or inappropriate activation of leg muscles

Swing—Early and Late

Atypical leg muscle firing patterns
Lack of proper initiation
  Loss of ankle and foot dorsiflexion
  Inability to control trunk and lower extremity initiation pattern
  Initiation pattern
Inability of the body to continue to move forward as leg swings
Foot posturing

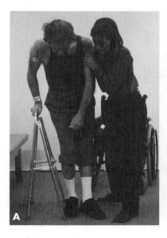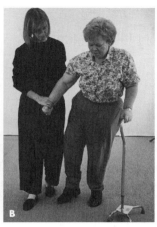

FIGURE 15-25 (*A*) Patient with a long standing severe hemiplegia walking precariously with a quad cane and the assistance of one. (*B*) Patient with a right hemiplegia and strong extensor hypertonicity of the leg. She is unable to walk safely with a quad cane because of loss of balance.

UNDESIRABLE COMPENSATORY PATTERNS

Compensatory patterns in walking result from severe problems of trunk control, weakness in the extremities, and strong hypertonicity. Undesirable compensatory patterns during walking usually develop when the patient uses a balance assist, such as a quad cane or hemiwalker. Common patterns include

1. Loss of control of trunk and leg resulting in complete reliance on a quad cane and an inability to walk safely, even with assistance (Fig. 15-25A).

2. Strong extensor hypertonicity of the leg resulting in an inability to move the leg without loss of balance (Fig. 15-25B).

ASSESSMENT GUIDELINES

The boxes below outline procedures for assessing the patient's abilities and weaknesses in forward progression, single/double limb support, and swing.

Forward Progression

I. From the step/stance position, with the involved leg forward, ask the patient to move the body forward and keep both feet on the ground. During the forward weight shift, describe the position of the trunk and the involved leg.

II. Assess the control of the upper trunk over the lower trunk as the patient moves forward.

III. Can the lower extremity initiate the movement? Does the ankle have range to move into dorsiflexion as the body moves forward? Can the hip extend toward neutral from flexion?

IV. Use your hands on the patient's trunk to correct the alignment and assist the movement. What improves when you put your hands on? What problems require further treatment.

V. List the trunk impairments that are interfering with forward progression.

VI. List the proximal leg impairments.

VII. List the ankle and foot impairments.

Single/Double Limb Support

I. From the step/stance position with the affected leg forward, ask the patient to step the unaffected leg forward. Describe the position of the trunk during single limb support.

II. Describe the position of the affected hip, knee, and ankle during single limb support

III. Use your hands on the patient's trunk to correct alignment and/or control problems. What improves when you put your hands on the patient? What problems require further treatment?

IV. Use your hands on the patient's hip to correct alignment and/or control problems. What improves when you put your hands on the patient? What problems require further treatment?

V. Use your hands on the patient's lower leg and femur/lower leg and ankle to assess knee control and to correct alignment and/or control problems. What improves when you put your hands on the patient?

VI. Describe the position of the trunk and leg at heel off.

VII. Use your hands on the patient's trunk to correct alignment and/or control problems. What improves when you put your hands on the patient? What problems require further treatment?

VIII. Use your hands on the patient's leg to correct alignment and/or control problems. What improves when you put your hands on the patient? What problems require further treatment?

IX. List the major impairments in the trunk that are interfering with this period of stance.

X. List the major impairments in the leg that are interfering with this period of stance.

Swing

I. Describe the position of the trunk and leg in early swing and in late swing as the body continues to move forward.

II. Assess the control of the hemiplegic leg as it swings through. Identify the movements that are missing or are performed with repeated atypical patterns.

III. Use your hands on the patient's leg to correct the alignment and/or assist the movements. What improves when you put your hands on the patient to correct asymmetries or assist the movement? What problems require further treatment?

IV. List the trunk impairments that are interfering with swing.

THERAPY GOALS

Functional Goals

The ability to walk independently means the ability to walk forwards, backwards, sideways. Functional walking allows us to walk and stop or turn and walk again. The ability to walk independently means being able to walk to where you need to go: to the next room, upstairs, downstairs, over carpets, and around chairs, outside, down a curb, across an open space, through a crowd of people, into an elevator, up an escalator. It also includes the ability to walk into the bathroom at night without needing to put on a brace.

The training of walking is necessary to help the patient meet the following functional goals:

1. Walk with assistance in therapy
2. Walk without assistance in therapy
3. Walk with assistance at home
4. Walk without assistance at home
5. Walk up and down stairs
6. Walk outdoors with assistance
7. Walk outdoors without assistance
8. Walk in social gatherings or in business settings
9. Walk and carry objects with either arm or both arms
10. Walk without use of brace or cane

Treatment Goals and Techniques

Treatment Goal: Correct alignment and increase symmetry and control of trunk during anterior/posterior weight shifts.

Treatment Technique: Reestablish alignment and control of upper trunk over lower trunk in step/stance position through the use of bilateral symmetric upper extremity grip (Fig. 15-26A–D).

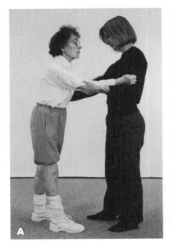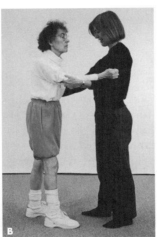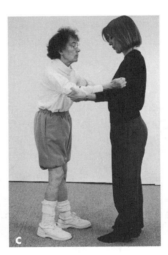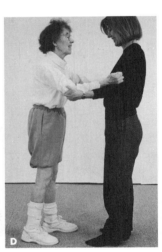

FIGURE 15-26 (*A*) Starting position, patient with a right hemiplegia in right step/stance. She cannot ambulate independently. Patient places her left arm on therapist's right arm. (*B*) Therapist places her right arm on the posterolateral aspect of the patient's left pelvis and holds the patient's humerus while supporting the forearm against her arm. Therapist corrects the upper trunk position by directing a backward and upward message through the patient's right arm and uses her right arm to direct a lateral message to help the patient keep her weight between her two legs. The therapist teaches the patient to shift forward over her hemiplegic right leg. (*C & D*) Patient steps her left leg forward and practices anterior/posterior lower-extremity-initiated weight shifts. Therapist moves her right hand to the patient's left arm to allow the patient to practice keeping her weight centered as she shifts forward/backward. (*Figure continues.*)

Treatment Technique: Practice of anterior/posterior weight shifts with a cane. Provide alignment to trunk and teach control of trunk over legs with unilateral upper trunk support (Fig. 15-26E–G).

Treatment Technique: Teaching the patient the movement memory of walking with a symmetric trunk using an axillary grip (Fig. 15-26H–J).

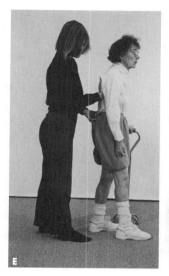
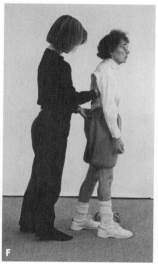
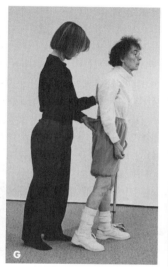
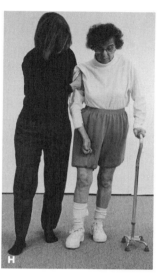

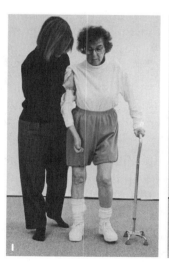
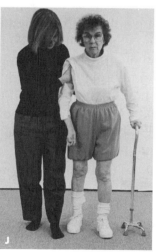

FIGURE 15-26 (*Continued*) (*E*) Therapist uses an axillary grip with her right arm and lifts the upper trunk up and back. Patient was previously trained to use a quad cane. As she gains control, a straight cane can be introduced. (*F*) She uses her left hand to assist the patient to initiate the movements from her legs in right step/stance. It is important to teach the patient how to shift over both legs without excessive leaning onto the quad cane. (*G*) As patient practices the same movements in left step/stance, she cannot keep her right heel on the floor because of overshifting to the cane, insufficient hip extension range/control, or insufficient ankle dorsiflexion range. This activity is practiced repeatedly without walking, but with forward/backward movements in right and left step/stance positions. (*H*) Therapist's right hand uses an axillary grip to support the upper trunk while her left hand is on the posterolateral side of the patient's left rib cage. (*I*) The therapist reminds the patient to keep her upper trunk extended as she shifts her trunk and hip forward. Note how the therapist's feet step in parallel with the patient's. (*J*) The therapist must be careful to time her corrections and assistance to the patient's initiation pattern.

Treatment Goal: Train forward weight shifts and increase lateral hip stability during single/double limb support.

Treatment Technique: Therapist corrects leg asymmetries and lengthens shortened muscles during single/double limb support (Fig. 15-27A–E).

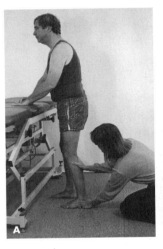
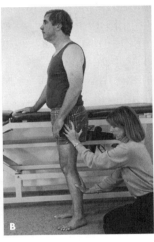
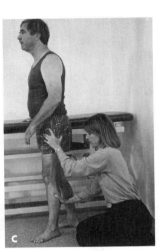
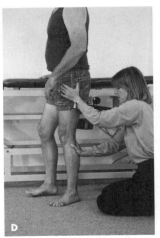
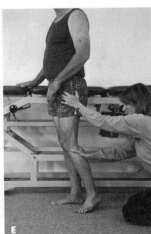

FIGURE 15-27 (*A*) Patient with a left hemiplegia in right step/stance. Therapist uses extended arm weight bearing to help provide upper body support while she lengthens his posterior calf muscles. The web space of her left hand holds the rearfoot while her right hand internally rotates his tibia to neutral and gives a downward pressure into his heel. She maintains correction of alignment and asks him to shift forward/backward from his legs. She asks him to stop or reverse the movement when she feels muscle resistance and waits for the tightened tissue to release. (*B*) When the patient has enough length in his ankle for the demands of single/double limb support, the therapist asks the patient to turn sideways. She places her left hand over his hip joint and her right hand on the back of the calf. Her left hand rotates the pelvis back to neutral and her right hand internally rotates the tibia to neutral and keeps weight evenly distributed over the foot. (*C–E*) As she asks the patient to step his right leg backward and then forward, she uses both hands to keep the knee from moving into recurvatum and to teach the patient the feeling of moving over his foot. She corrects the tendency of the pelvis to rotate forward in single limb support with her right hand and the tendency of the foot to supinate at heel off with her left hand. (*Figure continues.*)

Treatment Technique: Using verbal reminders for more independent practice in preparation for home program (Fig. 15-27F–H).

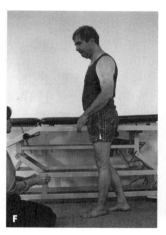
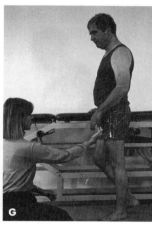
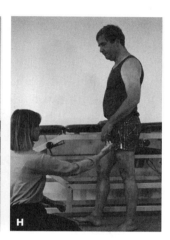

FIGURE 15-27 (*Continued*) (*F–H*) Patient practices moving over his affected leg in single double limb support with the therapist using verbal reminders and relating them to the manual messages previously experienced. Before taking both hands off, the therapist decides which hand is controlling the impairment that is most significant, leaves that hand on, uses verbal reminders and a manual message for a few repetitions.

Treatment Goal: To control severe knee recurvatum during stance phase of walking.

Treatment Technique: Correction of ankle and hip asymmetries and reeducation of leg control throughout stance phase (Fig. 15-28).

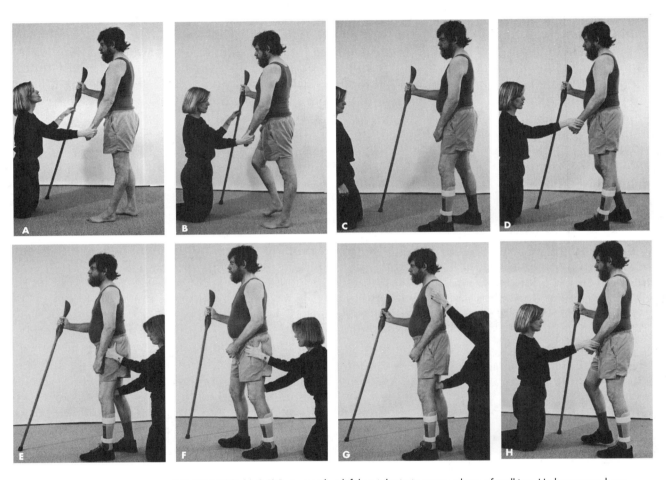

FIGURE 15-28 (*A & B*) Patient with a left hemiplegia in stance phase of walking. He has severe knee recurvatum at heel contact and during single limb support. (*C & D*) Therapist uses a polypropylene solid ankle brace with foot control and asks patient to practice shifting onto his leg. The recurvatum is less in left step/stance but still present as he tries to shift forward onto his left leg. (*E*) With the brace assisting ankle alignment and control, the therapist corrects pelvis and femoral rotation. With the thumb and palm of her left hand, she rotates his pelvis forward, and with her right hand she externally rotates his femur to neutral. (*F*) As she corrects these two rotational asymmetries, the hyperextension force at the knee decreases, and he shifts forward with no hyperextension. (*G*) The therapist moves more proximally and gives him a reminder to keep his upper trunk moving with his pelvis as she continues to control the femoral rotational component. (*H*) Patient practices with minimal manual assistance and verbal reminders.

Treatment Goal: Reeducate foot and ankle muscles in early swing phase.

Treatment Technique: Correction of leg asymmetries and active assistive reeducation to the ankle and foot (Fig. 15-29).

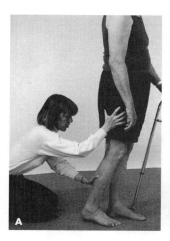 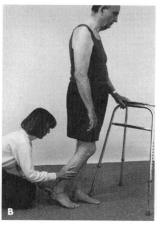 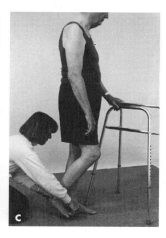

FIGURE 15-29 (A) Patient with a right hemiplegia standing with the support of a walker in left step/stance. Therapist places her right hand on his femur and her left hand on the tibia and externally rotates both leg segments to neutral as she asks him to shift forward onto his left leg. (B) She moves both hands more distally and her left hand now controls the rearfoot. Her control of the rearfoot helps prevent toe clawing. She uses both hands to help him learn how to move his heel gradually off the floor without losing control of depression so that he can shift forward onto the ball of the right foot. (C) As he shifts further forward and begins to swing his leg, she has him practice lifting his toes and ankle into dorsiflexion while the leg moves. Note the small size of the step/stance position. This decreases the demands on the hip and lower trunk so she can focus on ankle and foot reeducation.

Treatment Goal: Train trunk and leg movements during swing phase.

Treatment Technique: Correct trunk alignment and teach patient to continue moving over stance leg (Fig. 15-30A–E).

Treatment Technique: Alternate hand placements for assisting trunk alignment and control during swing (Fig. 15-30F–H).

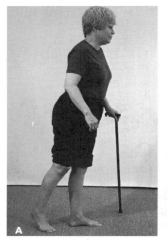
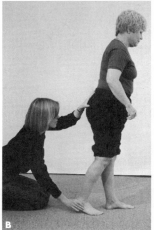
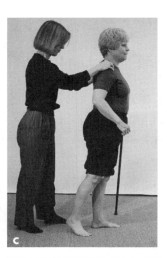
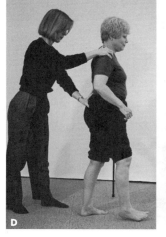
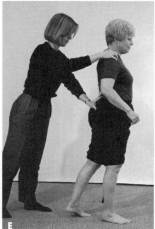

FIGURE 15-30 (*A*) Patient with a right hemiplegia with her right leg at the end of stance. Her lower trunk and pelvis are rotated backward excessively, and her right lower leg and foot are spinning out. Her hip is flexed instead of extended and her thumb is inclined forward. (*B*) Therapist corrects the rotational component of the lower trunk and leg. Patient practices moving forward into hip extension. (*C*) Patient practices lower trunk and leg movements while therapist helps her align the upper trunk over the lower trunk and leg. (*D & E*) Therapist assists upper trunk extension and lower trunk rotation and teaches the patient to continue moving forward as her leg swings. They practice continuing to shift forward onto the foot in forward progression. (*Figure continues.*)

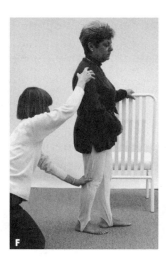

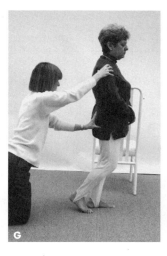

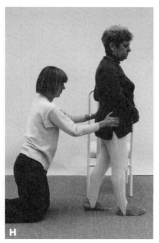

FIGURE 15-30 (*Continued*) (*F*) Therapist's hands are teaching the patient to stay balanced over both feet as the body moves forward and the hip extends. This helps keep the foot on the floor at the end of stance in preparation for swing. (*G*) The therapist's right hand reminds the upper trunk to stay aligned over the lower trunk and her left hand assists the lower-extremity-initiated forward weight shift by giving a message diagonally and down toward the left foot. (*H*) Therapist uses a bilateral pelvic grip to teach the patient to shift both sides of her lower trunk forward.

Treatment Technique: Reeducating leg movements during swing (Fig. 15-31).

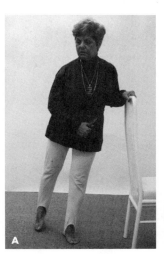

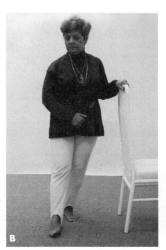

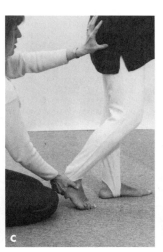

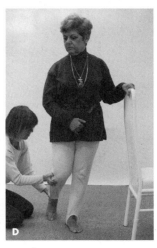

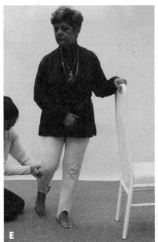

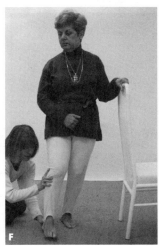

FIGURE 15-31 (*A & B*) Patient with a right hemiplegia moving her leg in swing phase. She initiates swing with pelvis elevation and rotation backward. Her right foot plantarflexes and inverts during swing. (*C*) Therapist's left hand is on the back of the pelvis as a reminder not to rotate backward (she does not rotate the pelvis forward). Her right hand holds the rearfoot to assist ankle movement, to correct rearfoot varus, and to help the patient grade the weight shift over the forefoot. (*D–F*) As the patient shifts forward over her left leg, the therapist corrects lower leg and rearfoot alignment as the patient swings her leg through. The therapist holds the heel by placing the web space of her left hand behind the heel with her thumb on the outside and her fingers on the inside. Her right hand guides the rotational components of the lower leg.

Treatment Goal: Reeducate trunk and leg components in a progression.

Treatment Technique: Upper trunk symmetric support for alignment and control of trunk and legs, unilateral trunk support while training use of a standard cane, upper extremity support while turning and walking with a cane (Fig. 15-32).

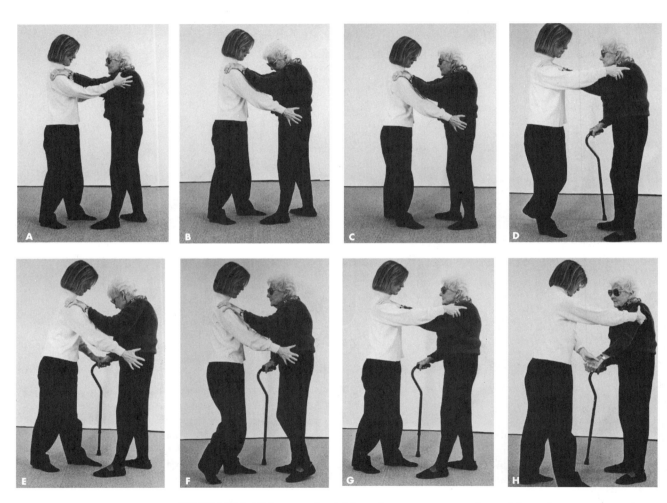

FIGURE 15-32 (A) Patient with a left hemiplegia practicing standing in left step/stance position. Therapist uses her hands on the patient's upper trunk to assist with alignment of trunk over the legs. (B & C) Therapist moves her right hand to the patient's hip to assist as the patient begins to walk. (D) Patient begins to walk with a standard cane. Therapist uses her right hand to align the upper trunk over the pelvis and allows the patient to practice balancing. (E) Patient's left arm remains on the therapist's shoulder as an assist for the upper trunk as the therapist helps her practice moving the cane forward. (F & G) Therapist's left hand moves from the pelvis to the upper trunk to assist with balance or strength needs as the patient walks. (H–J) Therapist supports the upper trunk with a unilateral axillary hand grip as the patient practices turning to the affected side. This helps the patient maintain alignment of the upper trunk over the pelvis and teaches her to avoid placing excessive weight on the cane. (*Figure continues.*)

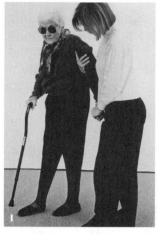
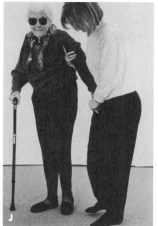
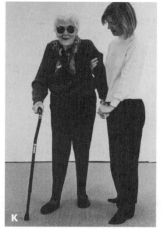
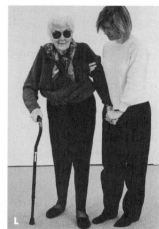

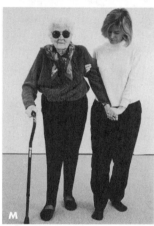
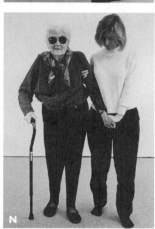

FIGURE 15-32 (*Continued*) (*K–N*) Therapist continues to use this grip to encourage alignment of the upper trunk over the left leg as the patient practices walking with equal step lengths and an even cadence.

ACTIVITIES REQUIRING HIGHER LEVELS OF FUNCTIONING

Activities such as stair climbing, walking while changing direction, carrying, pushing or pulling while walking, jumping, running, and sports push the demands of the trunk and limbs (Fig. 15-33A–C). Higher level activities require increased strength, increased control of functional trunk/limb sequences, and increased balance. When we use are arms to swing a tennis racquet or a golf club, when we jump or kick a ball, or when we push or pull a heavy object across a floor, we need more precise timing, sequencing, and coordination between trunk and limb movement components. Through the practice of these activities, the arm and leg increase their ability to produce power and to refine the timing of movements.

In the functional chapters, we analyzed movement components of the trunk with coordinated components of an arm or a leg and stressed the importance of combining trunk components with either arm or leg components in treatment sequences to ensure carryover from treatment into daily life. As we begin to train higher-level activities, we need to plan treatment sequences that combine the coordination of the trunk with both the arm and the leg.

FIGURE 15-33 (A–C) Normal subject walking, turning, carrying objects while walking. (D & E) Patient with a left hemiplegia practicing carrying objects with his uninvolved arm while walking. (F) Patient uses an upper-body-initiated anterior weight shift to bend forward and hold a chair. The therapist assists with the arm portion of the task. (G) She teaches him the arm/trunk sequence as he lifts it up, and he then practices walking and moving it across the room.

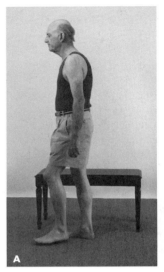
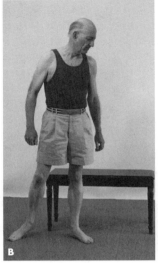
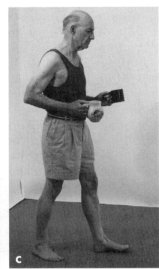
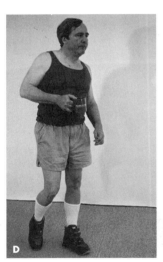
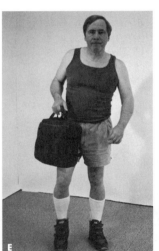
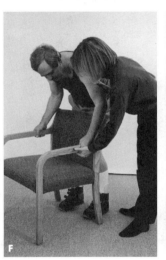
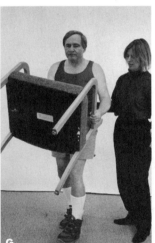

As the demand on the arm or leg increases, so does the demand on the trunk. During treatment, therapists organize their treatment plan to use arm or leg movements to push the demands on the trunk. During practice of these activities in treatment, as the therapist assists with alignment or stability of an arm or leg and asks the patient to initiate or perform part of the task, the trunk becomes stronger and trunk/limb control increases. Likewise, if the therapist corrects or assists alignment of the trunk and asks the arms and/or legs to work, the limbs become stronger and trunk/limb control increases (Fig. 15-33D–G).

Activities of higher level functioning are necessary to continue to push the level of movement control and recovery. The impairments that are present during walking become more noticeable as the difficulty of the task increases, but as the higher skill is practiced and learned, the impairments decrease and functional abilities increase.

Stair Climbing

Stair climbing is a higher-level task than walking because it requires significantly more trunk control and leg strength. Patients with hemiplegia learn to perform stair climbing independently and safely after they walk independently with a cane. The leg pattern used to lift a leg up onto a stair step or to reach it down to a stair step differs from the leg pattern used in walking. To move the leg up a step, we use a forward lift pattern. To step down a step, we use a forward reach pattern (see Ch. 9). As the photo sequences show, normal stair climbing requires leg strength to push and lift the body up, while descending stairs requires leg control to lower the body down slowly. The upper trunk remains aligned while the lower trunk adjusts to provide stability for the leg or follows the movement of the leg.

Stair climbing is initiated by strong ankle dorsiflexion as the left leg lifts up to the step. The left hip and knee flex, and the right leg supports weight in hip and knee extension with ankle dorsiflexion. The legs initiate a forward weight shift from a left step/stance position. As the left leg lifts the body up the step, the left hip and knee extend as the right leg moves up to the next step with hip, knee, and ankle flexion. The trunk remains upright over the pelvis (Fig. 15-34)

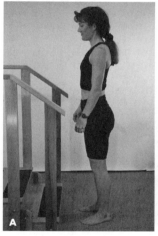
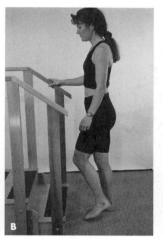
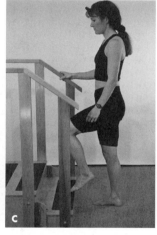
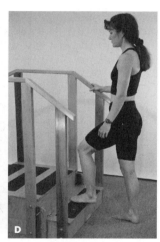
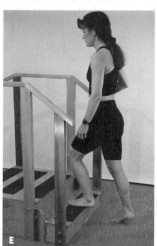
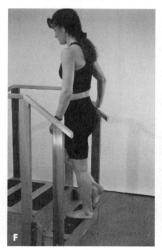
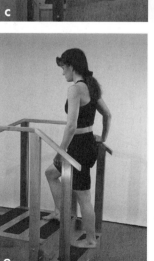

FIGURE 15-34 (A–G) Normal stair climbing.

To descend stairs, we shift weight to the right leg and initiate the stepping movement with slight hip, knee, and ankle dorsiflexion to clear the leg from the top step. As the left leg uses a forward reach pattern (hip flexion, knee extension, ankle plantarflexion), the right leg flexes and controls the descent of the body. The left foot is plantarflexed at foot contact. The left forefoot supports weight and the ankle dorsiflexes until the foot is flat on the step. As weight moves down on the left foot, the right leg flexes to clear the step, and the pattern repeats itself (Fig. 15-35).

FIGURE 15-35 (A–G) Normal stair descending.

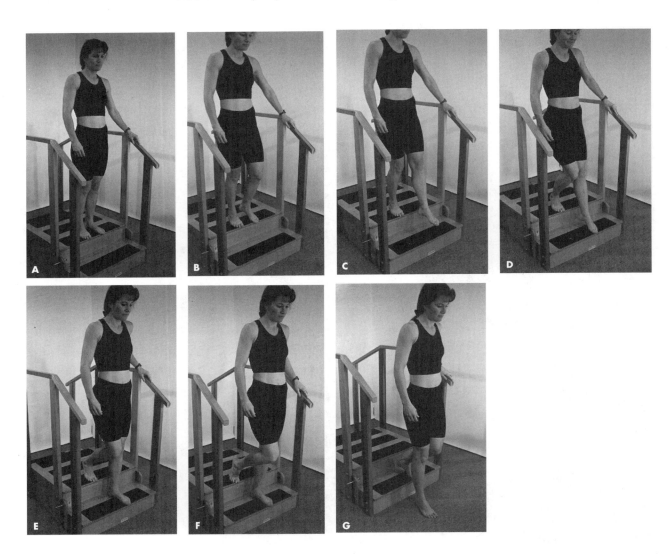

Treatment in Stair Climbing

The impairments that interfere with going up and down stairs are loss of trunk control and inadequate strength and control in the legs. Trunk asymmetries are more obvious as the patient tries to initiate and move the leg. Leg weakness is apparent as the patient tries to lift the body up or control weight as the body moves down (Fig. 15-36). Descending stairs with the affected leg leading often results in leg adduction/internal rotation. Leg adduction/internal rotation is due to poor trunk con-

FIGURE 15-36 (*A & B*) Patient with a right hemiplegia initiating the leg lift onto a step. She initiates the pattern with pelvic elevation and a strong overshift of her trunk to the left as she circumducts and lifts her leg with knee extension. (*C*) Therapist uses her left hand in an axillary grip to correct trunk alignment and uses her right hand to help the patient learn to lift her right leg with hip and knee flexion. (*D & E*) The therapist uses her right hand on the distal femur to teach the patient to move forward over her extending right leg. The therapist's left hand moves the trunk forward and up as the leg extends and the patient lifts her left leg up. Notice the patient does not overshift and rely on her left arm as the therapist helps her learn to use her right leg.

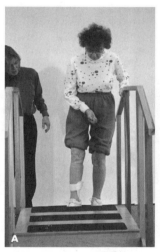
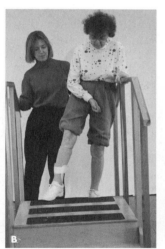
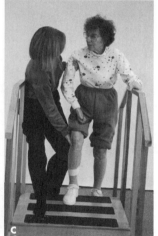
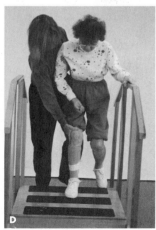
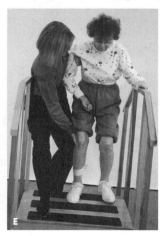

trol and loss of control of trunk/pelvis movement components. The therapist corrects the leg position by reestablishing alignment in the trunk and pelvis; as the affected leg leads the descent, the pelvis should depress. However, in hemiplegic patients the pelvis depresses, not actively, eccentrically, but "falls down" because of loss of trunk and pelvis control. It is this "passive" lowering/forward rotation of the pelvis that accompanies the pattern of leg adduction (Fig. 15-37A–E). When patients learn to descend stairs with their uninvolved side leading, they have difficulty controlling body weight on their hemiplegic leg, which is flexing. Loss of trunk control becomes evident as they attempt this pattern (Fig. 15-37F–I).

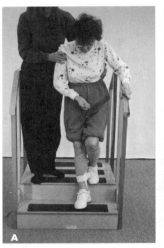
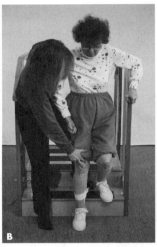
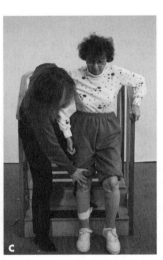
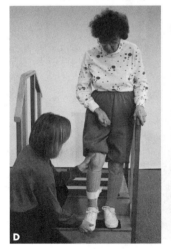
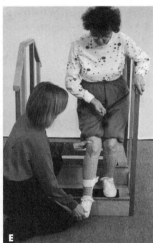

FIGURE 15-37 (A) Patient leads with her right leg. The right leg is adducting as it reaches to the step. This leg adduction contributes to the feeling of "falling" to the hemiplegic side. (B & C) The therapist uses her left hand in an axillary grip to support the trunk and pelvis. She reminds the patient to keep the upper trunk extended over the pelvis as the right foot reaches to the floor and the left foot steps down. (D & E) Therapist lets the patient control trunk as she reeducates the forward reach pattern of the right leg. (*Figure continues.*)

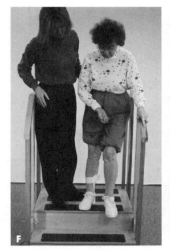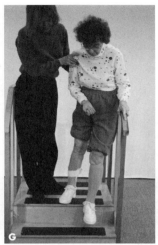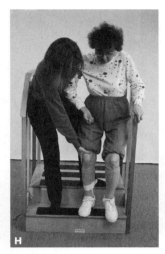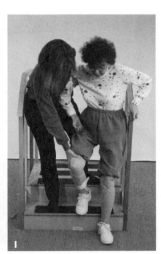

FIGURE 15-37 (*Continued*) (*F & G*) Patient attempting to descend stairs with her uninvolved leg leading. She is unable to actively bend the right leg as she steps with the left. (*H & I*) Therapist uses an axillary/leg grip similar to the one she used in Figure D to assist the alignment of the trunk and leg as the patient moves down with her left leg leading. When patients learn to descend stairs with their uninvolved side leading, they have difficulty controlling body weight on their hemiplegic leg, which is flexing. Loss of trunk and leg control becomes evident as they attempt this pattern.

Jumping

Jumping is trained in therapy to prepare for jogging and running, to increase strength in the leg, especially the foot and toes, and to improve control of trunk/leg movement sequences. Treatment begins by ensuring upper trunk symmetry and stability through upper-extremity extended-arm weight-bearing support. This support makes it easier for the lower trunk and legs to practice increasing their strength, timing, and coordination. The weight bearing arms may also assist the lift as the trunk and legs leave the floor. Practice begins with bouncing movements, then moves to single jumps, single jumps with alternating foot movements, and later adds jogging. Jumping and jogging/running require that you take off and land on the ball of the foot. Control and support of the ankle and foot during the activity is important to prevent spraining. Even if jogging is not a functional goal for the patient, practice in jumping increases the trunk and leg strength needed for independent walking without the use of a cane or brace.

Treatment in Preparation for Jumping

The mini-trampoline can be used in treatment in preparation for jumping (Fig. 15-38).

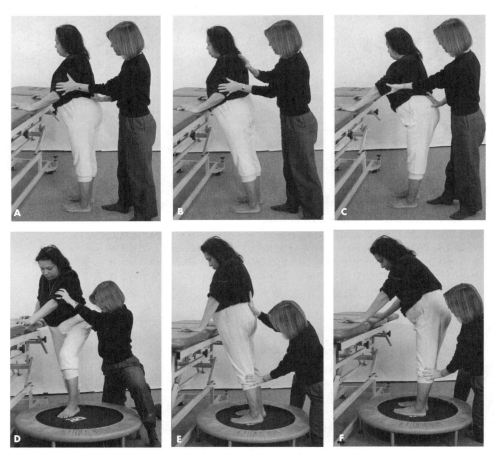

FIGURE 15-38 (*A–C*) Patient with a left hemiplegia who walks without a cane or brace but cannot jump. The therapist prepares for the activity by reviewing the arm, trunk, and leg sequences in extended-arm weight bearing. (*D–F*) Patient uses arm support to step onto the trampoline, and the therapist reviews the leg and trunk movements that will later be combined with bouncing. The therapist's left hand is on the posterior aspect of her calf to correct tibial rotation and to teach the patient how to push down and bounce into the surface. (Foot posturing often increases in this higher-level activity; tibial external rotation accompanies unwanted inversion of the foot.) (*Figure continues.*)

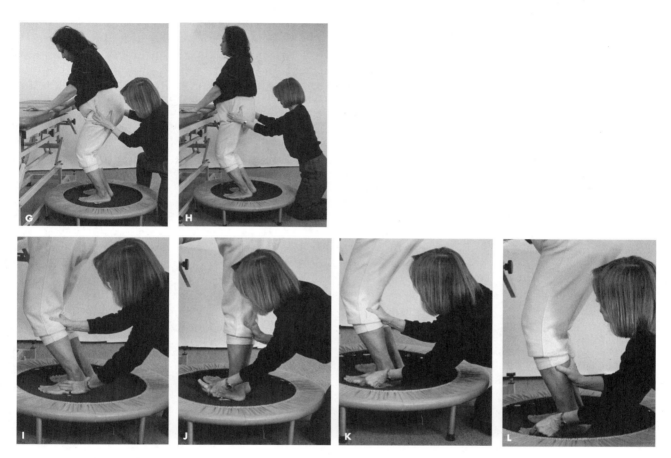

FIGURE 15-38 (*Continued*) (*G & H*) Patient practices bouncing. The therapist uses a bilateral symmetric pelvic grip to teach the patient how to bounce down. Bouncing is practiced with the knees and ankles flexed. This activity pushes the demands on the trunk and is tiring for patients when they step off the trampoline. One treatment session may stop here. (*I–L*) The therapist uses foot/lower leg grips to assist with foot/ankle alignment as the patient practices bouncing on her forefoot and on her heels. This distal treatment is very useful for increasing muscle strength in ankle and toe muscles.

Treatment In Preparation for Jogging/Running

Treatment for jogging/running adds the changing movement of the legs and trunk. From the trampoline, the patient practices jumping without arm support and then jumps on the ground without arm support. As the level of activity increases, it is necessary to add arm support to assist trunk alignment as the trunk/leg sequences are practiced (Fig. 15-39).

FIGURE 15-39 (*A–E*) Patient with a right hemiplegia who walks without a cane or brace. He stands with arm support as the therapist teaches him to swing his legs repetitively. She assists the leg and removes her manual assistance as he learns the task. (*F–H*) Therapist assists the trunk alignment as the patient practices jumping while changing leg step/stance position. He practices taking off and landing with bent knees. (*Figure continues.*)

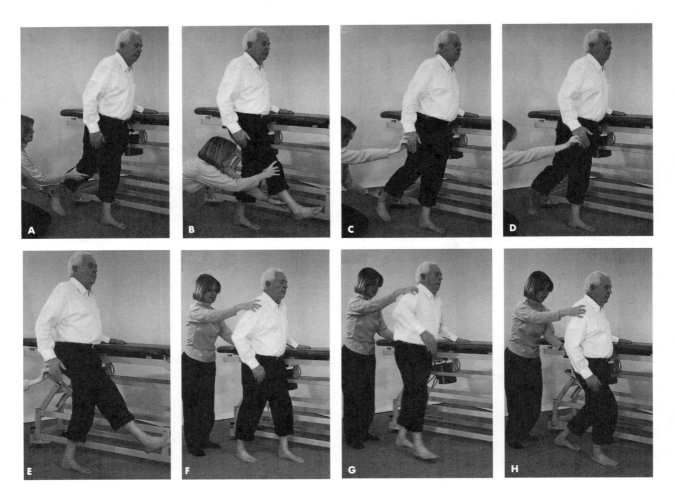

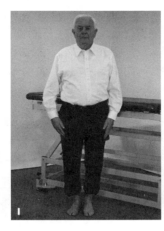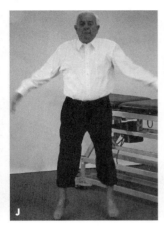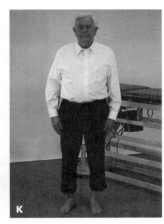

FIGURE 15-39 (*Continued*)   (*I–K*) Patient practices stationary jumping without arm support.

REFERENCES

1. Smidt G: Rudiments of gait. p. 1. In Smidt GL (ed): Gait in Rehabilitation. Churchill Livingstone, New York, 1990

2. Inman VT, Ralston HJ, Todd F: Human Walking. Williams & Wilkins, Baltimore, 1981

3. Smidt G: Rudiments of gait. In Smidt GL (ed): Gait in Rehabilitation. Churchill Livingstone, New York, 1990

4. Perry J: The mechanics of walking. Phys Ther 47:778, 1967

5. Winter D: Biomechanical and Motor Control Factors in Gait. Waterloo Press, Toronto, 1989

6. Knutsson E: Gait control in hemiparesis. Scand J Rehabil Med 13: 101, 1981

7. Brandstater ME, Bruin H, Gowland C et al: Hemiplegic gait: analysis of temporal variables. Arch Phys Med Rehabil 64: 585, 1983

8. Winter D: The Mechanics of Walking. Waterloo Press, Toronto, 1989

ADDITIONAL READING

Giuliani C. Adult hemiplegic gait. In Smidt GL (ed): Gait in Rehabilitation. Churchill Livingstone, New York, 1990

Index

A

Activities of daily living
  compensatory training in, 85
  movement analysis of, 1
  muscle strength and, 20
Alignment
  changes in, 31–32
    treatment interventions for, 81
  of trunk, loss of, 33
Alignment correction, 60–61, 64
  for legs
    in standing, 299–300, 310–311
    during transfers, 430
  for subluxed shoulder and arm, 164–165
    in sit to stand, 409
  in supine, 346–347, 351–352
  for trunk
    in sit to stand, 401–403
    in standing, 272–274
    in transfers, 428–429
  for trunk and hip, in sitting, 236–239
  during walking, 458–459
Ankle
  eversion of, 267, 268
  inversion of, 267, 268
  loss of range in
    in sit to stand, 405
    in transfers, 421
    in walking, 445–446
Ankle dorsiflexion
  insufficient, in walking, 452
  restoration/maintenance of, in sit to
    stand, 410
  in standing, 271–272
Ankle plantarflexion, in standing, 271–272
Arm(s). *See also* Upper extremity
  alignment changes in, 31–32
  atypical movements of, 44
  chronic pain in, treatment of, 160–161
  distal, alignment changes in, 152–154

equilibrium responses in, 4
hemiplegic. *See* Hemiplegic arm
hypertonicity of
  in sidelying to sitting, 387–388
  in walking, 453
involuntary posturing of, 45, 47
loss of functional performance in, 162
movement deficits in, 43
muscle weakness in, 142
positioning of, for comfort, in supine,
  322
unbalanced muscle strength in, 143–145
weakness of, in walking, 452–453
Arm movement(s)
  atypical, 44
  in extended arm forward reach, 11
  functional, reeducation of, 180–181
  generalized, 8
  loss of, 131–132
  non-weight bearing, 6–7
  postural control during, 9
  reach patterns of, 131
  in space, 131
    increasing strength and control of,
    174–179
Arm muscles, in equilibrium reactions, 4
Assessment, 55–69
  documenting efficacy of, 55–56
  establishing baselines for, 55
  of functional level, 56
  of intact motor abilities, 56
  of movement deficits and compensatory
    patterns, 56
  process of, 56–71
  purpose of, 55–56
  of relevant impairments, 56
  of response to manual therapy, 56–57
  stage I: initial impressions and establish-
    ing rapport, 58
  stage II: observation of posture and
    movement control, 58–60

  stage III: hands-on assistance, 60–63
  stage IV: assessment of relevant impair-
    ments, 63–64
  stage V: analysis of information and
    problem solving, 64–69. *See also*
    Problem solving
  stages of, 57–64
  understanding trunk-extremity relation-
    ships in, 55
Asymmetry(ies)
  in anterior/posterior trunk movements,
    108
  lateral flexion, of trunk, 108, 110–111
  in lower extremities, in sit to stand, 404
  from undesirable compensations, 84–85

B

Backward reach, 137
Balance control
  loss of
    scooting and, 255
    in standing, 262
  in standing, 293–294
Bed mobility, 327–328
Biceps brachii muscle, hypertonicity of, 23
Body
  lower. *See also* Lower extremity(ies);
    Lower extremity movement(s)
    defined, 88
  upper. *See also* Upper extremity(ies);
    Upper extremity movement(s)
    defined, 88

C

Carrying, 467–468
Clavicular movement(s), 134
Climbing, stair. *See* Stair climbing

Closed-chain kinetic activity, 5
Codman's shoulder girdle rhythm, 134
Compensation(s), 47–49
  appropriate, teaching, 84–86
  assessment of, 56
  bilateral, 48–49
  defined, 38
  undesirable, 84–85
    in rolling pattern, 366
    in scooting, 256
    in sidelying to sitting, 388–389
    in sit to stand, 407
    in transfers, 423–424
Composite movement impairment(s), 38–49
  atypical movements, 43–47
  compensations, 47–49
    bilateral, 48
    undesirable, 48–49
  movement deficits, 40–43
Contracture, defined, 34

D

Daily activities. *See* Activities of daily living
Disability(ies), 49–50
  defined, 16, 49
  definitions of, 15–17
  functional behaviors and, 50
  intervention in, 51–52
Disablement
  role of therapy in treatment of, 50–52
  WHO classification of, 16
  WHO definition of, 15
Disease, WHO classification of, 16
Dressing, compensatory training in, 85

E

Edema, 37–38, 161
  treatment interventions for, 81
Elbow flexion
  reeducation of, 74
  with shoulder extension, 139–140
  with shoulder internal/external rotation, 140
Elbow flexion/extension, 138
Elbow movement(s), reeducation of, 172–174
Elbow/shoulder flexion
  elevation combining, 139
  reach combining, 138–139
Equilibrium reactions, defined, 4
Eversion, 267, 268
Exercise, for secondary impairments, 82
Extended-arm weight bearing, 183, 207–226

  assessment of, 218–219
  components of, 208–215
    lower-trunk-initiated, 210–213
    rotational movements, 213–215
    upper-trunk-initiated, 209–210
  concepts and principles in, 207–208
  versus forearm weight bearing, 207
  impairments interfering with, 215–218
    soft tissue restrictions, 218
    upper extremity hypertonicity, 215–216
    upper extremity weakness, 216–218
  treatment applications of, 208
  treatment goals and techniques for, 219–226
    incorporating functional patterns, 226
    reducing flexor hypertonicity and/or lengthening shortened tissues, 224–225
    reeducating components of, 220–223
  uses of, 207
Extension rotation patterns
  lower-trunk-initiated, 96
  upper-trunk-initiated, 96
Extremity(ies). *See also* Lower extremity(ies); Lower extremity movement(s); Upper extremity(ies); Upper extremity movement(s)
  hypertonicity of, in sidelying to sitting, 387–388
  inability to accept weight on, in sidelying to sitting, 386–387
  loss of alignment of, in sidelying to sitting, 385–386
  trunk relationships to, 55
  weakness of, in sidelying to sitting, 381–385
Extremity control
  loss of, 42
  skilled, defined, 5
Extremity movement(s)
  atypical, 43–44
  closed-chain kinetic activity in, 5
  open-chain kinetic activity in, 7
  trunk's role in, 3

F

Flaccidity, defined, 18
Flexion, forward
  0 to 60 degrees, 134–135
  60 to 90 degrees, 135
  90 to 120 degrees, 135
  120 to 180 degrees, 135
Flexion rotation patterns
  lower-trunk-initiated, 94–95
  upper-trunk-initiated, 94
    in sidelying to sitting, 375–377

Flexor hypertonicity, reducing, 102–103
Foot
  eversion of, 267, 268
  hypermobility in, 32
  inversion of, 267, 268
  lack of joint range in, in transfers, 421
Foot movement(s), analysis of, 267
Foot posturing, in walking, 452
Forearm, pronation of, 140–141
Forearm movement(s), reeducation of, 172–174
Forearm weight bearing, 183–206
  assessment of, 196–197
  concepts and principles of, 183–184
  versus extended-arm weight bearing, 207
  functional applications of, 191
    in sit to stand, 191
    in stabilization of objects, 191
  impairments interfering with, 192–196
    abnormal upper extremity alignment, 195–196
    loss of control of critical trunk movements, 192–193
    upper extremity hypertonicity, 194–195
    upper extremity weakness/paralysis, 193–194
  movement components of, 184–190
    lower trunk-initiated patterns, 185–186, 187
    rotational patterns, 190
    upper-trunk-initiated patterns, 186–190
  for reducing hypertonicity, 195
  in sitting, functional goals for, 197
  in supine, 323
  treatment applications of, 184
  treatment goals and techniques for 198–206
Forward reach, 134–136
  0 to 60 degrees of forward flexion, 134–135
  60 to 90 degrees, 135
  60 to 90 degrees of forward flexion, 135
  90 to 120 degrees, 135
  120 to 180 degrees, 135
  reeducation in, 170–172
  shoulder protraction, 135–136
Function
  defined, 2
  loss of, 15–53
Functional level, assessment of, 56
Functional movement(s). *See also* Movement(s); *specific body part movements*
  compensatory, 9
  defined, 2
  extremity control, 5
  non-weight bearing, 7–8

versus normal movement, 13
parts of, 3–9
    extremity control, 5
    non-weight bearing movements, 7–9
    trunk control, 3–5
    weight bearing, 5–7
Functional movement reeducation
    approach of, 1
    basics of, 79–81
Functional training, task-specific, 82–86

G

Gait. *See also* Walking
    functional segments of, 436–440
        forward progression, 437–438
        single/double limb support, 438–439
        swing, 440
    hemiplegic, characteristics of, 433
Glenohumeral joint. *See* Shoulder
Glenohumeral joint subluxation. *See* Shoulder subluxation
Goal setting, 66–69
    functional, 66–67
    long-term, 67–69
    treatment, 67

H

Hand(s)
    bringing to body, in supine, 321–322
    edema in, 37, 161
    in forearm weight bearing, 185
    functional movement reeducation for, 79–80
    movement deficits in, 43
    positioning of, for function, 140–142
Handicap(s), defined, 16, 50
Hemiplegia
    flexor hypertonicity in, 24
    gait characteristics in, 433
    right, 20, 21, 22
    trunk postures associated with, 104
Hemiplegic arm
    and changes in distal alignment, 152–154
    movement problems in, 132
    reducing flexor hypertonicity in, 203–205
    treatment goals and techniques for
        increasing scapula mobility and decreasing hypertonicity, 166–169
        increasing strength and control of arm movements in space, 174–179
        preparing for functional use of, 180–181

reeducating functional movements, 170–173
restoring alignment to subluxed shoulder and arm, 164–165
treatment goals and techniques in, 164–181
treatment of, 132
Hemiplegic side, inappropriate rotation of, 109–111
Hip(s)
    instability of, in walking, 446
    loss of control of, in weight bearing, 106–107
Hip abduction, with knee extension, in standing, 270
Hip adduction, with knee extension, in standing, 270–271
Hip control, lack of, and lower extremity movements in sitting, 231–232
Hip extension, in standing
    with knee extension, 269
    with knee flexion, 269
Hip flexion
    decreases in, with posterior weight shift in sitting, 229
    increases in, with anterior weight shift in sitting, 228, 230
    with knee flexion, in standing, 268, 269
Humeral movement(s), 134
Hypermobility, defined, 32
Hypersensitivity, pain due to, 36
Hypertonicity, 23–26
    of arms, during walking, 453
    assessment of, 24
    defined, 21
    extensor, in leg, in transfers, 421
    of extremities, in sidelying to sitting, 387–388
    flexor, 24, 26
        reducing, 102–103, 203–205
        forearm weight bearing for reducing, 195
    in lower extremities, in rolling pattern, 360–361
    in lower extremity extension, in sit to stand, 406
    and lower extremity movements in sitting, 234
    and lower extremity movements in standing, 274, 276, 278–279
    mechanisms of, 23–24
    and non-weight bearing leg movements in sitting, 245–247
    permanent changes in, 26
    in upper extremities
        development of, in hemiplegic arm, 154–157
        and extended-arm weight bearing, 215–216
        and forearm weight bearing, 194–195

in sit to stand, 406–407
in treatment of, 157
Hypomobility
    defined, 32
    soft tissue tightness and, 32–33
Hypotonicity
    defined, 21
    of hemiplegic arm, 154
    permanent changes in, 26
    sensory deficits in, 29

I

Impairment(s), 17–49. *See also under specific movements*
    assessment of, 56
    categories of, 38
    changes in, 17–18
    of composite movement, 38–49. *See also* Composite movement impairment(s)
    defined, 16
    definitions of, 15–17
    primary, 18–30
        atypical movement development and, 45
        changes in muscle activation, 26–28
        changes in muscle strength, 18–20
        changes in muscle tone, 20–26
        deficits in kinesthetic memory, 30
        deficits in sensory awareness, 28–29
        deficits in sensory interpretation, 29–30
        definition and example of, 17
        role of therapy in treatment of, 51
        sensory changes, 28
    secondary, 30–38
        atypical movement development and, 45–46
        changes in muscle and soft tissue length, 33–35
        definition and example of, 17
        edema, 37–38, 161
        orthopedic changes in alignment, 31–32
        orthopedic changes in joint mobility, 32–33
        pain, 35–37. *See also* Pain
        prevention of, 81
        role of therapy in treatment of, 51
        treatment of, 81–82
        types of, 30–31
    testing of, 63–64
Independence, increasing, task-specific training for, 82–86
Independent movement, 77–78
Infants, weight bearing in, 6
Inversion, 267

J

Jogging, treatment in preparation for, 476–477
Joint mobility. *See also specific joints*
    changes in, 32–33
        treatment interventions for, 81
Joint pain, definition and causes of, 35
Jumping, 467, 473–475
    treatment in preparation for, 473–475

K

Kinesthetic memory, deficits in, 30
Knee, hyperextension of, 267, 447–448
Knee extension
    early, 405
    excessive, 405
    loss of control of, in sit to stand, 405
Knee flexion, excessive, in walking, 448–449

L

Leg(s). *See also* Lower extremity(ies)
    atypical movement sequencing in, 45
    atypical movements of, 44
    extensor hypertonicity of, in transfers, 421
    functional movement reeducation for, 79
    hypertonicity of, 23–24
        in rolling pattern, 360–361
        in sidelying to sitting, 387–388
    inability to step, in standing, during transfers, 422–423
    movement components of, 10
    postural role of, 9
    reestablishing alignment of, in transfers, 430
    reestablishing control of, in transfers, 430
    weight-bearing movement of, 6
Leg initiation patterns, reeducation for, 274
Leg movement(s), non-weight bearing, 240–243
Lower body, defined, 88
Lower extremity(ies). *See also* Ankle; Hip(s); Knee(s); Leg(s)
    alignment changes in, 31–32
    edema in, 37–38
    loss of control in, in weight bearing, 106–107
    muscle shortening in, in rolling pattern, 363–364
    muscle weakness of, in rolling pattern, 361–362
    pain in, 35
    in sitting, 87

weakness and asymmetry in, in sit to stand, 404
    weight bearing role of, 6
Lower extremity extension, hypertonicity in, in sit to stand, 406
Lower extremity movement(s)
    categories of, 131
    integration of trunk movements with, 8–9
    non-weight bearing, 7–8
        generalized, 8
        task specific, 8
    in sitting, 227–259
        non-weight bearing. *See* Sitting, non-weight bearing leg movements in
        scooting. *See* Scooting
        therapy goals and techniques for, 235–239
        weight bearing. *See* Sitting, lower extremity weight bearing in
    in standing, 261–316. *See also* Standing, lower extremity movements in
Lower trunk
    anterior weight shift of, 92
    in initiation of forearm weight bearing patterns, 185–186, 187
    lateral weight shift of, 93
    posterior weight shift of, 93
    in sitting, movements initiated from, 92–94

M

Manual assistance, techniques of, 61–63
Manual therapy, response to, assessment of, 56–57
Memory, kinesthetic, deficits in, 30
Mobility, joint, changes in, 32–33
Motor ability(ies), assessment of, 56
Motor control
    defined, 2
    recovery of, role of therapy in, 51
Motor deficits, residual, teaching appropriate compensations in, 84–86
Motor recovery
    complete, 39
    defined, 39
    and development of atypical movement patterns, 45
    incomplete, 39–40
    incomplete distal, 39
    incomplete proximal, 40
    process of, 39–40
    unbalanced motor return, 40
Movement(s). *See also entries under specific body parts;* Functional movement(s)
    analysis of, in activities of daily living, 1
    assisted, during assessment, 61–62
    atypical, 43–47

defined, 38
    and patterns of motor recovery, 45
    categories of, 131
    components of, 10
    coordinated, atypical patterns of, 44
    functional
        defined, 2
        definitions of, 2
        versus normal, 13
    independent, 77–78
    loss of, 15–53. *See also* Impairment
        manifestations of, 15
    normal
        versus abnormal, in functional performance, 1
        analysis of, 10–12
        defined, 2
        in neurologic treatment, 1
        sequences of, 10
    undesirable, blocking, during assessment, 62–63
Movement analysis
    completion phase of, 11–12
    initiation phase in, 11
    transition phase of, 11
Movement control
    loss of, abnormal muscle tone and, 25
    observation of, 58–60
Movement deficit(s), 40–43
    assessment of, 56
    defined, 38
Movement dysfunction, 38. *See also* Composite movement impairment(s)
Movement problems
    definitions of, 15–17
    types of, 16
Movement reeducation, 12–13, 71–81
    functional. *See* Functional movement reeducation
    and problems with muscle activation, 28
    stages of, 73–81
        assisted practice: muscle activation, 75–77
        functional movement reeducation and practice, 79–81
        independent movement, 77–78
        sensory education, 73–75
Movement sequences, 10
    mobility, 10
    task-related, 10, 12
    transitional, 10
Muscle, changes in length of, 33–35
Muscle activation
    assisted practice for, 75–77
    changes in, 26–28
    excessive, in hemiplegic arm, 155–156
    excessive cocontraction in, 27–28
    excessive force production in, 27–28
    inappropriate muscle substitution in, 27–28

inappropriate pattern of initiation of, 27
inappropriate patterns of, 27
synergistic patterns of, 76
Muscle contraction(s), inappropriate, 76
Muscle deficit(s), defined, 41
Muscle firing, atypical, in swing phase of walking, 451
Muscle length, loss of, treatment interventions for, 81
Muscle pain, definition and causes of, 35–36
Muscle restriction, defined, 34
Muscle shifting, defined, 34
Muscle shortening
   in lower extremities, in rolling pattern, 363–364
   in lower extremity movements in sitting, 234–235
   in lower extremity movements in standing, 277
   in trunk, in rolling pattern, 363–364
Muscle strength
   changes in, 18–20
   imbalance in, 20
   loss of, 20
   unbalanced, in arm, 143–145
Muscle tightness, in lower extremities, in sit to stand, 406
Muscle tone
   abnormal
      and hemiplegic arm, 154–157
      and loss of movement control, 25
   changes in, 20–26
   defined, 20
   distribution of, 22
   variation in, and type of brain lesion, 22–23
Muscle weakness, 19–20
   in arm, 142
   and loss of initiation patterns in standing, 278
   in lower extremities
      in rolling pattern, 362–363
      in sit to stand, 404
   in upper extremities, in rolling pattern, 361–362

O

Open-chain kinetic movement, 7

P

Pain
   from altered sensitivity, 36
   from edema, 37
   in hemiplegic upper extremity, 158–161
   joint, 35

muscle, 35–36
   treatment interventions for, 81
Paralysis
   defined, 18
   flaccid, sensory deficits in, 29
   and forearm weight bearing, 193–194
   total, in all upper extremity muscle groups, 142
Paresis, 18
   defined, 19
Pelvis, in sitting *versus* standing, 88
Postural control, 9
   during arm movement, 9
Postural response, defined, 3
Postural tone, defined, 20
Posture
   changes in, 31–32
      in hemiplegia, 104
   establishment of, 6
   observation of, 58–59
Problem solving, 64–69
   establishing goals in, 66–69
      functional, 66–67
      long-term, 67–69
      treatment, 67
   list of functional limitations in, 65
   list of movement problems and impairments in, 65
   problem list in, 65–66
Pulling, 467
Pushing, 467

R

Rapport, establishing, 58
Reaching movement(s), 131
   abducted, 136
   across midline, 137–138
   away from midline, 137
   backward, 137
   forward. *See* Forward reach
Rib cage, hypomobility of, in forearm weight bearing, 202–203
Rolling, 355–374
   assessment of, 367
   atypical, 46
      inappropriate spinal extension, 364, 366
      inappropriate spinal flexion, 366
   components of, 357–360
   concepts and principles of, 355–357
   impairments interfering with, 360–366
      hypertonicity, 360–361
      loss of alignment due to muscle shortening, 363–364
      loss of trunk control, 361
      lower extremity weakness, 362–363
      shoulder pain, 364–365
      upper extremity weakness, 361–362

initiated from lower body, 358–359
   initiated from upper body, 357–358
   initiated with nonsegmental, 359
   to involved side, 355
   movement summary of, 360
   treatment goals and techniques in, 367–374
      increasing strength and control in trunk and limb muscles, 374
      providing pain-free arm movement during, 368
      reeducating and strengthening leg and arm components, 372
      reeducating lower-body-initiated rolling, 370
      reeducating nonsegmental rolling in patient with right hemiplegia and loss of trunk and arm control, 369
      reeducating upper-body-initiated rolling, 371
      reestablishing or maintaining shoulder and pelvic girdle musculature, 371
      unassisted practice without undesirable compensations, 373
      undesirable compensatory patterns in, 366–367
   to uninvolved side, 355
Rotational movement(s)
   with arm movement across midline, 190
   with arm movement away from midline, 190
   in extended-arm weight bearing, 213–215
      on stable lower trunk, 213
      with trunk extension, 214–215
      with trunk flexion, 214
   in scooting, 252–253
   in standing, 286–287
   in supine, of lower body, 320
Running, 467
   treatment in preparation for, 476–477

S

Scapula
   hemiplegic, 148
   increasing mobility and decreasing hypertonicity of, 166–169
   normal resting position of, 148
Scapula movement(s), 132–133
   in forearm weight bearing, reeducation of, 200
Scapula winging, correction of, 196
Scooting, 252–259
   assessment of, 256
   components of, 252–254
   concepts and principles of, 252
   impairments interfering with, 254–256

Scooting (*Continued*)
    loss of balance control, 255
    trunk and leg weakness, 254–255
    undesirable compensatory patterns, 256
    lower-body-initiated patterns of, 252–253
        lateral weight shift, 252
        partial stand, 254
        rotational weight shift, 252–253
    therapy goals and techniques for,
        256–259
        correcting trunk asymmetries and
            reeducating trunk control, 258
        practicing trunk component with ver-
            bal reminders and leg movements
            with assistance, 259
        providing model for task, 257
Sensitivity, altered, pain due to, 36
Sensory awareness, deficits in, 28–29
Sensory education, 73–75
    for elbow flexion, 74
    in severe weakness or paralysis, 74–75
Sensory interpretation, deficits in, 29–30
Shoulder
    loss of alignment of, 147–148
    subluxation of, 32
Shoulder/elbow flexion
    elevation combining, 139
    reach combining, 138–139
Shoulder extension, with elbow flexion,
    139–140
Shoulder girdle
    hemiplegic, abnormal positioning of,
        194
    rhythms of, 134
Shoulder-hand syndrome
    pain due to, 36–37
    symptoms of, 160
Shoulder movement(s), assessing, 162–163
Shoulder pain
    acute *versus* chronic, 160–161
    due to changes in joint alignment and
        mobility, 158
    due to changes in muscle tone and
        length, 158–159
    due to changes in sensation, 159
    rolling and, 355, 364–365
    in shoulder-hand syndrome, 160
Shoulder rotation, with elbow flexion, 140
Shoulder subluxation, 147–152
    anterior, 150–151
        biceps hypertonicity due to, 23
    correction of, in sit to stand, 409
    inferior, 148–150
        correction of, 196
    superior, 150–152
    treatment goals and techniques for,
        164–165
Sidelying to sitting, 375–396
    assessment of, 389

concepts and principles of, 375
impairments interfering with, 381–388
    hypertonicity of extremities, 387–388
    inability to accept weight on extremi-
        ties, 386–387
    loss of trunk and extremity alignment,
        385–386
    trunk and extremity weakness, 381–385
movement components in, 375–381
    lower trunk lateral initiation/ex-
        tended arm, 377–379
    upper-trunk-initiated flexion rotation,
        375–377
    upper trunk lateral initiation/flexed
        arm, 379–381
treatment goals and techniques for,
    390–396
    combining reeducation of active arm
        use and trunk components,
        392–393
    reeducating and strengthening leg
        components, 394
    reeducating and strengthening trunk
        component, 390–391
    reeducating trunk and arm compo-
        nents, 395–396
undesirable compensatory patterns in,
    388–389
Sitting
atypical trunk movements in, 108–111
    asymmetric performance of ante-
        rior/posterior movements, 108
    lateral flexion asymmetry, 108,
        110–111
    in performance of lateral movements,
        109–111
extended-arm weight bearing in. *See*
    Extended-arm weight bearing
forearm weight bearing in, functional
    goals for, 197
function of legs in, 227
and loss of lower extremity/hip control
    in weight bearing, 106–107
lower extremity weight bearing in, 6,
    228–239
    assessment of, 235
    components of, 228–231
    concepts and principles of, 227–228
    correcting trunk and hip alignment
        in, 236
    functional task reeducation in, 239
    functions of, 227
    with hypertonicity, 234
    impairments interfering with,
        231–239
    with lack of hip control and weakness,
        231–232
    lengthening shortened muscles in,
        237–238

    with loss of trunk control and align-
        ment, 232–234
    lower-trunk-initiated weight bearing
        patterns, 228–230
    with muscle shortening and abnormal
        hip alignment, 234–235
    upper-trunk-initiated weight bearing
        patterns, 230–231
non-weight bearing leg movements in,
    240–251
    abduction and adduction, 241
    assessment of, 247
    combined, 242–243
    components of, 240–242
    concepts and principles of, 240
    hip flexion, 240–241
    hypertonicity and, 245–247
    impairments interfering with, 243–247
    increasing trunk symmetry and length-
        ening tight leg muscles in, 250
    knee and ankle flexion and extension,
        241–242
    leg weakness and, 243–244
    and loss of trunk control and align-
        ment, 244–245
    reeducating proximal and distal leg
        movements in, 248–249
    selecting efficient movement pattern
        for, 251
    therapy goals and techniques for,
        247–251
pelvis in, 88
and poor trunk control during task per-
    formance, 108
reeducating for normal trunk move-
    ments in, 13, 113–120
    by activating equilibrium responses in
        trunk and extremities, 126–127
    by combining trunk and extremity
        movements in functional tasks, 129
    for compatible trunk and arm move-
        ments, 123–124
    for compatible trunk and leg move-
        ments, 125
    with cotreatment by two therapists,
        120
    by increasing independent function-
        ing in sitting, 128
    problem solving for determining opti-
        mal hand placements in, 121–122
    with rib cage or rib cage/pelvis grip,
        113–115
    with support of hemiplegic arm
        during trunk movements, 113,
        116–117
    using upper trunk/rib cage grip,
        118–119
role of trunk in, 3–4
task performance in, 88, 90

trunk control in, 96–99
  summary of, 99
trunk movements in, 87–130
  assessment guidelines for, 112
  concepts and principles of, 87–88
  functional goals for, 112
  impairments interfering with, 100–108
  and loss of alignment and stability in
    upper extremity, 102–104
  and loss of trunk alignment with soft
    tissue/joint restrictions, 104–106
  muscle weakness and, 100–102
  therapy goals and techniques for,
    112–129
upper extremity weight bearing in, 183.
    See also Upper extremity move-
    ment(s), weight bearing
Sitting to sidelying
  lower trunk lateral initiation/extended
    arm in, 377–378
  in trunk rotation, 377
  upper trunk lateral initiation/flexed arm
    in, 379–380
Sitting up, without use of hemiplegic side,
    47
Sit to stand, 397–413
  assessment of, 407
  completion of, defined, 398
  components of, 398–401
  concepts and principles of, 397-398
  extended arm weight bearing in, 226
  forearm weight bearing in, 191
  impairment interfering with
    inefficient trunk initiation patterns, 403
    loss of ankle joint range, 405
    loss of knee extension control, 405
    loss of trunk control and alignment,
      401–403
    lower extremity extension hypertonic-
      ity, 406
    lower extremity weakness and asym-
      metry, 404
    muscle and soft tissue tightness, 406
    upper extremity hypertonicity, 406–407
  impairments interfering with, 401–407
  increasing functional use of forearm
    weight bearing in, 206
  initiation in lower trunk, 398–399
  initiation in lower trunk/pelvis, 399–400
  initiation in upper trunk, 400–401
  initiation of, defined, 397–398
  kinesiology of, 397–398
  movement summary of, 401
  transition in, defined, 398
  treatment goals and techniques for,
    408–413
    correcting glenohumeral joint sublux-
      ation and maintaining arm align-
      ment on trunk, 409

decreasing secondary impairments,
    410–411
  maintaining symmetric weight bearing
    through legs, 412–413
  training components of task, 408
  undesirable compensatory patterns in, 407
Skin, loss of mobility in, 34
Soft tissue
  changes in length of, 33–35
  shortening of, in hemiplegic arm, 157
Soft tissue restriction, defined, 34
Soft tissue tightness, in lower extremities, in
    sit to stand, 406
Spasticity
  defined, 21–22
  versus excessive force production during
    movements, 27
Spinal extension, inappropriate, in rolling
    pattern, 364–366
Spinal flexion, inappropriate, in rolling pat-
    tern, 366
Spine
  excessive extension in, 146
  hypomobility of, in forearm weight bear-
    ing, 202–203
  inappropriate straightness of, 109–111
  thoracic, excessive flexion in, 146
Sports, 467
Stair climbing, 467, 469–473
  initiation pattern in, 469
  treatment in, 471–473
Stair descending, 470
Stand, partial, as scooting pattern, 254
Standing
  balance control in, 293–294
    weight shift, equilibrium, and protec-
      tion, 293–294
  inability to step affected leg in, during
    transfers, 422–423
  kinesiology of, 262–267
    in ankle and foot movements, 266–267
    in hip movements, 266
    in knee movements, 266
    in pelvic movements, 263–266
  lower extremity movements in, 261–283
    abduction with knee extension, 270
    adduction with knee extension,
      270–271
    ankle dorsiflexion, 271–272
    ankle plantarflexion, 271–272
    assessment of, 279
    components of, 267–271
    concepts and principles of, 261–262
    correcting trunk alignment and reestab-
      lishing trunk control in, 280–281
    with flexor hypertonicity, 278–279
    hip extension with knee extension,
      269, 270
    hip extension with knee flexion, 269

hip flexion with knee extension, 269
  hip flexion with knee flexion, 268, 269
  with hypertonicity, 274, 276
  impairments interfering with, 272–279
  and loss of trunk control and align-
    ment, 272–274
  with muscle shortening and tightness,
    277
  reeducating ankle and foot muscles
    for, 282–284
  therapy goals and techniques for,
    280–284
  training trunk and leg movement pat-
    terns for, 281–282
  with weakness and improper initiation
    patterns, 274–275
  with weakness and loss of initiation
    patterns, 278
lower extremity weight bearing move-
    ments in, 284–315
  in abducted stance, 287–288
  assessment of, 304
  balance control in, 293–294
  combining and reeducating trunk and
    leg components of unilateral
    stance, 313–314
  components of, 284–294
  concepts and principles of, 284
  correcting leg alignment and practic-
    ing leg components of, 310–311
  correcting trunk alignment and reedu-
    cating trunk and leg control during,
    305–306
  facilitating automatic leg responses to
    upper body movements in, 315
  with feet parallel, 285–287
  impairments interfering with, 294–304
  lengthening tight leg muscles, 306–309
  and loss of lower extremity alignment,
    299–300
  and loss of trunk control, 294–297
  and lower extremity hypertonicity,
    300–304
  lower extremity initiated, 284–285
  and lower extremity weakness, 297–299
  providing trunk support and reeduca-
    tion, 306
  in step/stance, 290
  in step/stance position, 288–290
  teaching upper-trunk-initiated move-
    ments for, 312–313
  therapy goals and techniques for,
    305–315
  upper-trunk-initiated, 290–293
pelvis in, 88
role of trunk in, 3–4
trunk control in, 261–262
weight bearing in, 7
Step length, defined, 435–436

Stride length, defined, 435
Supine
    bed mobility in, 327–328
        sliding down, 328
        sliding sideways, 328
        sliding up, 327
    restoring trunk/extremity movements in
        by maintaining/restoring normal rest-
            ing alignment and tissue mobility,
            337–342
        by reeducating patterns of movement
            in hemiplegic arm, 343–345
        treatment goals and techniques for,
            337–354
    restoring trunk/lower movements in
        by maintaining or restoring normal
            alignment and tissue length in
            hemiplegic leg, 346–347
        by reeducating normal movement pat-
            terns in hemiplegic leg, 348–350
        by reeducating normal trunk move-
            ments, 353
        by restoring alignment and symmetry
            in trunk, 351–352
        by training bed mobility, 353–354
    treatment of patient in, 317–318
    trunk/extremity movements in, 318–321,
        324–328
        assessment of, 336–337
        on bed surface, 324
        bilateral weight bearing: bridging,
            324–325
        bilateral weight bearing: with lower
            trunk rotation, 326
        and changes in alignment, 333–335
        components of, 318–329
        concepts and principles of, 317–318
        hypertonicity and, 330–333
        impairments interfering with, 329–335
        initiated from lower body, 319–320
        initiated from upper body, 318–319
        lower body rotation, 320
        moving off bed or back on, 324
        and undesirable compensatory pat-
            terns, 335
        unilateral bridging, 326
        weakness/movement deficits and,
            329–330
        weight bearing patterns, 324–326
    upper extremity functional movements
        in, 321–323
        bringing hand to body, 321–322
        positioning arm for comfort, 322
        weight bearing on forearms, 323

T

Task performance, retraining, 83–84
Tendon(s), changes in length of, 33–34

Thoracic spine, excessive flexion in, 146
Tibialis muscle, anterior, muscle deficit in,
    41
Tissue length, loss of, treatment interven-
    tions for, 81
Toe clawing, in walking, 449–450
Toe curling, in walking, 449–450
Transfers, 415–431
    assessment of, 425
    concepts and principles of, 415
    full stand, 417–420
    impairments interfering with, 421–423
        extensor hypertonicity in leg, 421
        inability to step affected leg in stand-
            ing, 422–423
        lack of ankle/foot joint range, 421
    movement components of, 416–420
    partial stand, 416–418
        lower-trunk-initiated, 416–417
        teaching, 426
        upper-trunk-initiated, 417, 418
    pivoting in, 415
    treatment goals and techniques for,
        425–431
        aligning upper trunk over lower
            trunk, 428–429
        increasing independence in task, 431
        providing model of movement,
            426–427
        reeducating movement components
            of leg, 430–431
    undesirable compensatory patterns in,
        423–424
Treatment interventions, 71–86. *See also
    under specific movements*
    goal of, 71
    movement reeducation in, 71–81. *See also*
        Movement reeducation
    parts of, 71–86
    for relevant secondary impairments,
        81–82
Treatment plan, implementation of, 69
Trunk
    in activities requiring higher level of
        functioning, 468
    alignment changes in, 31
    asymmetry of, 273
        in sitting, treatment intervention for,
            82
    atypical movement sequencing in, 45
    atypical movements of, 43–44
        during sitting. *See* Sitting, atypical
            trunk movements in
    defined, 88
    dynamic role of, 3, 5
    in equilibrium reactions, 4
    extension rotation patterns of
        lower-trunk-initiated, 96
        upper-trunk-initiated, 96

in extremity movement, 3–4
    extremity relationship to, 55
    flexion rotation patterns of
        lower-trunk-initiated, 94–95
        upper-trunk-initiated, 94
    loss of alignment of, 33
        secondary impairments associated
            with, 104, 106
        in sidelying to sitting, 385–386
        in sitting, correction of, 236–239
        with soft tissue/joint restrictions, sit-
            ting and, 104–106
        and upper extremity movements,
            145–146
        during walking, 42
    lower, 88. *See also* Lower trunk
    muscle shortening in, in rolling pattern,
        363–364
    muscle weakness in, effect on sitting,
        100–102
    postural role of, 3–4, 9
    reeducation of, in sitting, 13
    rotational movements of, 94
        in sitting, 87–130. *See also* Sitting, trunk
            movements in
        planes of movement of, 89, 90
    upper, 88. *See also* Upper trunk
    weakness of
        scooting and, 254–255
        in sidelying to sitting, 381–385
Trunk alignment, reestablishing, in trans-
    fers, 428–429
Trunk control, 3–5
    defined, 3
    loss of, 41–42
        as factor in forearm weight bearing,
            192–193
        and lower extremity movements in sit-
            ting, 232–234
        and non-weight bearing leg move-
            ments in sitting, 244–245
        in rolling pattern, 361
        in sit to stand, 401–403
        in standing, 272–274
        during swing phase of walking, 443
        and upper extremity movements,
            145–147
    reestablishing
        in scooting, 258
        in sit to stand, 408
        in transfers, 426–427
    in sit to stand, 397
    in standing, 261–262
        loss of, 294–297
    during task performance while sitting,
        108
    upper over lower, loss of, in walking,
        441–443
Trunk flexion, lateral, 146

Trunk initiation, inefficient patterns of, 403

Trunk movement(s)
in forearm weight bearing, reeducation of, 198–199
integration of extremity movements with, 8–9
in supine
initiated from upper body, 318–319
in lower body rotation, 320–321

Trunk postures, associated with hemiplegia, 104

Trunk stability, poor, in hemiplegic arm, 155–156

Turning, 467–468

U

Upper body, defined, 88

Upper extremity(ies). *See also* Arm(s); Elbow *entries;* Shoulder *entries*
edema in, 37–38, 161
hypertonicity of, in sit to stand, 406–407
loss of alignment and stability in, effect on trunk movements in sitting, 102–104
muscle weakness of, in rolling pattern, 361–362
paralysis, and forearm weight bearing, 193–194
weakness of, in walking, 452–453
in weight bearing, 6–7

Upper extremity movement(s), 131–182
categories of, 131
complex patterns of, 138–140
components of, 132–134
clavicular, 134
humeral, 134
scapular, 132–133
concepts and principles of, 131–142
elbow flexion/extension, 138
elbow flexion with shoulder extension, 139–140
elbow flexion with shoulder internal/external rotation, 140
elevation combining shoulder and elbow flexion, 139
in functional performance, 140–142
impairments interfering with performance of, 142–181
muscle weakness in arm, 142
unbalanced muscle strength, 143–145
integration of trunk movements with, 8–9
non-weight bearing, 7–8
generalized, 8
task specific, 8
reaching combining shoulder and elbow flexion, 138–139

in supine, 321–323. *See also* Supine, upper extremity functional movements in
treatment goals and techniques for, 164–181. *See also* Hemiplegic arm, treatment goals and techniques for
weight bearing, 6–7, 183–226. *See also* Extended-arm weight bearing; Forearm weight bearing
uses of, 183

Upper trunk
anterior weight shift of, 90
excessive flexion of, during forearm weight bearing, 192
excessive lateral movement of, 109–111
in initiation of forearm weight bearing patterns, 186–190
lateral weight shift of, 91–92
posterior weight shift of, 91
in sitting, movements initiated from, 90–92

W

Walking, 433–477. *See also* Gait
assessment of, 455–457
in forward progression, 455
for single/double limb support, 456
in swing, 457
components of, 440
concepts and principles of, 433–436
defined, 433
definitions and kinematics of, 434–436
distance and time dimensions of, 434
gait. *See* Gait
higher level activities during, 467–477
impairments interfering with, 441–454
summary of, 454
loss of trunk alignment and stability during, 42
lower extremity impairments in, 444–452
atypical muscle firing, 451
double limb support-heel off, 450–451
excessive knee flexion, 448–449
foot posturing, 452
inability to keep foot on floor, 450–451
instability of hip, 446
insufficient ankle dorsiflexion, 452
knee hyperextension, 447–448
loss of ankle joint range and control, 445–446
loss of knee control, 447–448
loss of lower-extremity-initiated forward weight shift, 444–445
single limb support, 446–450
stance-forward progession, 444–445

in swing, 451–452
toe curling and clawing, 449–450
stance phase of, 434–435
swing phase of, 451–452
treatment goals and techniques for, 457–467
controlling severe knee recurvatum during stance phase, 462
correcting alignment and increasing symmetry and control of trunk, 458–459
reeducating foot and ankle muscles in early swing phase, 463
reeducating trunk and leg components in a progression, 466–467
training forward weight shifts and increasing lateral hip stability, 460–461
training trunk and leg movements during swing phase, 464–465
trunk impairments in, 441–443
loss of control of upper trunk over lower trunk, 441–443
stance, 441–443
swing, 443
undesirable compensatory patterns in, 455
upper extremity impairments in, 452–454
in stance and swing, 452–453

Walking cycle
defined, 434
double and single limb support in, 435
measurement of, 435

Walking cycle times, 435–436

Weight bearing
extended arm. *See* Extended-arm weight bearing
forearm. *See* Forearm weight bearing
in infants, 6
loss of lower extremity/hip control in, 106–107
lower extremity in, 6
upper-trunk initiated, 230
in sitting. *See* Sitting, weight bearing in
in supine
on forearms, 323
lower extremity patterns, 324–326
symmetric, in lower extremities, in sit to stand, 412–413
upper extremity in, 6–7

Weight shift
anterior
in extended-arm weight bearing, 210, 211–212
and increased ankle dorsiflexion, in standing, 285
in sitting, 228, 230
in step/stance position, 288–289

Weight shift *(Continued)*
    in upper-trunk-initiated movements in standing, 290
  in balance control in standing, 293–294
  with feet unsupported, in sitting, 229
  flexion rotation, in upper-trunk-initiated movements in standing, 291–293
  in forearm weight bearing
    anterior, 185, 187–188
    lateral, 189–190, 192
  forward, lower-extremity-initiated, loss of, in walking, 444–445
  lateral
    in abducted stance, 287–288

    in extended-arm weight bearing, 210, 212
    and increased abduction/adduction, in standing, 286
    in scooting, 252
    in sitting, 229, 230–231
    in upper-trunk-initiated movements in standing, 291
  lower-extremity–initiated, in standing, 284–285
  posterior
    in extended-arm weight bearing, 212
    in forearm weight bearing, 186, 188–189

    and increased ankle plantarflexion, in standing, 285–286
    in sitting, 229, 230
    in step/stance position, 289
    in upper-trunk-initiated movements in standing, 290
  rotational, in standing, 286–287
  in standing, 272–273
World Health Organization
  classification of disease and disablement, 16
  terminology of, 15–17
Wrist movement(s), 141